MW00714078

Breast Pathology

Breast Pathology

A Volume in the Series
Foundations in Diagnostic Pathology

Edited by

Frances P O'Malley, MB, FRCPC
Surgical Pathologist
Department of Pathology and Laboratory Medicine
Mount Sinai Hospital
Associate Professor
University of Toronto
Toronto, Ontario
Canada

Sarah E Pinder, MB ChB, FRCPath
Consultant Breast Pathologist
Addenbrooke's Hospital
Cambridge University Hospitals NHS Foundation Trust
Cambridge
United Kingdom

Series Editor

John R Goldblum, MD, FCAP, FASCP, FACG
Chairman, Department of Anatomical Pathology
The Cleveland Clinic Foundation
Cleveland Clinic Lerner College of Medicine
Case Western Reserve University
Cleveland, Ohio
United States of America

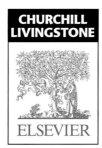

CHURCHILL
LIVINGSTONE

ELSEVIER

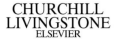

An imprint of Elsevier Inc.
© 2006, Elsevier Inc. All rights reserved.

ISBN-13: 978-0-443-06680-1
ISBN-10: 0-443-06680-9

No part of this publication may be reproduced, stored in a retrieval system, or transmitted in any form or by any means, electronic, mechanical, photocopying, recording or otherwise, without the prior permission of the Publishers. Permissions may be sought directly from Elsevier's Health Sciences Rights Department, 1600 John F. Kennedy Boulevard, Suite 1800, Philadelphia, PA 19103-2899, USA: phone: (+1) 215 239 3804; fax: (+1) 215 239 3805; or, e-mail: *healthpermissions@elsevier.com*. You may also complete your request on-line via the Elsevier homepage (http://www.elsevier.com), by selecting 'Support and contact' and then 'Copyright and Permission'.

NOTICE

Medical knowledge is constantly changing. Standard safety precautions must be followed, but as new research and clinical experience broaden our knowledge, changes in treatment and drug therapy may become necessary or appropriate. Readers are advised to check the most current product information provided by the manufacturer of each drug to be administered to verify the recommended dose, the method and duration of administration, and contraindications. It is the responsibility of the practitioner, relying on experience and knowledge of the patient, to determine dosages and the best treatment for each individual patient. Neither the Publisher nor the author assume any liability for any injury and/or damage to persons or property arising from this publication.

The Publisher

First published 2006

British Library Cataloguing in Publication Data
A catalogue record for this book is available from the British Library

Library of Congress Cataloging in Publication Data
A catalog record for this book is available from the Library of Congress

Commissioning Editor: Belinda Kuhn
Project Development Manager: Heather Krehling
Project Manager: Cheryl Brant
Design Manager: Louis Forgione
Marketing Manager(s) (UK/USA): Lisa Damico/Leontine Treur

Printed in China

Last digit is the print number: 9 8 7 6 5 4 3 2 1

Working together to grow
libraries in developing countries

www.elsevier.com | www.bookaid.org | www.sabre.org

ELSEVIER   BOOK AID International   Sabre Foundation

"(T)he student begins with the patient, continues with the patient, and ends his studies with the patient, using books and lectures as tools, as means to an end."
Sir William Osler (1849–1919)

To my family, Siobhan and Paul
and to my friend and mentor, David L Page
Frances P O'Malley

To my parents, Arthur and Sheila Pinder;
thanks for everything.
To Ian Ellis and Chris Elston;
thanks for being friends and mentors.
To J, J, A, H, J & R and to Watford & LCFC;
thanks for the sense of perspective!
Sarah E Pinder

Contributors

Sunil Badve, MD
Pathologist
Department of Surgical Pathology
University Medical Center
Indianapolis, IN
USA

Anita Bane, MB, MRCPath
Pathology Fellow, PhD Student
Department of Pathology and Laboratory Medicine
Mount Sinai Hospital
Toronto, Ontario
Canada

Beverly A Carter, MD
Surgical Pathologist
St Clare's Mercy Hospital
St Johns, Newfoundland
Canada

Ian O Ellis, BM BS, FRCPath
Professor of Cancer Pathology
Histopathology Department
Nottingham City Hospital NHS Trust
Nottingham
United Kingdom

Christopher WS Elston, MBBS, MD FRCPath
Professor of Tumour Pathology
Department of Histopathology
Nottingham City Hospital NHS Trust
Nottingham
United Kingdom

Andrew J Evans, FRCF
Consultant Radiologist
Nottingham Breast Unit
Nottingham City Hospital NHS Trust
Nottingham
United Kingdom

James J Going, MB, PhD, FRCPath
Senior Lecturer/Consultant Pathologist
University Department of Pathology
Glasgow Royal Infirmary
Glasgow
United Kingdom

Michael A Gonzalez, B Med Sci, BM BS, PhD, MRCP(UK)
MRC Clinical Research Fellow
MRC Cancer Cell Unit
Cambridge
United Kingdom

Gavin Harris, BM BS, MRCPath
Consultant Anatomical Pathologist
Canterbury Health Laboratories
Christchurch,
New Zealand

Timothy W Jacobs, MD
Pathologist
Department of Pathology
Virginia Mason Medical Center
Seattle, WA
USA

Jonathan J James, FRCR
Consultant Radiologist
Nottingham Breast Unit
Nottingham City Hospital NHS Trust
Nottingham
United Kingdom

Andrew HS Lee, MB BChir, MRCP, MRCPath
Consultant Histopathologist
Histopathology Department
Nottingham City Hospital NHS Trust
Nottingham
United Kingdom

Sunil R Lakhani, BSc, MBBS, MD, FRCPath, FRCPA
Professor of Pathology
Head, Molecular and Cellular Pathology
School of Medicine
The University of Queensland Mayne Medical School
Herston, Queensland
Australia

R Douglas MacMillan, MD, FRCS
Consultant Surgeon and Associate Clinical Director
Nottingham Breast Unit
Nottingham City Hospital NHS Trust
Nottingham
United Kingdom

Syed K Moshin, MD
Staff Pathologist
Riverside Methodist Hospital
Columbus, OH
USA

Anna Marie Mulligan, MB, MSc, MRCPath
Breast Pathology Fellow
Department of Pathology and Laboratory Medicine
Mount Sinai Hospital Toronto, Ontario
Canada

Frances P O'Malley, MB, FRCPC
Surgical Pathologist
Department of Pathology and Laboratory Medicine
Mount Sinai Hospital
Associate Professor
Department of Laboratory Medicine and Pathobiology
University of Toronto
Toronto, Ontario
Canada

David L Page, MD
Professor of Pathology
Division of Anatomical Pathology
Vanderbilt University School of Medicine
Nashville, TN
USA

Sarah E Pinder, MBChB, FRCPath
Consultant Breast Pathologist
Department of Histopathology
Addenbrooke's Hospital
Cambridge University Hospitals NHS Foundation Trust
Cambridge
United Kingdom

Jorge S Reis-Filho, MD
Clinical Fellow
Breakthrough Breast Cancer Research Centre
Institute of Cancer Research
London
United Kingdom

Jean F Simpson, MD
Professor of Pathology
Division of Anatomical Pathology
Vanderbilt University School of Medicine
Nashville, TN
USA

Nour Sneige, MD
Professor of Pathology
Chief, Sector of Cytopathology
Department of Pathology
University of Texas MD Anderson Cancer Center
Houston, TX
USA

Gregg Staerkel, MD
Professor of Pathology
Director, Cytopathology Fellowship
Medical Director, Cytotechnology Program
Department of Pathology
University of Texas MD Anderson Cancer Center
Houston, TX
USA

Donald L Weaver, MD
Professor of Pathology
Department of Pathology
University of Vermont College of Medicine
Burlington, VT
USA

Bruce J Youngson, MSc, MD, FRCP(C)
Staff Pathologist
Department of Pathology
Princess Margaret Hospital University Health Network
Toronto, Ontario
Canada

Foreword

The study and practice of anatomic pathology are both exciting and overwhelming. Surgical pathology, with all of the subspecialties it encompasses, and cytopathology have become increasingly complex and sophisticated, and it is not possible for any individual to master the skills and knowledge required to perform all of these tasks at the highest level. Simply being able to make a correct diagnosis is challenging enough, but the standard of care has far surpassed merely providing a diagnosis. Pathologists are now asked to provide large amounts of ancillary information, both diagnostic and prognostic, often on small amounts of tissue, a task that can be daunting even to the most experienced pathologist.

Although large general surgical pathology textbooks are useful resources, they by necessity could not possibly cover many of the aspects that pathologists need to know and include in their reports. As such, the concept behind Foundation in Diagnostic Pathology was born. This series is designed to cover the major areas of surgical and cytopathology, and each edition is focused on one major topic. The goal of every book in this series is to provide the essential information that any pathologist, whether general or subspecialized, in training or in practice, would find useful in the evaluation of virtually any type of specimen encountered.

Drs Frances O'Malley and Sarah Pinder, superb breast pathologists from Mount Sinai Hospital in Toronto, Canada, and Addenbrooke NHS Trust in Cambridge, UK, respectively, have edited what I believe to be an outstanding, state-of-the-art book on the essentials of breast pathology. The list of contributors is most impressive and includes renowned pathologists from the United States, Canada and the United Kingdom, all of whom have built a national and international reputa-

tion in the field of breast pathology. The content in each chapter is extremely practical, well organized and concisely written, focusing on the thorough evaluation of all types of specimens including fine needle aspirates, core biopsies, wire localization biopsies and resection specimens. There are overviews of the clinical and radiological aspects of breast diseases, which provide a thoughtful background for the practicing pathologist, since these aspects go hand in hand.

This edition of the series is organized into 27 chapters covering all the major problems encountered in breast pathology. There are separate chapters that describe the normal breast, inflammatory conditions, the always-difficult sclerosing lesions of the breast, papillary lesions, fibroadenomas and phyllodes tumors, stromal lesions, diseases of the nipple and fibrocystic changes. Chapters 14 through 20 are entirely dedicated to the ductal and lobular proliferations of the breast, describing in great detail the subtle changes that occur in the spectrum from hyperplasia to atypical hyperplasia to in-situ and invasive carcinoma. Separate chapters are dedicated to describing the molecular genetics of ductal and lobular neoplasia, including pre-invasive lesions. A thoroughly updated discussion on sentinel lymph node biopsies is also provided, as well as an overview of the use of immunohistochemistry in breast disease.

I wish to extend my sincerest gratitude to Drs O'Malley and Pinder as well as all the authors who contributed to this outstanding edition of *Foundations in Diagnostic Pathology*. I sincerely hope you enjoy this volume of the series as much as I did.

JOHN R. GOLDBLUM, M.D.

The practice of breast pathology is an exciting and varied one with new developments in the understanding of breast disease biology and genetics occurring seemingly daily. It is therefore difficult to keep up to date and the field can appear somewhat baffling to the trainee histopathologist. Similarly, the classification of breast lesions is undergoing regular changes, as exemplified by columnar cell lesions, and this can be challenging to even the most experienced pathologist. For these reasons we are pleased to act as joint editors for *Foundations in Diagnostic Pathology – Breast Pathology*. We believe that the standard, ordered format that is used, where appropriate, throughout the book, makes it particularly "user-friendly". Following on from initial chapters on diagnosis on cytology and core biopsy samples and handling of breast specimens macroscopically, we have aimed to cover the range of appearances of normal breast as well as the broad spectrum of breast lesions, both epithelial and stromal, benign and malignant. In our discussion of these topics we have focused on the most practical and clinically relevant information.

The role of the surgical pathologist in the area of breast diseases has expanded from that of diagnostician to one of prognostication. We provide information on the important histologic and biologic prognostic factors in breast cancer and we also cover in detail the complex and challenging issues associated with sentinel lymph node biopsies.

We are fortunate to have had many internationally renowned experts in breast pathology contribute to this book. We extend a sincere thanks to all for their time and effort. We hope that our readers will enjoy their words of wisdom, as we have done. We anticipate that the information in this book will provide a valuable resource for all those interested in breast pathology.

FRANCES P O'MALLEY, MB, FRCPC
SARAH E PINDER, MB CHB, FRCPATH

Acknowledgments

We acknowledge the support and patience of the staff at Elsevier, particularly Heather Krehling and Belinda Kuhn, who kept us on track. Special thanks goes to Dr Anna-Marie Mulligan for her help with photography, and to Colette Devlin and Marie Maguire at Mount Sinai Hospital, who provided excellent secretarial assistance.

Contents

1

Diagnostic Methodologies: Fine Needle Aspiration Cytology

Gregg Staerkel · Nour Sneige

Improvements in healthcare today typically come with the drawback of increased time and cost due to the greater complexity of the evolved procedure and/or the need for highly trained personnel to maintain and run high priced equipment. Consequently, it comes as a pleasant surprise that fine needle aspiration is the antithesis to this trend and, because of its ease of operation, it is a do-anywhere procedure. An aspiration can be performed during a routine doctor's office or clinic visit or at the patient's bedside. It utilizes inexpensive equipment and can typically be performed, interpreted and reported in a matter of minutes thereby accelerating a patient's entry into treatment. An intra-operative/pre-operative aspiration can negate the need for a frozen section/histologic examination of tissue, respectively, the first step in a traditional 'two step surgical procedure' or eliminate the time, cost and morbidity associated with the additional surgical exploration and incision of secondarily disclosed nodules.

It is largely accepted that the first individuals credited for laying the foundation for the development of today's needle aspiration were the surgeon Hayes Martin, Edward Ellis (pathologist James Ewing's laboratory technologist), and the pathologist Fred Stewart at The Memorial Center for Cancer and Allied Diseases in New York. In the late 1920s and 1930s, they demonstrated the utility of needle aspiration in the diagnosis of a large number of cases and detailed the procedure, which mirrors in large part the technique still used today. Unfortunately, despite these early reports, the use of needle aspiration did not catch on. This setback was thought to be due, in part, to a lack of communicating its efficacy and not incorporating the merits of needle aspiration into the training programs of surgical and pathology trainees. Also, contributing to the setback was the unsubstantiated belief, by some prominent individuals, that the acquisition of a small amount of tissue resulted in difficult/less than complete interpretations and that puncturing a tumor with needles carried a significant danger of tumor tract seeding and induction of metastatic disease. Needle aspirations would not make a comeback until the clinicians and pathologists at The Karolinska Institute in Stockholm, Sweden, reported their findings for needle aspirations performed from approximately 1950 to 1980. These reports documented the overwhelming efficacy and accuracy of this technique in the diagnosis of tumors at differing body sites. The utilization of a much smaller gauge needle than the individuals at The Memorial Center for Cancer and

Allied Diseases led to the use of the term thin-needle aspiration and later fine needle aspiration.

ROLE AND LIMITATION

For the evaluation of most lesions of the breast, fine needle aspiration represents a near perfect test. It is relatively easy to perform requiring no high-tech gadgetry; costs are as low as core biopsy and substantially more cost-effective than open biopsy. The procedure is safe, yielding tissues that provide for a high diagnostic accuracy in an extremely short timeframe. The main competition to the fine needle aspiration in breast is the cutting needle biopsy. Both of these techniques can be performed as an outpatient procedure with little significant negative cosmetic effect, e.g., scarring, dimpling of the breast due to loss of tissue.

Advantages of aspiration over cutting needle biopsy are as follows:
- Ability to immediately and accurately assess the adequacy of the specimen obtained (while some individuals endorse making touch preparations of cutting needle biopsies for an immediate assessment of adequacy, these preparations taken prior to processing the tissue for histologic examination, do not consistently reflect the final content of tissue seen).
- Greater mobility allowing for an increased area of sampling (the core biopsy obtains tissue in one plane only);
- Processing times are significantly less when compared to both paraffin embedded and frozen section cutting needle biopsies, thereby permitting a more timely immediate assessment and the processing of a larger number of patients;
- Greater sensitivity of the physical nature of the lesion and therefore better needle localization;
- Enhanced appreciation of the lesion's texture which helps determine the need for additional needle passes and diagnosis. e.g., a gritty, rubbery or no firm resistance feel suggests the possibilities of carcinoma, fibroadenoma and fat necrosis, respectively;
- Increased sensitivity; and
- Shorter time to final diagnosis.

Disadvantages of aspiration when compared to cutting needle biopsy include:

- Limited tissue available for ancillary studies and research endeavors (paraffin embedded, cutting needle cores of tissue can yield hundreds of slides for analysis whereas the average aspirate might have between four and ten slides);
- Less familiarity/experience among pathologists;
- Low cellular yield due to the nature of the lesion, despite the performance of an appropriate aspiration, e.g., desmoplastic stroma seen in a some types of carcinoma;
- Difficulty in classifying proliferative lesions that have a degree of atypia but lack unequivocal features of malignancy, i.e., minimal nuclear atypia and/or absence of single malignant cells;
- Inability to give an absolute assessment of the presence of *in-situ* versus invasive disease, a significant drawback when pre-operative chemotherapy or sentinel lymph node biopsy is considered;
- Slightly less specificity; and
- High rate of insufficiency when aspirating microcalcifications under imaging guidance due to the paucity of epithelial tissues present.

These drawbacks have led to a decline in breast fine needle aspirations, particularly for the evaluation of a patient's primary lesion. However, with the development of new treatment protocols for the care of breast cancer patients, fine needle aspiration of lesions, other than the index cancer, are increasingly used to rule in or out multicentric disease. In combination with regional lymph node and distant site aspirations, the staging of a patient's disease and planning of suitable therapy can be more quickly and economically achieved. Lastly, fine needle aspiration is now being used in obtaining tissues to assess proliferative breast changes and for the performance of marker studies to better assess patient risk for the development of breast cancer. The ability to perform either fine needle aspiration or cutting needle biopsy, based on a given set of clinical/radiologic/pathologic findings, allows one to take advantage of the benefits that both procedures have to offer.

FINE NEEDLE ASPIRATION PROCEDURE

Fine needle aspiration (FNA) of the breast requires simple and inexpensive equipment (Table 1-1). Most lesions are painless when aspirated with the patient feeling only the initial pinprick through the skin. Anesthesia is not required for most breast aspirations, however when used, it should be used sparingly as too much may infiltrate the connective tissue and, particularly with a small nodule, can mask it to palpation. Notable exceptions are gynecomastia and any nodule in close proximity to the nipple or areola. Preferably the aspirator should access a subareolar mass through an extreme lateral approach avoiding the nipple and areola altogether. Key to performing an adequate aspiration is the immobilization of the mass by the aspirator's free

---

TABLE 1-1

Equipment requirements for breast fine needle aspiration

Disposable needles with transparent plastic hubs
   23 to 25 gauge, 1 and 1.5″ in length (longer and more
   rigid needles, 20 to 22 gauge, may be needed for the rare
   more deeply seated lesion)
Disposable plastic syringes (10 or 20 cc)
Syringe holder (optional)
Glass slides
Fixative (optional if pathologist desires only air dried tissue
   for interpretation)
Rinse solution (optional)
Anesthetic agent for local anesthesia (optional)
Ethanol pads
Gauze pads

---

hand as better cutting or coring of the mass can be achieved. The needle, with syringe and holder attached, is then inserted into the mass. The syringe plunger is pulled back, creating negative pressure, as the needle is advanced forward and backward. It is not the suction that directly results in obtaining a sample but rather the cutting action of the needle. The suction helps to pull tissue into the cutting path of the needle and to move resulting fragments up into the needle's shaft. Pumping the syringe plunger does not enhance sampling; in fact, sampling can be reduced as a result of increased bleeding. Moving the needle in different directions, other than in an up and down manner, reduces cell yield due to the increased bleeding that results from the laceration of small capillaries. In general, needle movements that are more frequent, longer in length and kept within the tumor during the entire aspiration yield more tissue. Movement and frequency will depend on the size of the lesion and the aspirator's ability to maintain control. Typically, 30 to 50 excursions with the needle are made over a 10 to 20 second period. A blood-tinged specimen will appear in the hub of the needle. Suction is then released and the needle is withdrawn (Figure 1-1).

Although little bleeding occurs in a fine needle aspiration, it is best to eliminate all bleeding, as cellular yield decreases and lesion localization/demarcation is less distinct with increased soft tissue hemorrhage. Therefore, after withdrawing the needle, applying a gauze pad with one's fingertips pressing directly over the puncture site for one to three minutes is recommended (a longer time is applied for individuals with an easy bruising history or for those currently taking blood-thinning agents).

After removing the needle from the patient, the syringe is detached from the needle, filled with air and reattached. The aspirator expresses a drop of the sample acquired onto one or more slides. The drop is then smeared, fixed with 95% ethanol or air-dried, stained and interpreted. Acquisition of material to interpretation can take as little as 15 minutes. Non-palpable masses require radiologic imaging (via sonography or

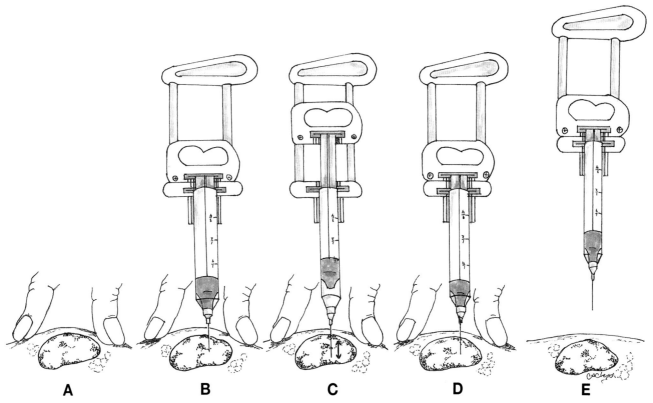

FIGURE 1-1

Fine needle biopsy with aspiration and syringe holder attached. (A) Immobilize the mass to be aspirated with fingers of free hand. (B) Insert needle into mass. (C) Apply suction while moving the needle upwards and downwards within the mass. (D) Suction is released after blood appears in the hub of the needle. (E) The needle is withdrawn from the mass and smears are prepared.

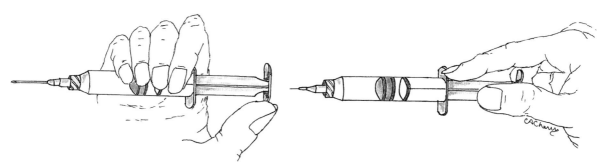

FIGURE 1-2

Fine needle biopsy with aspiration but without syringe holder attached. The procedure for aspiration is identical to the steps outlined in Figure 1-1, differing only in the holding of the syringe. The non-immobilizing hand either grasps the barrel with the fingers while the thumb pushes upward on the plunger or places the index finger on the wing of the syringe with the thumb and middle fingers pulling the plunger backward.

stereotaxic instrument) for correct needle placement; however, the procedure from acquisition to interpretation remains the same.

Although requiring greater manual dexterity, it is possible to perform a fine needle aspiration with suction, but without the aid of a syringe holder. One hand immobilizes the nodule to be aspirated while the other hand grabs the barrel of the syringe which is attached to the needle. The thumb of the syringe-grasping hand then pushes up on the syringe plunger. An alternate method for this procedure is to grasp the plunger with the thumb and all fingers, except the index finger. The thumb and fingers pull back on the plunger

while the index finger pushes on the end of the syringe barrel in the opposite direction (Figure 1-2).

FINE NEEDLE BIOPSY WITHOUT ASPIRATION

A modification of this aspiration technique is the acquisition of tissue using a needle only, the so-called 'capillary method.' The syringe with holder is not applied

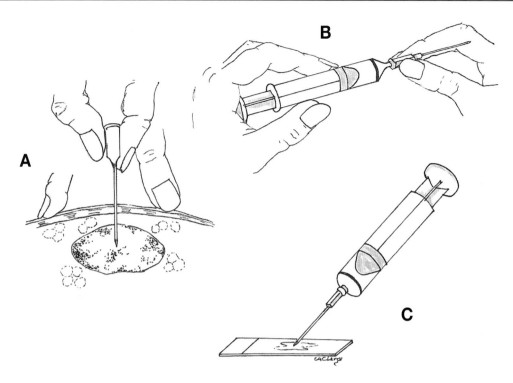

FIGURE 1-3

Fine needle biopsy without aspiration. (A) Immobilize the mass to be aspirated with free hand. With thumb and forefinger grasping hub of needle, advance the needle into the mass. Move the needle rapidly up and down within the mass. If a flash of blood or liquid appears in the hub of the needle or after 15–20 seconds, movement is stopped and the needle is removed. (B) An air-filled syringe is attached and (C) the acquired specimen is then expelled onto a slide and smeared.

(Figure 1-3). This modification allows greater sensitivity for the aspirator. Fingers are placed on the hub of the needle, allowing for a heightened appreciation of density changes within the subcutaneous soft tissues of the breast. Virtually no bleeding occurs and a pure sample, devoid of diluting blood is obtained. Because of the lack of suction, frequently no material is seen in the needle's hub, yet tissue will have been collected within the lumen of the needle. Consequently, the aspiration is voluntarily stopped after 15 to 20 seconds. The needle is withdrawn and an air-filled syringe is attached. Material is expelled onto a slide. Disadvantages of this method include the low cellular yield with fibrotic and sparsely cellular lesions and the rapid leakage of fluid from the end of the needle due to the pressure associated with most fluid-filled cysts.

FINE NEEDLE BIOPSY: ASPIRATION VERSUS WITHOUT ASPIRATION

To take advantage of the benefits of both methods and to minimize their disadvantages, it is recommended that the first and possibly second aspiration be performed using a needle only, while the syringe and holder set-up should be used for subsequent aspirations or initially when a cyst is suspected. If an immediate assessment is performed after each aspiration, the most advantageous method can be selected for all subsequent procurements.

MAXIMIZING THE FINE NEEDLE ASPIRATE

EXAMINING/POSITIONING OF PATIENT FOR LESION LOCALIZATION

If the primary physician has inked the skin overlying the nodule to be aspirated, it is important to place the patient in the original position in which the mark was made. After identification of the nodule in question, the patient may be shifted as necessary for the aspiration procedure. When the site of aspiration is not inked and the mass is not visually obvious, a thorough palpation of the breast is indicated. In this situation, it is best to examine the patient in the supine position, forearm up and underneath the head. Examine the breast systematically, nipple to axillary tail in a circular fashion or vice versa. The examining hand should be kept flat with no spacing between fingers (spacing between fingers can give a false impression of a nodule). A pillow or towel placed under the shoulder can aid in the appreciation of a subtle nodule.

It may be easier to palpate masses deep within the breast or close to the chest wall when the patient is supine with the arm of the side being aspirated raised above and under the head. However, aspiration in this position can at times be more difficult. This difficulty is due to the fact that the breast in this position will flatten out, which in turn places the nodule in question closer to the chest wall. The aspirator senses the added risk for pneumothorax and has a tendency to take a more tangential approach to the mass, which in turn carries a greater risk for insufficient sampling. Instead, it may be easier to locate the nodule in the supine position and then place the patient in an upright position for aspiration. This is due, in part, to the fact that a mass within the breast when in an upright position will become suspended (pulled downward by gravity) becoming more tethered to the surrounding connective tissue. This added immobilization of the mass enhances tissue acquisition. In addition, the nodule moves away from the chest wall, so the risk for pneumothorax decreases and the comfort zone for the aspirator is improved.

INCREASING CELLULAR YIELD

In contrast to deep organ sites, breast aspirations benefit from the fact that they are not impeded by overlying structures such as muscle. On the other hand, aspiration of deep-seated nodules can yield significant cellularity due to their fixation to surrounding tissues. Masses within the breast are often found within adipose tissue and are therefore mobile. It is this feature that frequently hinders adequate sampling. Consequently, it is imperative to completely immobilize the mass so that when a needle is introduced, a coring action is achieved. Nodules, which are permitted to move within the breast, move with the needle, reducing the yield of tissue. To achieve total immobilization, one should flatten the breast tissue between the mass and overlying skin by stretching the skin between the immobilizing fingers on each side of the mass. If properly done, almost any mass can be reached with a one or one-and-a-half inch needle. When possible, the mass should be fixed with the fingers along the axis of greatest mobility.

Infrequently, an aspirator is faced with a mass that mammographically suggests a concern for malignancy. However, because of the tumor's depth within the breast, the large size of the breast and/or the infiltrative nature of the mass, the lesion lacks definition. On palpation, only a vague firmness may be appreciated over a large portion of the breast. Multiple aspirations yield little significant tissue. The problem typically encountered here is that the aspirator has not placed the needle deep enough. The aspirator erroneously thinks that most of the deeply seated firmness is chest wall instead of tumor and not wanting to risk a pneumothorax, the individual stays too superficial.

NUMBER OF NEEDLE PASSES

A minimum of two to three aspirations per mass is recommended if an immediate assessment of the aspirate is not employed. More aspirations than this typically result in less and less tissue being obtained, as bleeding

and clotting ensues. Under the following conditions, additional aspirations are suggested:
- Lesions that are exceptionally fibrous in nature with non-discrete margins; this may represent a desmoplastic carcinoma which will have a low cell yield;
- Small lesions in which the risk of missing the target is great;
- A specimen that clots immediately when placed on a glass slide; evidence that significant bleeding has occurred and a diluted/hypocellular sample has been obtained;
- If the sample looks as smooth as a peripheral blood smear, without visible particles, chances are high that it will lack microscopic cellularity; or
- The aspirate is yellow and slightly oily in appearance; this specimen is primarily composed of adipose tissue with frequently little or no epithelium; this situation would be acceptable if one is relatively confident that a non-malignant process is being evaluated, i.e., a nodule which is soft on palpation and offers no resistance to needle penetration.

HANDLING BREAST CYSTS

Often a cyst within the breast will present as a firm mass, giving a concern for malignancy, due to the buildup of pressure within the cyst from fluid accumulation. When using a needle only (no attached syringe), the aspirator should always have a cup or syringe immediately available to capture the fluid which will otherwise rapidly leak onto the patient. Breast cysts require complete drainage. The drained area should be repalpated for any residual solid mass, which will in turn require a separate needle aspiration. Papillomas, papillary carcinomas and other significant lesions can be masked this way. The published guidelines from The National Cancer Institute – sponsored conference (September 9–10, 1996) states that any brown or red discolored aspirate, not traumatic in nature, should be examined cytologically. Cyst aspirations that are thin, watery, green-gray in color with no identifiable residual mass may be discarded at the discretion of an experienced aspirator.

HANDLING INFLAMMATORY SKIN CHANGES AND DERMAL INFILTRATES

Breast patients with slightly raised skin nodules or presumed inflammatory breast carcinoma may not be amenable to fine needle aspiration. Aspirations attempted in these patients are frequently scant in cellularity. If the few tumor cells obtained also lack significant cytologic atypia they will be difficult to separate from inadvertently acquired benign skin adnexal structures. These situations are best handled via a skin punch biopsy. Proficiency with this latter procedure also can be beneficial to both patient and aspirator alike. The

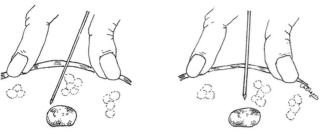

FIGURE 1-4
Aspiration of small deep-seated breast nodules. A tangential needle placement (left side) rather than a near vertical approach (right side) can result in a missed aspiration and a false negative result.

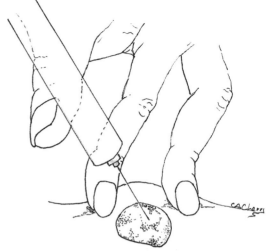

FIGURE 1-5
Enhancing control of fine needle aspiration. An alternative to immobilizing a mass with the thumb and index fingers of the free hand is to use the index and middle fingers. This permits the syringe to be placed across the thumb giving excellent control even to those individuals with intention tremors. It will be necessary to flex the immobilizing fingers so that the syringe and needle can penetrate the skin/mass at a near vertical angle.

patient ultimately receives a diagnosis, although not as timely, from a sample that can easily be taken at the same clinic visit as the originally scheduled aspiration.

HANDLING THE DEEPLY PLACED BREAST NODULE

An additional difficulty arises from the tendency for most aspirators to approach lesions with the needle positioned tangentially to the skin, rather than with a near vertical or perpendicular approach. This position is more comfortable to the aspirator but may not be optimal for small deep seated nodules. The problem that can occur with this approach is, that by the time the needle has reached the level of the lesion, little of the nodule is in the path of the needle (Figure 1-4). Consequently, a more vertical approach is recommended, albeit uncomfortable for some aspirators. This is especially true for individuals with intention tremors, specifically when a syringe holder is used in the aspiration, when the distance from hand to nodule is greatest. These individuals carry an added risk for a needle-stick injury of their fingers, particularly with small lesions where immobilizing fingers are not widely spaced. With greater focus on achieving accurate needle placement with the tremorring hand, there is often an inadvertent relaxation of the fingers fixing the nodule to be aspirated. Thus, the once immobilized mass unknowingly slips away. This scenario can be prevented by using the middle and index fingers, instead of the commonly used thumb and index finger, for immobilization. The aspirator's intention tremor can be controlled by resting the barrel of the syringe on the freed-up and extended thumb (Figure 1-5).

SMEAR PREPARATION

From each aspiration, one to three slides should be made with consideration given to an additional three slides if the specimen is particularly bloody. Aspirates in which more slides can be made rarely yield additional diagnostic tissue. Ideally, a single drop of sample, about 0.5 cm in diameter, is placed on each slide. Leftover tissue should be flushed into a rinse solution of normal saline or tissue media, e.g., RPMI growth media (if processed immediately), an equal parts mixture of 95 % ethanol and water (if the specimen is to be transported to an outside facility or if any other delay in processing is expected) or proprietary fixative of any of the monolayer preparation companies. From this rinse solution, cytospin, filter or monolayer preparations can be made, thereby providing additional cytologic material for review.

When smearing, three methods are commonly practiced. The first method yields one slide per drop of specimen. The preparation is excellent for cytologic viewing and minimizes the number of resulting slides. For this method, a specimen drop is placed at the top of the slide, 1 cm below the label area of the slide. With three to four fingers along the slide's backside, thumb at the top, a firm base is established. A second slide is moved downward using a minimal amount of pressure to guard against smearing artifacts (Figure 1-6).

The second method results in two identical slides and is the preferred method when extra slides are needed for special stains, e.g., mucin, immunoperoxidase, HER-2/neu testing via fluorescence *in-situ* hybridization etc. For this method, a small drop of specimen is placed on the lower third of the slide. A second slide, upside down and parallel, is moved over the specimen drop. With both slides held at one end, the slides are pressed together lightly and slid apart, smearing the drop. Even pressure is maintained in both hands so that the resulting slides have identical cell yields (Figure 1-7).

The third method is the same technique used frequently in preparing blood films. A drop of a specimen

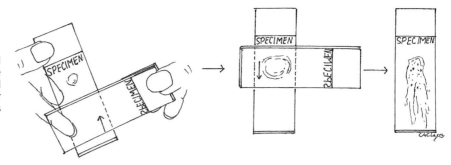

FIGURE 1-6
Smear method I. A specimen drop is placed 1 cm below the label. Fingers and thumb brace the slide for support. A second slide is placed perpendicular to the first slide and moved over the sample. As the drop flattens out, it is smeared in one smooth motion.

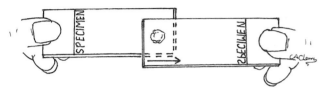

FIGURE 1-7
Smear method II. A drop of specimen is placed on the lower third of the slide. A second, parallel slide is moved over the sample drop. Thumb and forefingers are positioned at the ends of both slides. As the drop flattens out, it is smeared in one smooth motion.

is placed at the top of the slide, 1 cm below the labeling area. The edge of a second slide is placed between the specimen drop and label area; this slide is inclined to about 45°. The edge of the second slide is then moved toward the specimen drop. Upon contact the specimen becomes aligned along the slide's edge. The second slide is then advanced to the opposite end of the first slide, smearing the sample (Figure 1-8). The efficacy of this smear method decreases when clotting is present in the sample acquired. A clotted sample does not align well and a smooth dispersed smear is difficult to achieve. A totally frosted slide should never be used as a smearing slide, as significant cell distortion can be induced. Occasionally, too large a specimen drop is placed on a slide. This can be corrected by lightly touching, but not compressing the drop of specimen with a second slide. Specimen from the first slide will transfer to the second slide creating two slides that can be smeared and evaluated.

Clotted specimens are best handled by the first or second technique where compression of the overlapping slide can loosen up the clot, freeing once trapped cells for optimal microscopic review. Occasionally, an aspiration will acquire a small core of tissue. Attempting to smear this out frequently results in a non-diagnostic specimen due to artefacts induced by intense compression needed to spread this kind of specimen flat and/or because of poor microscopic visualization of cells due to the specimen's thickness. Tissue cores are usually better suited to histologic review. This can be achieved by pipetting or using the tip of a needle to pick up and transfer these tissue fragments to the rinse solution. Instead of a cytology preparation, a cell block (histologic preparation) can be made.

With fatty or sparsely cellular lesions, consider using totally frosted slides. While these slides are more costly and leave your specimen more susceptible to air-drying and smear artefacts, they provide superb cell adherence.

FIGURE 1-8
Smear method III. A sample drop is placed 1 cm below the label. The edge of a second slide is placed on the slide with the sample, between the drop of specimen and label. This top slide is advanced to the specimen drop which will spread along its edge. The sample is then spread across the bottom slide in one smooth motion.

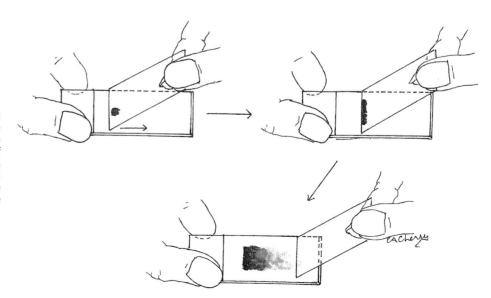

There is virtually no loss of tissue to subsequent processing.

Prepared slides that are to be fixed, should be done so immediately. This can be accomplished by either spraying the slide with fixative, e.g., gynecologic spray fixative or high alcohol content hairspray) or immersing slides in 95 % ethanol or modified Carnoy's solution (preferred), as it will lyse obscuring blood. Modified Carnoy's solution consists of six parts 70 % ethanol to one part glacial acetic acid. If immediate assessment is being performed between aspirations, staining may be speeded by a modification of the Papanicolaou stain:

Water	10 dips
Harris Hematoxylin	5–7 seconds
Water	10 dips
95 % ETOH	10 dips
OG-6	5 dips

(only if squamous cell carcinoma is suspected, otherwise skip OG-6 to further speed staining)

95 % ETOH	10 dips
EA modified	2 minutes
95 % ETOH	10 dips
95 % ETOH	10 dips
100 % ETOH	10 dips
100 % ETOH	10 dips
Xylene	10 dips
Coverslip	

In addition or in deference to ethanol fixation and the Papanicolaou stain, tissues acquired through aspiration can be air-dried and then Diff-Quik stained (proprietary staining kit). This method employs three steps which include fixation (10 dips) and two different stains requiring 10 and 20 dips, respectively. Following the last stain, the slide is rinsed in tap water. To save time, a layer of water should be left over the top of the slide, drying only the back of the slide with a paper towel or gauze (the latter is necessary to facilitate movement of the slide on the microscope stage). This process will permit microscopic evaluation from low to high power despite the lack of a coverslip. When time permits, the slide can be dried, placed into 100 % ethanol then xylene and finally coverslipped.

COMPLICATIONS OF FINE NEEDLE ASPIRATION

Potential complications occurring in breast aspirations are the same as those for any aspiration taken from around the thorax: bleeding, infection and pneumothorax. The most likely complication is soft tissue bleeding with a resulting hematoma; however, this can be avoided if, after aspiration, firm directed pressure is placed over the puncture site. The less clot that develops at the site of aspiration the better the cell yield will be for subsequent aspirations taken. Infection is uncommon, but when present is of little consequence and can be treated with antibiotics. Pneumothorax is extremely rare but, when present, may require chest tube insertion. In individuals with small breasts where an underlying rib can be palpated, one can position a mobile nodule over a rib for protection. Also, for deep-seated lesions adjacent to the chest wall, the use of a 25 gauge needle instead of a larger bore needle minimizes injury and therefore the risk of pneumothorax.

DIAGNOSTIC ACCURACY

To enhance diagnostic accuracy, it is important to obtain the following clinical information when evaluating an aspirate, this can affect the number of aspirations performed and one's threshold for a specific diagnosis:

- Patient age, e.g., advancing age increases suspicion for carcinoma and decreases the likelihood of fibroadenoma;
- Mass location, e.g., if subareolar consider possibility of a papillary neoplasm;
- A cystic lesion (seen radiologically or recognized by the acquisition of fluid on aspiration) suggests fibrocystic disease unless it is seen microscopically that the aspirate is markedly cellular with single columnar cells then one should consider a papillary neoplasm. In addition, the acquisition of thin, watery green-gray fluid typical of benign cyst fluid of fibrocystic change should caution an individual against an overdiagnosis of cells showing degenerated nuclear atypia as carcinoma;
- Tumor growth rate, e.g., large, rapidly growing mass suggests a phyllodes tumor; steadily growing lesion raises concern for carcinoma; static or regressing mass favors benign fibroepithelial lesion or fat necrosis, respectively;
- Previous trauma or surgery at the aspiration site requires one to exclude a reactive/reparative process;
- History of prior therapy, e.g., individuals who have undergone lumpectomy with radiotherapy can show residual fat necrosis and extreme epithelial nuclear atypia;
- Past history of another malignancy, e.g., the breast can be a recipient of metastatic disease;
- Needle penetration findings, e.g., soft, low resistance suggests benign disease, fat necrosis or mucinous carcinoma, a firm, rubbery texture favors fibrocystic change or fibroadenoma whereas a firm, gritty feel suggests carcinoma.

It should be noted that when immediate assessment of the aspiration does not take place, when communication between the patient's evaluator and aspirator is poor or the aspirator lacks experience, the non-diagnostic rate and negative predicative value significantly increase and decrease, respectively. These situations should therefore be avoided.

Lastly, as recommended at the National Cancer Institute sponsored conference in Bethesda, Maryland, the diagnosis derived from the fine needle aspiration of breast should be correlated with both clinical and radiologic imaging findings to determine patient management (a so-called 'triple test' approach). A benign triplet results in the patient being followed clinically with a return visit in six months. A patient with a malignant triplet is referred for definitive therapy. A mixed (inconclusive) triplet requires excisional biopsy of the lesion in question. An extension of this idea can be made for those patients who undergo fine needle aspiration with immediate assessment performed on each needle aspirate made. At the time of aspiration, the need for additional aspirations or the necessity of a surgical core biopsy can be made and performed on the spot when aspiration results together with clinical and/or imaging findings yield a mixed or inconclusive triplet (i.e., an aspiration diagnosis that does not suitably explain the clinical/imaging findings). Several studies have documented a marked reduction in both false negative and false positive cases when this approach is employed.

ACKNOWLEDGMENT

The authors wish to thank Carol Cherry, CT (ASCP), cytotechnologist at The University of Texas M. D. Anderson Cancer Center, for her artistic contributions to this article.

SUGGESTED READING

Ballo MS, Sneige N. Can core needle biopsy replace fine-needle aspiration cytology in the diagnosis of palpable breast carcinoma. Cancer 1996;78: 773–777.

De May RM. Fine Needle Aspiration Biopsy and Breast. In: The Art & Science of Cytopathology. Chicago: ASCP Pres; 1996, pp. 464–492, 805–853, 891–893 and 920–937.

Frable WJ. Introduction and History and Techniques of Thin-Needle Aspiration Biopsy. In: Thin-Needle Aspiration Biopsy. Vol. 14 in the Series, Major Problems in Pathology, Bennington JC, ed. Philadelphia: W.B. Saunders Co.; 1983, pp. 1–19.

Frable WJ. Needle aspiration of the breast. Cancer 1984;53:671–676.

Hermansen C, Poulsen HS, Jensen J, et al. Diagnostic reliability of combined physical examination, mammography, and fine-needle puncture ('triple-test') in breast tumors – a prospective study. Cancer 1987;60: 1866–1871.

Kline TS, Kline IK. Introduction and Clinical Laboratory Techniques. In: Guides to Clinical Aspiration Biopsy – Breast. New York: Igaku-Shoin; 1989, pp. 1–19.

Martin HE, Ellis EB. Aspiration biopsy. Surg Gynecol Obstet 1934;59: 578–589.

Martin HE, Ellis EB. Biopsy by needle puncture and aspiration. Ann Surg 1930;92:169–181.

National Cancer Institute Sponsored Conference. The uniform approach to breast fine-needle aspiration biopsy. Diagnostic Cytopathology 1997;16: 295–311.

Oertel YC. Introduction, Advantages and Disadvantages of Fine Needle Aspiration, Fine Needle Aspiration Technique and How to Succeed at Fine Needle Aspiration. In: Fine Needle Aspiration of the Breast. Boston: Butterworths; 1987, pp. 1–7 and 16–33.

Stanley MW, Lowhagen T. Equipment, Basic Techniques, and Staining Procedures. In: Fine Needle Aspiration of Palpable Masses. Boston, Butterworth-Heinemann, 1993, pp. 1–122.

Stewart FW. The diagnosis of tumors by aspiration biopsy. Am J Pathol 1933;9:801–812.

Zakowski MF. Fine-needle aspiration cytology of tumors: diagnostic accuracy and potential pitfalls. Cancer Investigation 1994;12:505–515.

2 Diagnostic Methodologies: Core Biopsy and Handling of Surgical Specimens

Sarah E Pinder · Frances P O'Malley

INTRODUCTION

There are some general principles in breast pathology histology that can be described whether one is handling and reporting non-operative/core biopsy samples, diagnostic open surgical or therapeutic specimens. Whatever the sample, good fixation of tissue and high quality processing and optimal standard hematoxylin and eosin (H&E) stained sections are essential. Indeed a small number of the more diagnostically difficult lesions which one may encounter in histopathology practice may be impossible to assess, if good fixation, processing, section cutting and staining have not been undertaken.

NON-OPERATIVE DIAGNOSIS/CORE BIOPSY

Core biopsies can be of differing sizes; these may range to up to 11 gauge samples, such as may be obtained by vacuum-assisted techniques. The number taken may also vary widely from a single core biopsy sample to more than 20. Large numbers may particularly be sampled from screen-detected microcalcifications. In some centers, the vacuum-assisted large bore needle technique is now being used as a method for excision of small benign lesions, such as fibroadenomas. Trials are also underway for excision of lesions such as papillomas and radial scars by large bore vacuum-assisted 'biopsy guns'.

Cores taken from radiographically detected microcalcifications will be radiographed by the radiologist to confirm that the lesion of mammographic concern has been adequately sampled. It is extremely useful if this core biopsy specimen radiograph is sent along with the specimen, which is in an adequate amount of fixative, to the pathology laboratory. It is then possible for the pathologist to confirm the site and extent of calcification in the tissue and to correlate this with the amount in the specimen radiograph. If, for example, only a small focal amount of microcalcification is seen in the initial levels of the tissue but abundant calcification is seen scattered in the specimen radiograph, additional tissue sections can be requested.

In some centers the radiologists will select the cores of interest in the clinic and place them in a separate container or capsule so that the laboratory can focus attention on this portion of the sample. For example, while a single H&E stained section may be examined for cores from clinically detected mass lesions, it is recommended that 3 or more levels should be assessed for cores taken from microcalcifications.

SURGICAL SAMPLES

Both in relation to the operation itself and in the laboratory, there are also some general comments that can be made. The type of surgery performed will be related to whether a pre-operative diagnosis has been made. A specific benign lesion such as a fibroadenoma may be excised within a tissue sample, which may not be orientated by the surgeon performing the procedure, as clearly the margin status of the disease will not be of particular importance. Similarly, if it has not been possible to achieve a pre-operative diagnosis but clinical suspicion is high that the lesion is malignant, then the surgical procedure will be in the form of a diagnostic open biopsy; the surgeon does not usually, in this circumstance, take a rim of surrounding tissue and frequently does not orientate the sample with sutures or clips. If, however, a pre-operative diagnosis of invasive carcinoma has been previously documented, then the surgeon will attempt to obtain a widely clear rim of normal/benign tissue and thorough and careful assessment of the tissue surrounding the cancer is essential.

The size, nature and site of the lesion will affect the nature of the surgery performed as well as the choice of the particular patient; thus, some patients will have carcinomas that are large and for which mastectomy may be prudent, whilst other patients will be suitable for, and will choose, a wide local excision. These two therapeutic options will clearly be handled in different ways in the laboratory. It is, however, also the case that surgeons will undertake wide local excision in differing ways and each laboratory/pathologist requires a knowledge of the operation performed for each patient, including the surgical method used and the anatomical boundaries of the resection (see wide local excision, below).

Both diagnostic and therapeutic surgical excisions may contain a nonpalpable lesion and resection may require image-guided localization using wire, dye or radioisotope. Whichever surgical technique is used, an understanding of this allows the pathologist to handle the specimen in such a way as to provide a high quality diagnosis and, in particular for cancer cases, the histologic minimum data set for breast carcinomas.

SURGICAL HANDLING

As described above, lesions are usually surgically excised according to a defined protocol, which is the standard in an individual surgical team. A therapeutic excision generally extends from the subcutis to remove all the breast tissue posteriorly down to the pectoral fascia.

The specimen should be received with the completed pathology requisition, having been orientated by the surgeon. Many surgeons perform this with sutures or clips of varying lengths or number, or ink of differing colors. Recent recommendations are that the margin nearest the nipple should be separately marked, particularly for cases of ductal carcinoma *in situ* (DCIS). Occasionally, more than one portion of tissue is excised in one surgical procedure; if this is done it must be clear how the samples are orientated with respect to each other in order to assess the size of the lesion (if present within both samples) and the margin distance.

Resection specimens that are from nonpalpable lesions should be radiographed and, in some cases, wide local excision specimens from palpable lesions are also radiographed. In this way, the presence of the lesion can be confirmed and the distance to the margins (if therapeutic) can be assessed and immediate re-excision performed if the lesion is too close to a margin. As with radiographs of core biopsy samples, radiographs of surgical excisions should also be available to the pathologist so that they can be certain of the nature and site of the lesion facilitating histologic sampling.

Ideally, the specimen should be sent immediately to the pathology laboratory in the fresh state. If this is not possible, it should be placed immediately in a sufficient volume of fixative. If the specimen cannot be sent directly to the laboratory it is possible for the surgeon to make a controlled single or cruciate pair of incisions into the lesion (usually from the posterior aspect) preserving the integrity of relevant margins, while allowing penetration of fixative. The benefits of optimal fixation (morphologic conservation, preservation of mitotic activity and retention of immunoreactivity of proteins such as hormone receptors) outweigh the misguided desire to preserve the posterior aspect of the specimen. This is particularly important in large mastectomy specimens as formalin penetration can be slow.

LABORATORY HANDLING

In the histopathology laboratory, the surface of the specimen should be inked so that the margins of excision can be easily determined histologically. Dipping the specimen in alcohol and drying can be valuable in mordanting the ink to the surface. An appropriate pigment, such as Indian ink, Alcian blue, dyed gelatine or a multiple ink technique can then be used.

DIAGNOSTIC LOCALIZATION BIOPSIES

The specimen should be measured and weighed and is then usually serially sliced at intervals of approximately 3–5 mm. If the specimen is small, it can be simpler and easier to block the sample in its entirety, e.g., if the sample is 30 mm or less in maximum dimension. Entire embedding of wire localization specimens containing non-palpable DCIS allows accurate assessment of the extent of the DCIS and also allows one to rule out associated invasive disease. If it is not feasible to embed the entire specimen, radiographs of the specimen slices can prove helpful, particularly if the lesion is associated with microcalcifications. Blocks can, in this way, be taken from the area of mammographic abnormality and the source sites of blocks marked on the radiographs. Specifically, portions should be sampled from the mammographic lesion and from the extremes of the lesion (in order to accurately determine lesion size). This is especially important for microcalcifications as not all of a DCIS lesion may undergo microcalcification and mammographic size is often an underestimate of true size of DCIS. Thus, apparently normal tissue at the periphery of the lesion should also be blocked and examined histologically.

THERAPEUTIC WIDE LOCAL EXCISIONS

As noted above, when performing a therapeutic procedure the surgeon typically removes all of the tissue from the subcutis to the pectoral fascia. If the operation is not performed in this way, the pathologist should be informed, as this will affect the specimen handling technique. In addition to orientation sutures/clips/ink, it is particularly helpful for cases of DCIS if the surgeon marks the margin nearest the nipple ducts; DCIS can extend some distance from the area of microcalcification and has a propensity to spread in this direction.

A degree of flexibility is required in specimen handling and it is impossible to provide proscriptive guidelines for laboratory technique. Several options are available (see Figures 2-1–2-3) but, whichever is used, the specimen should be weighed and measured in three dimensions. It is essential that the method used enables provision of the histologic minimum dataset for breast cancer. The pathologic features which should be reported are described elsewhere in this book and include tumor size, distance to margins, histologic grade, the presence of lymphovascular invasion and hormone receptor status. Ideally, this information should be provided in a synoptic report format.

Options for specimen handling of therapeutic wide local excision specimens include 'bread-slicing' from either medial to lateral or superficial to deep aspects (see Figures 2-1 and 2-2). Slicing can be performed either before or after fixation and marking of the excision margins, and should be at 3–5 mm intervals. Sampling

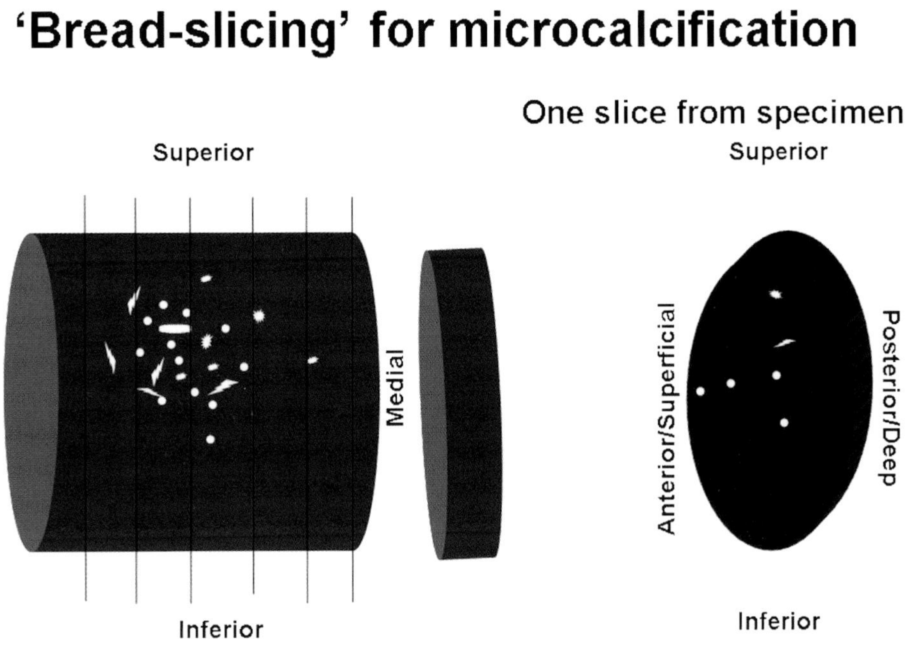

'Bread-slicing' for microcalcification

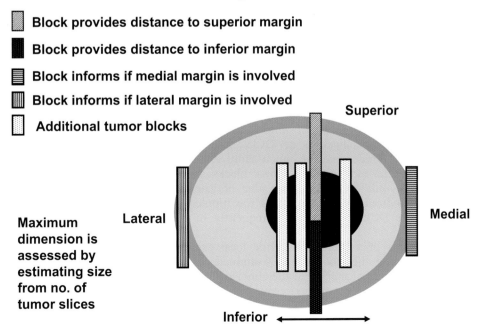

One slice from specimen

FIGURE 2-1

'Bread-slicing' of the specimen samples excised for microcalcification. This is the most frequent technique for handling samples excised for microcalcification (either therapeutic or diagnostic operations). The slices can then be laid out and re-radiographed so that histologic examination can be targeted to areas of concern.

Bread-slicing for mass lesion

FIGURE 2-2

Bread-slicing for breast masses. Wide local excision samples for breast masses can be handled in several ways according to the nature of the lesion and personal preference. This is one method of sampling mass lesions in wide local excisions. The sample is 'bread-sliced' as for microcalcification. The 'full face' of the tumor can often be included in one histologic section and the tumor size measured from this. If the maximum dimension does not correlate with the direction of slicing, however, it may not be possible to provide the maximum dimension by histologic measurement; thus in this figure, the maximum size is from medial to lateral which cannot be measured histologically from any one section. Similarly the distance to some of the margins, especially for nonpalpable lesions, must be estimated according to the thickness of the slices; in the example given the distance to the medial and lateral margins must be estimated.

▨ **Block provides distance to superior margin**

■ **Block provides distance to inferior margin**

▤ **Block informs if medial margin is involved**

▥ **Block informs if lateral margin is involved**

▢ **Additional tumor blocks**

Maximum dimension is assessed by estimating size from no. of tumor slices

Radial blocking technique

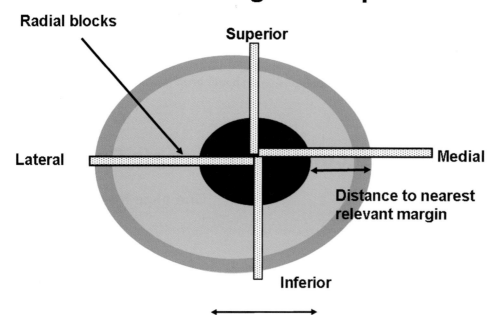

Maximum dimension is assessed by adding size from lateral radial and medial radial tumor blocks

FIGURE 2-3
Radial blocking technique for breast masses. This is an alternative method in which the mass is sampled with four 'radial' blocks that include tissue from the center of the tumor extending at right angles to include the margin. Thus the 'medial radial block' will include the medial portion of the tumor and the medial margin on the same section. The benefit of this method is that one can determine accurately the maximum dimension of the tumor (by addition of histologic size from two opposite sections (e.g., superior and inferior portions of tumor). A measurement of distance to each margin can also be provided.

should include the lesion of concern (either mass or areas of calcification as directed by the clinical history and macroscopic appearances). Some laboratories use large blocks to embed the entirety of therapeutic excisions, but such blocks require proper processing that can delay the reporting of the case and may be difficult to store. They are, nevertheless, very helpful for assessment of tumor size and distance to margins in wide local excision specimens and, if resources permit, can be valuable.

Specimen slice radiographic examination may not be absolutely essential for all samples but is undoubtedly very valuable for microcalcifications; in these cases, slicing and re-radiographing the slices will enable blocks to be taken accurately from the areas corresponding to the mammographic abnormality. As in the handling of diagnostic surgical samples, the sites of sampling can be marked on the specimen radiograph for radiologic–pathologic correlation. Blocks should be taken to include areas of fibrous breast tissue surrounding the calcification as DCIS, particularly of low nuclear grade, may be much more extensive than is suspected radiologically. Thus, blocks should be taken, not only from the main area of calcification, but also from the area towards the nipple and distal to it as DCIS extends most frequently in this plane.

The margins of a therapeutic wide local excision specimen should be thoroughly examined. As a minimum, the nearest margin to the abnormality must be sampled, but, ideally, more extensive blocking of the margins should be undertaken. The aim is to be able to provide an accurate assessment of the distance to the

nearest relevant margin. There is frequent confusion as to what is regarded 'relevant'; this is closely related to the methodology of the surgery performed. If all the tissue has been removed down to the pectoral fascia, this margin is not generally considered 'relevant' by the clinical team and the so-called 'radial' margins are those of clinical importance. The use of different color inks applied to the whole specimen or to individual histologic sections can assist in the identification of specific margins.

An alternative to slicing the entire specimen from one aspect to the other is to sample the lesion (often a mass) as a series of blocks taken at right angles in a cruciate fashion (Figure 2-3). This allows the tumor to be sampled as four blocks from the center of the tumor extending to the periphery towards the medial, lateral, superior and inferior aspects. Each block will include the anterior and posterior aspects although, as noted above, these are, according to the surgical procedure performed, often not 'relevant.'

It may be possible to take the four radial margins (superior, inferior, medial and lateral) and the lesion in one block from the center to the inked aspect of the specimen if the specimen is small. Larger samples may require two or more cassettes for the tumor and the radial margin. If this is the case, one block of, e.g., tumor from the center extending medially and one or more (contiguous) block to the medial margin will be required.

In addition to this 'radial' sampling technique, some laboratories process additional tissue from the circumferential edge of the specimen which is 'shaved' allowing more thorough examination of relevant surgical resection margins. It should be noted that these shave margins do not allow assessment of the distance to the margin, but the pathologist can determine from these whether disease is close to the external aspect (i.e., within the thickness of the block). In this system, all the radial (inferior, superior, medial and lateral) peripheral aspects of the specimen are shaved off in portions approximately 2–3 mm thick and embedded cut-side down in the cassettes which are labeled as superior, supero-medial, medial, infero-medial, inferior, etc. Thus, at least 8 additional cassettes of tissue are usually taken.

CAVITY SHAVES AND RE-EXCISION SPECIMENS

If the radiologic abnormality extends close to one or more margins as identified by specimen radiography, the surgeon may perform an immediate re-excision of that aspect. A separate re-excision specimen may, therefore, be taken either at the time of initial surgery, subsequent to the discovery of incomplete excision histologically or of the entire biopsy cavity site following diagnostic biopsy of a lesion which is discovered to be malignant. Thus, the aim is to remove either all of the previous surgical site and its margins or a specific aspect of the surgical site suspected to be involved by malignancy. Alternatively, some surgeons will routinely take additional samples from around the biopsy cavity in the form of 'cavity shaves'; these are very variable in size and range in some centers from pieces of tissue less than 10 mm in maximum extent (which should be all-embedded and examined) to large crescentic portions of tissue.

If sufficiently large, the surgeon should orientate the re-excision specimen; this is often done by the simple procedure of placing a suture on the cavity side of the specimen. If examination of the entire lesion is not feasible, the specimen may be bread-loafed and random transverse slices blocked with targeting of fibrous areas or, alternatively, the cavity aspect of the specimen and the new margin side can be shaved from the specimen at 2–3 mm thickness and examined; as with assessment of cavity shaves taken from the main specimen by the pathologist, it should be noted that this latter technique does not allow a measurement of the distance to the margin to be determined.

MASTECTOMY SPECIMENS

Mastectomy specimens should be orientated by the surgeon. This is usually done by positioning a suture in the fat of the axillary tail. Particularly if the lesion is small or impalpable, a diagram indicating the site of the lesion (or lesions) may be especially helpful to the pathologist. As for wide local excision specimens, fixation is of paramount importance and the lesion should be incised from the posterior aspect; it is important that mastectomy specimens are not placed into fixative without such an incision as formalin is a slow penetrant of adipose tissue and the tumor will invariably be poorly preserved with consequent difficulty in assessment of histologic grade, vascular invasion and hormone receptor status.

The tumor should be thoroughly sampled; it is impossible to give specific numbers of blocks that should be taken as this will clearly depend on the size of the lesion. As a rule of thumb, from a 'typical' invasive mass on average six blocks of tumor are taken either as transverse slices or in the cruciate/right angle technique as for wide local excision specimens. As well as this thorough sampling of the tumor, the macroscopically normal breast should be sliced at approximately 1 cm intervals and additional suspicious areas sampled. In addition, if resources permit, four quadrant blocks can be examined if fibrous areas are seen; there is little benefit in examining large numbers of blocks of mammary adipose tissue, as the likelihood of discovering unsuspected pathology is very low. If targeted on fibrous or suspicious areas, however, these additional blocks of the quadrants or any fibrous areas allow detection of unsuspected multifocal disease. It should be noted that even this finding is rarely of great clinical relevance and very infrequently impacts on patient management. If resources are limited, therefore, it is recommended that these are concentrated on careful examination of the tumor. Additional representative sampling of the nipple-areolar complex can be taken to determine the presence of Paget's disease of the nipple.

PATHOLOGIC EXAMINATION OF LYMPH NODES

Axillary lymph nodes that have been removed should be submitted for careful histologic examination. These may be axillary lymph node clearance/dissection specimens, lymph node samples or sentinel lymph node biopsies. Other lymph nodes may also, less commonly, be received such as internal mammary or intramammary nodes.

A few laboratories use clearing agents to remove fat and aid in identification of lymph nodes in axillary dissection specimens, but this is time-consuming and expensive and is not regarded as essential. Whatever the specimen, ideally, each lymph node should be examined and blocked independently for histologic examination. The methodology used should ensure the highest chance of finding metastatic disease by conventional microscopic examination of hematoxylin and eosin (H&E) stained tissue sections. Thus, a representative section of any grossly involved lymph node is adequate, with complete embedding of all remaining lymph nodes. Handling of sentinel lymph nodes is discussed in detail in

Chapter 22, thus will not be further addressed in this chapter.

SUGGESTED READING

Elston CW, Ellis IO, Evans AJ, Wilson ARM and Pinder SE. Diagnostic techniques and examination of pathologic specimens. In Elston CW, Ellis IO eds. The Breast Systemic Pathology Volume 13. Edinburgh: Churchill-Livingstone, 1998:21–46.

Holland R, Hendriks JHCL, Verbeek ALM, et al. Extent, distribution, and mammographic/histological correlations of breast ductal carcinoma in situ. Lancet 1990;335:519–522.

Lagios MD, Westdahl PR, Margolin FR, Roses MR. Duct carcinoma in situ; Relationship of extent of noninvasive disease to the frequency of occult invasion, multicentricity, lymph node metastases, and short-term treatment failures. Cancer 1982;50:1309–1314.

Schnitt SJ, Connolly JL. Processing and evaluation of breast excision specimens: a clinically oriented approach. Am J Clin Pathol 1992;98:125–137.

Schnitt SJ, Wang HH. Histologic sampling of grossly benign breast biopsies: how much is enough? Am J Surg Pathol 1989;13:505–512.

Smitt MC, Nowels KW, Zdeblick MJ, et al. The importance of the lumpectomy surgical margin status in long-term results of breast conservation. Cancer 1995;76:259–267.

3 Assessment of Fine Needle Aspiration Cytology and Core Biopsy Samples

Sarah E Pinder · Frances P O'Malley

FINE NEEDLE ASPIRATION CYTOLOGY (FNAC) REPORTING

Although the pathologist always attempts to make a definitive diagnosis on any specimen received, it should be recognized that fine needle aspiration cytology (FNAC) breast samples can, in some cases, be impossible to diagnose unequivocally as benign or malignant. The proportion of such problematic cases depends to some extent on the expertise of the pathologist, but is also closely related to the quality of the samples and thus the aspirator plays a central role both in obtaining sufficient cells and in providing good quality smear preparation. For those cases that simply cannot be unequivocally diagnosed on cytology preparations, the most appropriate approach is to use terms such as 'atypia – probably benign' or 'atypia – suspicious, probably malignant' (or, as recommended by a National Cancer Institute consensus conference on the reporting of FNA, as indeterminate/atypical or suspicious/probably malignant). If one recognizes the difficulty in histologic diagnosis of some breast lesions, such as atypical epithelial proliferations, then it is not surprising that some cases can be difficult to classify cytologically.

INADEQUATE SAMPLES

Despite experience and expertise in aspiration there are a proportion of cases where insufficient cells are obtained to achieve a diagnosis. Whether these samples are categorized as inadequate or insufficient is not of great importance. It is impossible to be prescriptive in defining a number of epithelial cells on a slide which falls below the threshold of 'adequate'. Although some authorities specify that one requires 6 to 10 epithelial cell clusters to qualify as 'adequate', it will to some extent depend on the clinical history, age of patient, quality of the cells which are present and also the background of the smear. If, for example, there are many epithelial cells present but these are obscured by blood, or are crushed or show preparation artefact, then the specimen is inadequate for assessment.

In general, a smear is inadequate for assessment if it is (a) insufficiently cellular; (b) obscured by red blood cells or other cells or debris; or (c) if the preparation of the sample is poor and there is artefact such that assessment is impossible.

It is important to note that in some instances, the absence of epithelial cells may not preclude diagnosis of another process or lesion and the smear may still be interpreted accurately. For example, abundant fragments of adipose tissue will be seen from a lipoma and a cellular smear with abundant polymorphic lymphoid cells may reflect an intramammary lymph node. Other examples of non-epithelial processes such as fat necrosis or an abscess may be identified by the presence of foamy macrophages and giant cells or abundant polymorphs and debris, respectively.

BENIGN SMEARS

A benign smear may represent a specific benign, non-epithelial process (as described above, for example, from an abscess), but more commonly contains regular, ductal epithelial cells. These should show no atypia and the specimen should contain sufficient epithelial cells for assessment. Benign smears are typically only poorly or moderately cellular and the epithelial cells are arranged in monolayers with evenly spaced regular small to moderately sized cells (Figure 3-1). An exception to this is the fibroadenoma which may provide abundant sheets and clumps of epithelial cells in large clusters with an irregularly shaped outline (Figure 3-2). It may not be possible to recognize a specific benign breast entity and the sample should be simply categorized as 'benign' in most cases.

Benign cells are not pleomorphic and have evenly spaced chromatin and nuclear features; the latter are more easily seen in Papanicoloau stains than in Giemsa-stained preparations, but the choice of preparation is usually related to the laboratory's and the pathologist's personal choice and experience. In fibrocystic change and cysts, apocrine cells and foamy macrophages may be noted. The former are seen as larger cells with abundant cytoplasm, granules and prominent nucleoli, as in histologic preparations.

In addition to the epithelial cell clusters, it is valuable to assess the background population in a breast aspiration cytology smear. This is usually composed of dispersed individual and naked (bare/stripped) nuclei

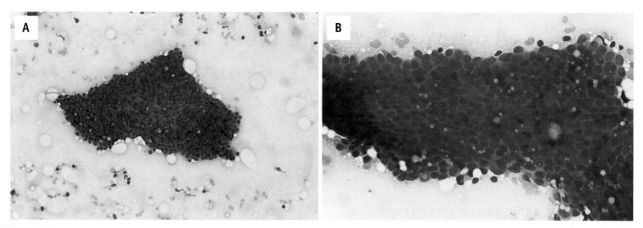

FIGURE 3-1

Benign epithelial cells in Giemsa-stained breast FNAC. These are seen as mild to moderate in size, evenly spaced cohesive sheets of cells.

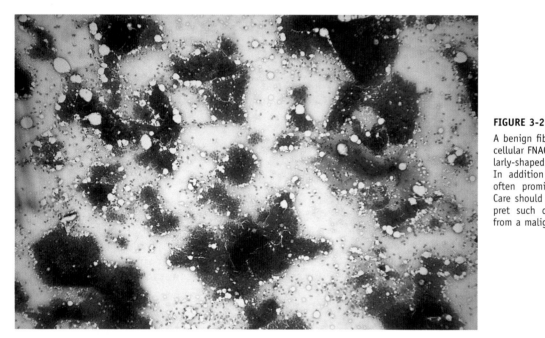

FIGURE 3-2

A benign fibroadenoma may provide a cellular FNAC sample with large irregularly-shaped sheets of epithelial cells. In addition stripped/bare nuclei are often prominent in the background. Care should be taken not to misinterpret such cellular samples as being from a malignant lesion.

along with scanty stromal fragments; both of these elements may be particularly prominent from a fibroadenoma and recognition of these components can be valuable in avoiding a false positive diagnosis from these cellular lesions.

ATYPIA – PROBABLY BENIGN

These samples, in general, have overall benign appearances but show additional features that are mildly atypical. This is usually either (a) a mild degree of nuclear atypia or pleomorphism; or (b) some loss of cohesion; or (c) increased cellularity with either (a) or (b).

ATYPIA – SUSPICIOUS, PROBABLY MALIGNANT

These smears have highly atypical features that are considered to almost certainly represent malignancy but on which definitive diagnosis is not possible. This may be (a) because there are very scanty, but highly atypical cells present which are insufficient in number for an unequivocal diagnosis; or (b) because there are marked preparation or preservation artefacts but very worrisome cells are seen; or (c) if the overall appearances are benign but a few highly atypical cells are present; or (d) if the cells present show some, but not unequivocally, malignant features. In essence this category is used if the pathologist assesses the specimen as highly suspicious of malignancy, but is not recommending definitive therapeutic surgery such as mastectomy.

MALIGNANT

These smears contain sufficient and sufficiently well-preserved cells for an unequivocal diagnosis of malignancy. In general these are epithelial cells that are large (comparison with red blood cells can be valuable for determination of cell size), invariably discohesive and pleomorphic to some extent (Figure 3-3). Particularly in Papanicoloau-stained smears, atypical nuclear features will be seen, including irregularly sized and shaped cells, often with multiple nucleoli and clumped chromatin.

DIAGNOSTIC PITFALLS IN BREAST FNAC

The histologic patterns seen in benign and malignant breast lesions are varied, as described elsewhere in this book, and this is, not surprisingly, reflected in the cytologic appearances. It is important for this reason to have knowledge of the patterns of breast histology, normal, benign and malignant, before reporting breast cytology samples; this will have a beneficial impact and lower the risk of false positive and false negative diagnoses. There are, however, some well-recognized pitfall lesions which can give worrisome cytologic appearances.

Excessive pressure during spreading of slides may produce discohesion of epithelial cells, particularly in fibroadenomas, but this can occur in any breast FNAC sample. This can often be recognized as most prominent at the peripheral or trailing edge of the smear, but if there is also air-drying artefact the cells can also be apparently pleomorphic but also appear somewhat smudged and rather flattened. Care should be taken in providing a definitive diagnosis on a sub-optimal cytology preparation.

The archetypical lesion which may be mistaken for malignancy in breast FNAC preparations is the fibroadenoma. This is because these smears may be highly cellular and there may be some epithelial pleomorphism and discohesion around the edges of the epithelial cell clumps; this is more common in younger women. Good clinical and radiologic correlation (the 'triple approach') is essential in avoiding errors in breast FNAC diagnosis. As noted above, the background population should be assessed and contains, usually abundant, bare nuclei in an FNAC from a fibroadenoma. The bare nuclei present should, however, be distinguished from stripped cancer nuclei; the latter will have similar nuclear features to those of the atypical epithelial cells that have retained their cytoplasm and that may be seen singly or in clumps.

Apocrine cells in FNAC samples may be derived from cysts or fibrocystic change and can thus show some degenerate features, including discohesion and some clumping of the chromatin. The nature of the cells should be correctly identified by the typical cytoplasm which is, as in histologic samples, relatively abundant and may be granular. The nucleus may bear prominent nucleoli, again as in histologic sections, and may appear

---

DIAGNOSTIC PITFALLS ON FNAC

Lesions that may lead to a false suspicious/malignant diagnosis
▶ Fibroadenoma
▶ Apocrine proliferations
▶ Papillomas
▶ Lactational change
▶ Fat necrosis

Lesions that may lead to a false benign diagnosis
▶ Paucicellular, low grade invasive ductal carcinoma, no special type
▶ Special type carcinomas, particularly tubular and lobular carcinomas

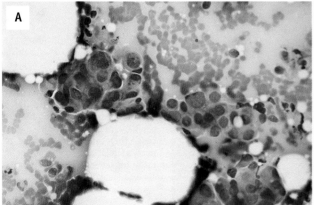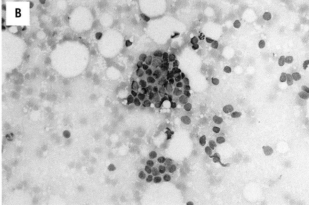

FIGURE 3-3

Medium (A) and high (B) power images of carcinoma cells in a breast FNAC sample are usually discohesive and show pleomorphism. The tumor cells are often, but not invariably, of moderate or large size. The degree of pleomorphism varies considerably between cases. The sample is most frequently cellular. Background stripped/bare nuclei are rare, although stripped tumor cell nuclei may be seen which should be recognized as being of similar appearance to the intact carcinoma cells.

somewhat pleomorphic; it is sometimes necessary to classify these lesions as 'atypia – probably benign' if the degree of this is worrisome but care should be taken not to overdiagnose apocrine cells as malignant unless unequivocal features are seen, such as marked pleomorphism and discohesion in a cellular sample.

Aspiration of papillomas often produces 3-D clusters of epithelial cells. These may look like the balls of cells which may be seen in ascitic fluid or pleural aspirates from metastatic carcinoma, which somewhat resemble aggregate fruit such as blackberries (Figure 3-4). It is often wise, in the presence of such clumps, to classify the lesion as 'papillary' and to recommend diagnostic excision as it can be impossible to distinguish a benign papilloma from papillary carcinoma *in situ*. Rarely nuclear pleomorphism and crowding can be seen in FNAC samples from benign papillomas.

It is not possible to distinguish with accuracy *in situ* carcinoma from invasive disease on FNAC whether a 'lobular' or 'ductal' process. The difference between atypical hyperplasia (either atypical lobular (ALH) or atypical ductal hyperplasia (ADH)) and *in situ* carcinoma is one of extent and degree of atypia histologically; evidently this cannot be determined on cytologic preparations. FNAC from lobular proliferations (ALH, lobular carcinoma *in situ* (LCIS) or invasive lobular carcinoma) may contain small to moderately sized epithelial cells which are seen singly or in small clumps. Clearly if the sample is cellular and composed entirely of such forms, a diagnosis of invasive lobular carcinoma can be made. Intracytoplasmic vacuoles may be present, but these can also be seen in benign epithelial cells. Similarly, low grade ductal carcinoma *in situ* (DCIS) cannot be differentiated from ADH on cytologic grounds. Conversely, high grade DCIS may be seen cytologically as large, pleomorphic epithelial cells that cannot be distinguished with any reliability on cytology specimens from

invasive carcinoma, although the sample is frequently paucicellular in the former and bears background necrotic debris. Thus, although some groups have described systems for distinguishing, for example ADH from low grade DCIS, a pragmatic approach is recommended and the use of the 'atypia' category highlights to clinical colleagues the need for further investigation.

Lactational changes produce dissociated cells with prominent nucleoli within cells with larger nuclei than 'typical' benign epithelial cells. It should be remembered that focal lactational change may occur in older women and indeed those who have never been pregnant. The epithelial cells have a pale blue or mauve vacuolated cytoplasm seen on Giemsa staining due to lipid droplets. A clinical history should be, but is not always, provided. Similarly a clinical history of previous surgery and radiotherapy can be invaluable in avoiding the pitfall of changes due to such previous treatment; cells from such samples may be moderately pleomorphic but are usually scanty.

Cellular smears may be obtained from lymphoid lesions, whether a benign intramammary or low axillary lymph node or a benign or malignant lymphoid process. The scanty cytoplasm and variety of morphology in the former should enable diagnosis. Lymphomas may be problematic but recognition of the nature of the cells should be possible. As well as the scanty cytoplasm, in general no clumps of cells will be present and the entire population will be discohesive, whereas in a malignant epithelial population at least some of the cells are usually seen in clusters. If there is doubt, a report of atypia (suspicious) can be issued and subsequent repeat FNAC or core biopsy will allow immunohistochemical confirmation of the nature of the malignant population. A similar course of action is recommended if the malignant cells may potentially be from metastasis from another epithelial malignancy or malignant melanoma.

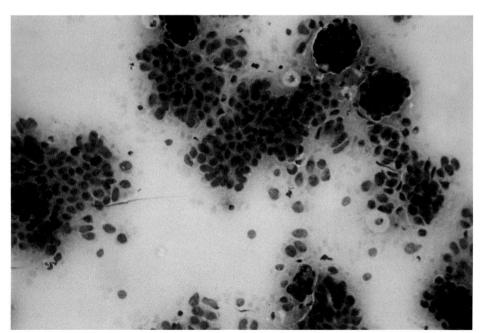

FIGURE 3-4

FNAC of papillary lesions. This technique may produce samples of the typical appearance shown here. The papillary cell clusters form 'balls' of cells. These specimens may be relatively cellular and should not be mistaken for carcinoma.

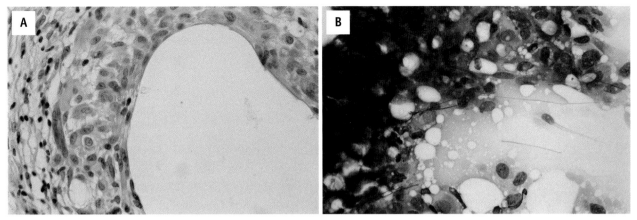

FIGURE 3-5

FNAC from fat necrosis may mimic carcinoma. The cells aspirated may be discohesive and large. Unless the more abundant cytoplasm and the variety of macrophage appearances which are present, for example including giant cells and foamy forms, are recognized, this may be mistaken for pleomorphism of an epithelial process.

Fat necrosis can mimic carcinoma cytologically (Figure 3-5). The smear is usually cellular and contains discohesive cells, but on scrutiny bears a mixed population including foamy macrophages and inflammatory cells. A search for overt foamy macrophage forms and multinucleated giant cells can be helpful.

False negative FNAC diagnoses are most commonly derived from low grade or special type carcinomas such as tubular carcinoma. Tubular carcinomas may, because of the desmoplastic stroma, provide only poorly cellular samples with mild to moderately atypical epithelial cells. The absence of typical bare nuclei, a degree of discohesion to at least some of the epithelial cells and stripped malignant nuclei may provide clues to the diagnosis. Tubular structures may be present, but these should not be interpreted as a diagnostic feature as they can rarely be derived from benign lesions.

CORE BIOPSY REPORTING GUIDELINES

As with cytology samples, good clinical and radiologic correlation is required for interpretation of core biopsy samples. Histologic assessment of the vast majority of such specimens can determine whether the lesion is normal, benign or malignant, but a very small proportion cannot. It should be noted that lesions that are diagnostically difficult in surgical open biopsies are likely to be more so on the limited tissue sampling that is undertaken with core biopsy and thus there are, as with FNAC, a variety of lesions that are problematic on such specimens. It is recommended that in such cases the pathologist does not make an unequivocal diagnosis and repeat core biopsy or diagnostic surgical open biopsy is obtained. The proportion of such 'atypical' cases is less with core biopsy than with FNAC in most breast pathology practices.

A normal portion of tissue may be received; this may contain normal fat or fat and fibrous tissue only or may bear breast parenchymal structures. The components present should be noted in the histology report. While this may reflect inadequate sampling of the lesion of clinical or radiologic concern, this may be appropriate from a lesion such as a lipoma or hamartoma. Microcalcification may be seen in normal breast cores, for example, within involutional change, although it is essential to discuss this finding with clinical colleagues to determine whether it is representative and whether indeed radiologically visible. Small foci of microcalcification may be seen histologically which cannot be identified radiologically (<100 micrometers) and the lesion may potentially have been missed (Figure 3-6).

A core may contain histologic features of a specific benign abnormality such as a fibroadenoma (Figure 3-7), fibrocystic changes or sclerosing adenosis (Figure 3-8) and can definitively be classified as 'benign'. There are, however, some lesions that are known to be associated with malignancy in the adjacent breast tissue or are themselves known to be heterogeneous. As described in Chapter 14, the diagnosis of ADH involves an assessment of extent of the proliferation that is often not possible to determine with accuracy on the limited tissue sampling undertaken by core biopsy. While some authorities have stated that limited ADH confined to 1 or 2 foci on a core biopsy may not require further surgery, particularly if the microcalcifications have been removed, others have reported that up to 50% of core biopsy samples with an atypical intraductal proliferation such as ADH may be 'up-graded' to DCIS in subsequent diagnostic excision samples; clearly this depends on the numbers and size of cores taken. Until further data becomes available, we recommend local excision for core biopsies containing atypical epithelial proliferations, particularly ADH.

There is no widespread agreement on the management of cases which bear lobular neoplasia in a core biopsy but clearly this does not have the same implication as a diagnosis of DCIS (see Chapter 15). As most lobular neoplastic lesions are mammographically silent, it is essential to determine if the histologic features in the core biopsy correlate with the mammographic find-

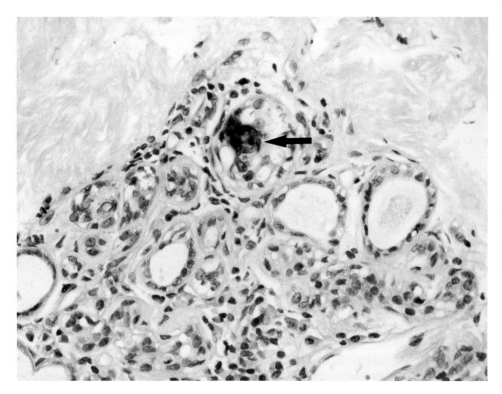

FIGURE 3-6

Microcalcification may be present within normal structures in the breast. Microcalcification is seen here within a lobular unit (arrow). It is essential that multidisciplinary discussion takes place to determine whether the histology and the radiologic features correlate and whether the microcalcification present histologically is (a) representative and (b) likely to be radiologically visible.

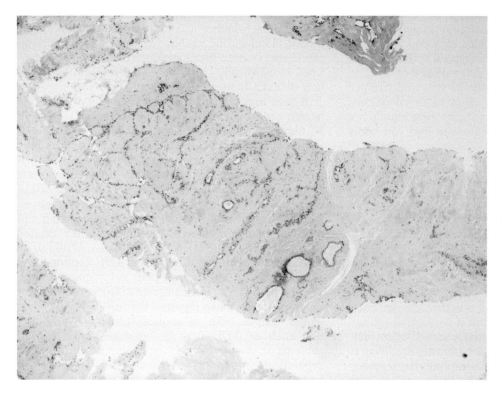

FIGURE 3-7

Core biopsy of a benign fibroadenoma. This can be unequivocally diagnosed as benign and will explain a clinical or radiologic well-defined mass in the breast.

ings in such cases. Clearly, if the core biopsy findings do not explain the mammographic abnormality, further tissue sampling is required.

Rarely, it may not be possible to classify a proliferation as either lobular neoplasia or low grade DCIS and the pathology report should describe this difficulty and further sampling be undertaken (see Chapter 15).

Columnar lesions are seen with increased frequency as a result of mammographic breast screening and the investigation of calcifications. Whilst benign columnar cell changes may be evident, degrees of architectural or cytologic atypia should be sought and may cause diagnostic difficulties. There is, at present, controversy regarding the appropriate management of such lesions

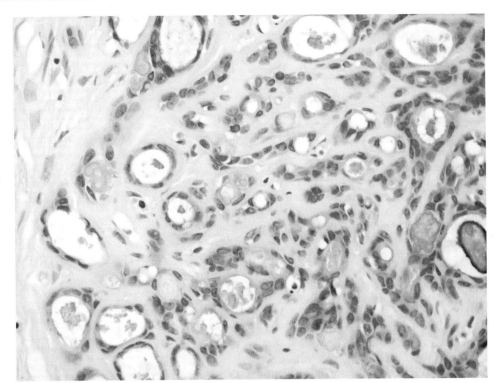

FIGURE 3-8

High power of H&E stained section of sclerosing adenosis. Note the lack of stromal reaction to the infiltrating cords of cells which should not be misinterpreted as invasive carcinoma. The presence of a myoepithelial layer could be confirmed immunohistochemically.

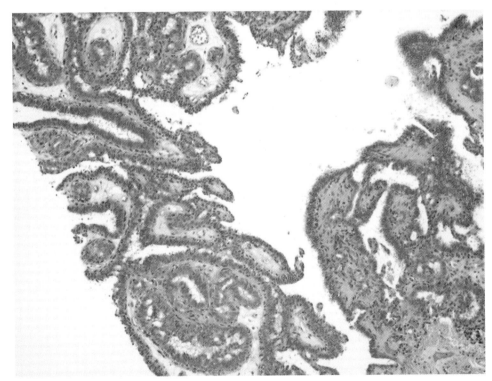

FIGURE 3-9

Core biopsy including a portion of benign papilloma. These lesions are known to show heterogeneity and on occasions to be difficult to assess due to fragmentation. Some authorities recommend excision of all papillary lesions identified on core biopsy, either by surgical excision or by vacuum-assisted wide bore core biopsy.

but, if there is atypia present, the majority of centers would recommend diagnostic excision at this time. (See also Chapter 13.)

Cores may bear features of a radial scar/complex sclerosing lesion such as areas of fibro-elastosis with entrapped tubules. Such lesions are believed by many authorities to be associated with malignancy. In the

majority of centers these lesions, once diagnosed on core biopsy, are excised; this may be by surgical open biopsy or by vacuum-assisted 11 gauge core biopsy.

Similarly, papillary lesions are difficult to assess in the relatively limited tissue obtained by core (Figure 3-9). They may fragment and are recognized to show heterogeneity. Thus, we recommend that these are reported as 'a papillary lesion' without comment about benignity or malignancy (unless unequivocally malignant); excision of such lesions by vacuum-assisted 11 gauge core or open surgical diagnostic biopsy should be undertaken.

Occasionally an unequivocal diagnosis of a phyllodes tumor can be made on core biopsy if the lesion is of borderline or malignant nature. More often a cellular fibroepithelial lesion is seen and it can be difficult to distinguish a cellular fibroadenoma from a benign phyllodes tumor. The features of a phyllodes tumor include the cellularity and degree of atypia of the stroma as well as stromal overgrowth and increased mitotic activity; often these features cannot be assessed on core biopsy and the lesion should be excised as a diagnostic procedure.

Very rarely in core biopsy samples, definitive diagnosis cannot be made because, despite the features of malignancy, the worrisome areas are on the edge of the core or have been crushed or fragmented. Occasionally only a portion of a duct with a suspicious epithelial proliferation is seen; the appearances can be reported as suspicious of DCIS if this is a high grade process and definitive diagnosis is not possible (Figure 3-10). Very small foci of highly atypical cells insufficient for confirmatory immunohistochemistry can also preclude definitive diagnosis. In such instances a report of 'suspicious of malignancy' is issued and repeat sampling undertaken.

In the majority of cases of breast carcinoma an unequivocal diagnosis can be made on core biopsy, whether it is DCIS or invasive cancer. Indeed one of the benefits of core biopsy as a pre-operative technique is that *in situ* can be distinguished from invasive disease

as the pathologist has the architecture available for assessment as well as the cytologic features. In difficult cases, such as DCIS/LCIS involving areas of sclerosing adenosis, immunohistochemistry can be undertaken to assess whether a myoepithelial and basement membrane layer is indeed present. The finding of pure DCIS in a core does not, of course, preclude the finding of an invasive focus in the subsequent surgical excision sample and in approximately 20% of cases it has been reported that a co-existing invasive carcinoma will be seen. One of the benefits of core biopsy is that the diagnosis of special type and low grade carcinomas is not as problematic as this may be on FNAC (Figure 3-11).

PITFALLS IN CORE BIOPSY ASSESSMENT

Pitfalls in the assessment of core biopsy samples are often due to the limited sampling that is inherent in the

---

DIAGNOSTIC PITFALLS ON CORE BIOPSIES

Lesions that can lead to false suspicious/malignant diagnosis
▶ Lobular neoplasia within sclerosing adenosis
▶ Entrapped benign glands within a radial scar
▶ Apocrine proliferations

Lesions that can lead to a false negative diagnosis
▶ Paucicellular, invasive lobular carcinoma

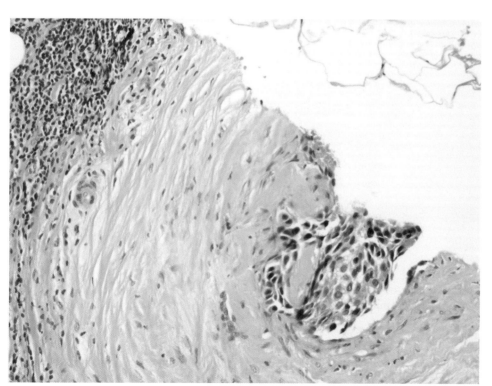

FIGURE 3-10

Although less frequent than with FNAC, some lesions cannot and should not be unequivocally diagnosed on core biopsy and are classified as 'suspicious of malignancy'. This is most often because the lesion has been insufficiently sampled. Here a portion of a duct space bears a worrisome epithelial proliferation. There is surrounding fibrosis and chronic inflammation and the appearances are suspicious of high grade DCIS.

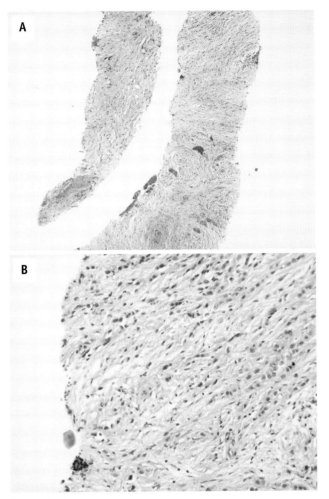

FIGURE 3-11
Core biopsy with invasive lobular carcinoma of classical type. (A) Low power and (B) high power images. Low grade and special type carcinomas, as well as *in situ* disease, may not be definitively diagnosed on FNAC, but definite diagnosis can be made on core.

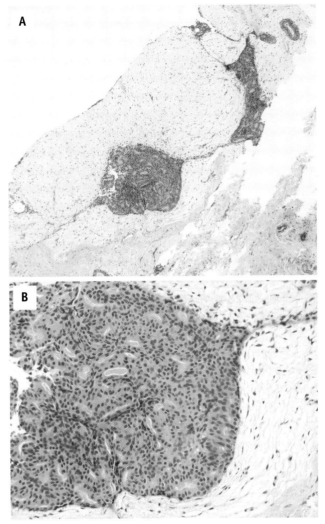

FIGURE 3-12
Particularly in core biopsy samples, usual epithelial hyperplasia in a fibroadenoma may be misdiagnosed as a more worrying process such as ADH or DCIS. The epithelium may 'telescope' from the duct wall during the sampling procedure and appear prominent and may be seen in clumped islands. As a rule, great care should be taken in the diagnosis of an atypical epithelial proliferation in a fibroepithelial lesion in core biopsy.

nature of the specimen. Particular problem lesions are those that utilize a low power histologic examination of the overall architecture of the disease process, which quite simply cannot be determined on smaller core biopsy specimens. Other pitfalls are associated with the high power examination of a few cells that in larger open surgical biopsies one would not assess in such a manner; a typical example of this is the high power examination of the epithelial cells in a fibroadenoma that the inexperienced pathologist may report as showing cytologic atypia (Figure 3-12). Indeed mild atypia of the epithelium often within lobular units is one of the commonest problems encountered in core biopsy samples, particularly if the lesion has undergone previous sampling and the epithelium shows reactive changes and mitoses may even (rarely) be prominent (Figure 3-13). Care must be taken not to overdiagnose such minimal degrees of atypia.

Specific difficulties inherent to core biopsy include sclerosing adenosis that may mimic invasive carcinoma, particularly as the low power normal lobular arrangement is not apparent in a limited sample (see Figure

3-8); if there is associated lobular neoplasia or apocrine change, the mimicry can be marked. However, immunohistochemical assessment with smooth muscle myosin or smooth muscle actin will show the myoepithelial layer and can be extremely valuable in cases of concern. Similarly, radial scars with entrapped tubular structures may mimic tubular carcinoma and the same immunohistochemistry will be helpful in difficult cases; the fibroblastic stroma usually present in tubular carcinomas should also be sought on routine hematoxylin and eosin (H&E) stains.

Conversely, paucicellular, low grade invasive lobular carcinomas may mimic a benign process such as chronic inflammation or stromal fibrosis. In such cases, one requires a high index of suspicion. Cytokeratin immunohistochemistry can be particularly helpful in resolving this differential diagnosis.

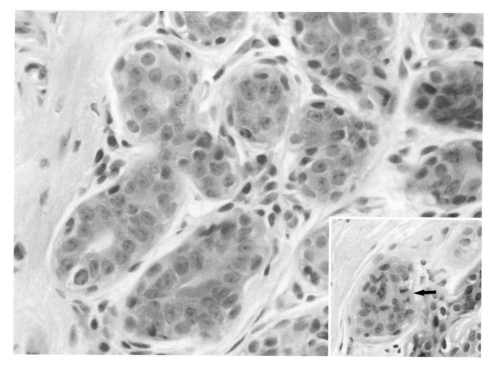

FIGURE 3-13

Minor degrees of atypia should not be overinterpreted in a core biopsy. Particularly if previous sampling has been undertaken the epithelium may show some reactive changes. Nucleoli may be present and even mitoses as shown here (arrow in inset) may be evident.

Apocrine proliferations, as noted above, particularly in association with sclerosing adenosis may be difficult to diagnose. In the limited sample received in a core biopsy, the large nuclei and prominent nucleoli may be mistaken for DCIS by the unwary. The archetypical abundant, eosinophilic granular cytoplasm provides a clue to the apocrine nature of the cells. Unless there is marked nuclear atypia, necrosis and mitoses in an apocrine proliferation in a core biopsy sample, the diagnosis of apocrine DCIS should be made with considerable caution.

Stromal proliferations in core biopsy samples may be difficult to diagnose. Repeat core biopsy that shows a spindled cell proliferation may reflect sampling of the previous core site with stromal fibrosis, but could also represent the lesion of concern clinically or radiologically. The search for fat necrosis seen as foamy macrophages with inflammatory cells may prove helpful and occasionally in core biopsies hemosiderin-laden macrophages can be present indicating that the process is reactive. A stromal proliferation may be seen that does not reflect core site, i.e, in a patient who has not undergone a previous needling procedure; such spindled cell proliferations can be problematic. Possible diagnoses include fibromatosis, nerve sheath tumor, myofibroblastoma, phyllodes tumor, metaplastic carcinoma or even primary sarcoma. Particularly in an older patient, a high index of suspicion of metaplastic carcinoma is appropriate and a low threshold for resorting to immunohistochemistry is advised. As described in Chapter 18, a range of anti-cytokeratin antibodies is often required for recognition of the epithelial nature of these lesions and if positive definitive diagnosis can be made. However, in some spindled cell processes on core biopsy samples, definitive diagnosis is not possible and diagnostic excision is prudent.

Malignant lymphomas are less difficult to recognize in core biopsy than they can be in FNAC samples. Most lymphomas in the breast are of high grade, diffuse large B-cell type and can be easily suspected and diagnosed with judicious immunohistochemistry (CD45, CD20, CD3, CD30, etc). Low grade lymphomas may mimic chronic inflammation and a panel of lymphoid markers may be necessary to confirm the immunophenotype and to allow correct diagnosis.

ASSESSMENT OF PROGNOSTIC INFORMATION ON CORE BIOPSY

Histologic grading can be performed on core biopsy samples and is requested by many clinicians. The system used is the same as in larger surgical excisions (see Chapter 19). It is reasonably accurate with concordance with subsequent excision in about 75% of cases. In particular, the mitotic count tends to be lower in the core than in the excision as the area of highest proliferation may not have been sampled. Thus there is a tendency to 'under-grade' on core biopsy. If, however, a carcinoma is classified as being of histologic grade 3, then this is very likely to be correct and it is unusual for an invasive cancer to be 'down-graded' in the subsequent subsequent excision. Tumors may also often be sub-typed but this is less accurate, as most types require assessment of the overall morphology of the lesion and determination of the proportion of 'purity' of the architectural phenotype. Vascular invasion cannot be assessed with any reliability on core biopsy as it is infrequently seen even when present in the surgical excision sample; when present this feature should be reported.

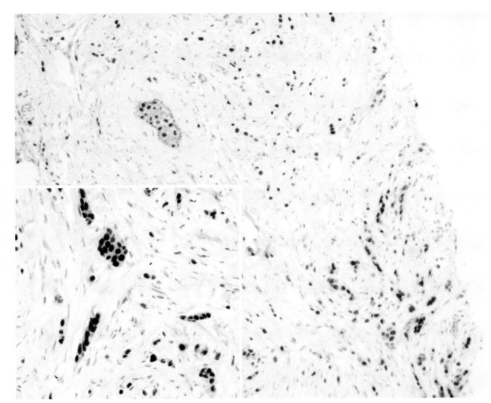

FIGURE 3-14

Assessment of prognostic information on core biopsy. One of the advantages of core biopsy is the relatively easier assessment of estrogen receptor (ER) status of a carcinoma compared to FNAC. Although ER can be determined on FNAC this requires an additional slide and is technically more difficult. This tumor shows predominantly strong reactivity in the majority of tumor cell nuclei (Allred score = 8, see Chapter 24).

Predictive factors, such as hormone receptor status (Figure 3-14), can be assessed reliably on core biopsy and the results correlate well with assessment on subsequent excision samples.

SUGGESTED READING

The uniform approach to breast fine-needle aspiration biopsy. National Cancer Institute Fine Needle Aspiration of Breast Workshop Subcommittees. Diagn Cytopathol 1997;16:295–311.

Boerner S, Fornage BD, Singletary E, Sneige N. Ultrasound-guided fine-needle aspiration (FNA) of nonpalpable breast lesions: a review of 1885 FNA cases using the National Cancer Institute-supported recommendations on the uniform approach to breast FNA. Cancer 1999; 87:19–24.

Best Practice No 179. Guidelines for breast needle core biopsy handling and reporting in breast screening assessment. Ellis IO, Humphreys S, Michell M, Pinder SE, Wells CA, Zakhour HD; UK National Coordinating Commmittee for Breast Screening Pathology; European Commission Working Group on Breast Screening Pathology. J Clin Pathol 2004; 57:897–902.

Berner A, Davidson B, Sigstad E, Risberg B. Fine-needle aspiration cytology vs. core biopsy in the diagnosis of breast lesions. Diagn Cytopathol 2003;29:344–8.

Overview of Clinical Aspects of Breast Disease

R Douglas MacMillan

CLINICAL FEATURES

Many benign breast disorders are not considered diseases but represent exaggerated forms of the normal state. Disorders of breast development include simple asymmetry, juvenile hypertrophy, fibroadenoma, hamartoma and accessory breasts. Disorders of cyclical hormonal change include mastalgia and nodularity. Disorders of breast involution include cysts, sclerosing lesions, hyperplasias and duct ectasia (Table 4-1).

At least 90 % of all women attending a specialist breast out-patient clinic will be symptomatic with such disorders and only approximately 10 % will be diagnosed with true breast 'diseases' of which the most important are obviously invasive breast cancer and ductal carcinoma *in situ* (DCIS). However, much time and effort is spent eliminating the possibility of a malignant diagnosis, whilst most benign breast disorders are managed by confident reassurance and few require treatment. For asymptomatic women recalled for assessment as part a screening program, a very small proportion will be diagnosed with malignant disease approximately 1 in 8.

ASSESSMENT OF BREAST LUMPS

A breast lump might be defined as a discrete mass palpably separate from surrounding tissue and invariably of different consistency. An experienced breast examiner can usually make a distinction between a definite breast lump and a generally lumpy breast. As a rule, all breast lumps require assessment.

Assessment of a breast lump includes clinical examination, imaging and some form of biopsy (fine needle aspiration (FNA), core or occasionally excisional). There is a trend towards performing ultrasound for all lumps, with mammography reserved for women over 40 years in whom clinical assessment or ultrasound is suspicious or uncertain.

Benign disorders that often require treatment or may be considered diseases are giant fibroadenoma, phyllodes tumor, duct papilloma, periductal mastitis, breast abscess, single duct nipple discharge and autoimmune mastitis.

LARGE FIBROADENOMAS AND PHYLLODES FUMORS

Fibroadenomas are classically smooth-surfaced, discrete from surrounding tissue, mobile, rubbery to the touch in young women but may be hard in older women due to sclerosis or calcification. They are only occasionally over 3 cm in diameter.

In a 2-year follow-up study of 163 fibroadenomas, 8 % increased in size, 12 % decreased in size, 26 % disappeared and 54 % did not change. Of the 8 % that increased in size, half of the patients were under age 20 years.

Juvenile or giant fibroadenomas are rare and usually occur in adolescence. An arbitrary definition would be a fibroadenoma greater than 5 cm. Growth is usually rapid and these lumps, which may reach 15–20 cm in size, require excision.

Phyllodes tumors may present with similar clinical (and imaging) characteristics to fibroadenomas. A preoperative diagnosis can be difficult. Suspicion of phyllodes tumor does, however, indicate that the lump should be excised with a margin of clearance (when compared to fibroadenomas which can be shelled out from the breast). For some large cases this may require mastectomy (for which a definitive diagnosis, sometimes by excision biopsy, is obviously required).

PAPILLARY LESIONS

These rarely present as breast lumps. Ductal papillomas more frequently present as nipple discharge and are discussed below. Larger papillomas occasionally present as a discrete hard lump beneath, or close to, the areola. Excision biopsy is indicated to identify possible papillary carcinoma or DCIS.

AUTOIMMUNE MASTITIS

Granulomatous mastitis is an uncommon condition usually presenting in the third or fourth decade. Etiology is largely unknown although may be associated with hyperprolactinaemia. It may present as an otherwise suspicious breast lump. Often, the clinical picture is fairly classical with multiple tender lumps forming sinuses at needle biopsy sites discharging sterile pus. Investigations to rule out systemic autoimmune disease are usually normal. Treatment is by immunosuppression (steroids and methotrexate) and the clinical course typically lasts 1–2 years before resolution. Surgery should be avoided. Other rare autoimmune diseases of the breast include lymphocytic lobulitis, which classically occurs in young insulin dependent diabetics. There is usually a history of poor diabetic control and

TABLE 4-1
Clinical/pathologic Associations

Clinical feature	Common cause	Rare cause
Benign-feeling lump	Fibroadenoma Cyst Lipoma Normal breast tissue	Papilloma Phyllodes tumor Hamartoma
Suspicious lump	Breast cancer	Scar tissue Fat necrosis Cyst Granulomatous mastitis Lymphocytic lobulitis Periductal mastitis
Tender lump	Normal breast Periductal mastitis Abscess Fibroadenoma	Inflammatory breast cancer Granulomatous mastitis Fat necrosis
Asymmetric thickening	Normal breast	DCIS Invasive lobular breast cancer
Multiduct discharge	Duct ectasia Physiologic	Drug-related
Single duct discharge	Papilloma Duct ectasia	DCIS
Scaling nipple	Dermatitis	Paget's disease of nipple

retinopathy. Clinical features are fibrous non-tender thickenings. Once a diagnosis is made (by core biopsy) the condition is managed conservatively. Spontaneous regression may occur over a few years.

INFLAMMATORY LUMPS

Breast abscess is most often seen either as a complication of periductal mastitis (anaerobic infection) or during lactation (staphlococcal infection). Abscesses are quite uncommon in post-menopausal women. First-line treatment is aspiration under ultrasound and appropriate antibiotics. It is now exceptional for a breast abscess to require surgery.

Periductal mastitis is a condition seen in young women (usually women in their early 30s) and is strongly associated with cigarette smoking. It presents with recurrent episodes of peri-areolar sepsis and clinical thickening. Associated complications include non-cyclical central breast pain, nipple retraction, nipple discharge and mammary fistula. Treatment is by antibiotics for acute episodes, encouragement to cease smoking and surgery (total duct excision) for chronic infection or mammary fistula.

NIPPLE DISCHARGE

Nipple discharge is uncommon but is often associated with considerable anxiety, especially if bloodstained.

Only approximately 5 % of all single duct discharges are due to DCIS and the more common causes are duct ectasia and ductal papilloma. In the assessment of nipple discharge a distinction is made between multiduct and single duct discharge. Multiduct discharge is frequently bilateral, requires no investigation and surgery (duct division/ligation) is only indicated if the discharge is profuse and troublesome. Single duct discharge always requires investigation. In some centres duct endoscopy is performed. Cytology of the discharge and mammography are usually performed. In the absence of suspicious findings, surgery (microdochectomy/microductectomy) is indicated only if the discharge is troublesome or persistent. Some cases will resolve spontaneously.

ASSOCIATION OF BENIGN BREAST DISORDERS WITH BREAST CANCER

Certain specific benign breast disorders are associated with a clinically relevant increased risk of subsequent development of breast cancer. Atypical lobular and atypical ductal hyperplasia (ALH and ADH, respectively) are both associated with an absolute risk of developing breast cancer over 10–15 years of approximately 10 %. The risk for ALH probably decreases dramatically after the menopause, a feature not recognized with ADH. They are invariably diagnosed as an incidental finding in breast biopsies performed for other reasons. No characteristic radiologic features are recognized. If a patient also has a family history of breast cancer the risk for ALH is additive and approximates that of low grade DCIS (20–25 % over 10–15 years). Both ADH and ALH indicate an increased risk of breast cancer in either breast although ipsilateral recurrences are more common.

Screening is indicated for ALH until the menopause and for ADH until at least ten years after diagnosis. If a family history is also present screening should continue beyond ten years.

DUCTAL CARCINOMA IN SITU

The incidence of DCIS has increased 6-fold over the past 15 years. This is entirely due to mammographic screening. In countries with a breast-screening program, the mode of presentation has also changed from a palpable mass, nipple discharge or Paget's disease of the nipple, to the current situation in which approximately 90 % of all DCIS cases present as clinically occult lesions on mammography. Approximately 80 % of these present as microcalcification. For women aged 50–65, 20 % of all screen-detected cancers are in the form of DCIS. If younger women are screened, this percentage is reportedly as high as 40 %.

The optimum management of DCIS is still debated. DCIS is increasingly recognized as a heterogeneous disease and management should perhaps reflect this and be individualized based upon a range of factors such as extent relative to breast size, mammographic appearance, grade, age of patient and co-morbidities.

Uncertainty remains about which women should be treated by mastectomy; which by wide local excision; who should have radiotherapy; and which patients should have hormone therapy. Whilst mastectomy is virtually curative, all series of wide local excision report a risk of local recurrence. Factors that predict this risk include close pathologic margin status, high grade and comedo histologic subtype, young age and large lesion size. Scoring systems have been developed which weight these factors to predict risk of recurrence and that proposed by the Van Nuys Group is perhaps the most widely known. There is general agreement that margin status is of paramount importance. In three randomized trials in which wide local excision alone has been compared with adjuvant radiotherapy, local recurrence rates are significantly reduced by radiotherapy. It is however clear that not all women require radiotherapy and some women will still get local recurrence after receiving it. Tamoxifen can also reduce the risk of local recurrence but this does not have the same magnitude of effect as radiotherapy, is likely only effective in ER positive DCIS, and may be expected to only have an influence on the incidence of ER positive recurrences.

High grade DCIS with comedo necrosis is a significant independent predictor of local recurrence risk. In addition, it is important to note that invasive cancer arising in high grade DCIS tends to be of histologic grade 3 (60%). Hence mortality from invasive recurrences of DCIS, although very small, will be greatest in those who have had high grade DCIS. In the EORTC trial, 11 of the 14 women (79%) who developed metastases following an invasive local recurrence had originally been treated for high grade DCIS. This may reflect short follow up (high grade recurrences tend to occur early) but if women with high grade DCIS are to be treated by breast-conserving surgery, adequate local treatment is particularly important. Young women are more likely to have high grade DCIS and are also at increased risk of local recurrence. It is this group who are perhaps most likely to choose breast-conserving surgery. Knowing pre-operatively that a woman is likely to have high grade DCIS may influence the extent of surgical excision which is recommended.

Currently, the mammographic extent of microcalcification is the main pre-operative determinant of suitability for breast-conserving surgery. However, a discrepancy between mammographic size and pathologic extent of DCIS measured at microscopy is well recognized. In addition, some cases operated on for DCIS will prove to have an invasive component. Extensive biopsy of microcalcification by mammotomy for example can minimize this surgical 'up-staging'.

Despite a widely held belief that DCIS is a contiguous disease process, all series of breast-conserving surgery report a rate of local recurrence despite apparently clear margins. Recurrences usually affect the site of previous excision. Clearly, the chance of obtaining clear margins is greater with increasing width of excision. There is an argument perhaps for recommending a wider margin for high grade DCIS, DCIS in young women and large areas of DCIS (30 mm) and it may be that fewer such cases of high grade DCIS in young women are suitable for breast-conserving surgery on this basis. Such women may be recommended mastectomy with reconstruction.

The treatment of DCIS is essentially preventative. Even in studies with high rates of local recurrence, mortality is very low (2% at 8 years). As a significant cause of death invasive cancer occurring after an initial diagnosis of DCIS is a much bigger problem in younger women (40% of all cause mortality) compared with women over age 60 (5% of all cause mortality). Radiotherapy is thus particularly indicated for high grade lesions and young women. Uncertain or involved margins should be re-excised. Currently, hormone therapy has no established role but chemoprevention may prove to have a role in the future.

INVASIVE BREAST CANCER

Invasive breast carcinoma is the most common malignancy to affect women worldwide; the incidence in western countries is approximately 2% by age 50 years and 10% over a lifetime. Although many factors are associated with increased risk, the most clinically relevant factors are increasing age, carriage of a known predisposing genetic mutation, a family history with no proven mutation, atypical hyperplasia (discussed above) and prior exposure to radiation. Other risk factors can usually be linked to various mechanisms of increased exposure to hormones and are individually of limited clinical value but may be additive.

GENETIC RISK

Two highly penetrant gene mutations have been identified (BRCA1 and BRCA2). The prevalence of each is low (about 1 in 800 women) but clinical significance rests with the risk of breast cancer (55–80% lifetime risk) and ovarian cancer (20–40% lifetime risk). BRCA1-associated breast cancer is usually high grade and HER2/neu negative and ER negative, whereas that associated with BRCA2 is more likely to be high grade, but ER/PR positive. Familial breast cancer is further discussed in Chapter 20.

DIAGNOSIS OF BREAST CANCER

Approximately 80% of women with breast cancer present symptomatically and 20% by screening. The majority of cancers will present as lumps. Other less common presentations include asymmetric thickening, peu-d'orange, axillary mass, inflammation and breast distortion. All lumps or other suspicious findings are investigated by triple assessment. Imaging by ultrasound in all cases, with ultrasound-guided core biopsy of lesions becoming the norm in many centers. Mammography is performed in women over age 40 or any age if a cancer is diagnosed. Breast MRI has no formally established role but is being assessed as a means of predicting multifocality of disease.

For malignant breast lesions, a pre-operative diagnosis is highly desirable for appropriate treatment planning. In certain cases repeat biopsy or mammotomy may be used to achieve this. Pre-operative staging of the axilla by ultrasound-guided axillary node biopsy is possible and is being investigated in some centers where over 40% of all node positive patients have been diagnosed prior to surgery in preliminary studies.

TREATMENT OF BREAST CANCER

The very large majority of breast cancers are operable and are treated by surgery in the first instance. Locally advanced and inflammatory cancers are treated initially by systemic therapy. In addition, pre-operative systemic therapy may be used with the aim of reducing the size of large carcinomas such that they are suitable for breast-conserving surgery. Overall local recurrence rates after such treatment scheduling are higher than after breast-conserving surgery for cancers, which present at a size suitable for this form of surgery in the first instance.

The strongest risk factors for local recurrence after breast-conserving surgery are margin involvement, omission of radiotherapy and young age. Other factors are high grade, lymphovascular invasion and an extensive intraduct component surrounding the invasive cancer. Size is not a risk factor. No study to date has identified a group of women for whom radiotherapy is not required after breast-conserving surgery but several series report low rates in older patients with ER positive cancers who are receiving hormone therapy.

SURGERY

The aim of surgery is to obtain prognostic information, achieve local disease control and leave an acceptable cosmetic result. Approximately two-thirds of all breast cancers are treatable by breast-conserving surgery. New oncoplastic techniques (such as therapeutic mammoplasty and latissimus dorsi miniflaps) are extending the indications for breast-conserving surgery and facilitating better cosmesis for suitable cases. Mastectomy is still however indicated where the disease is too extensive for an acceptable cosmetic result to be achieved by breast-

conserving surgery, or when there are multiple foci of disease. Mastectomy may be combined with breast reconstruction either as an immediate one-stage procedure or as a delayed operation after treatment is complete or even after some years.

Axillary node staging is required for all invasive breast cancer. Traditionally this has been achieved by axillary node clearance. Since in modern practice, less than 40% of all operable breast cancers will be node positive, axillary clearance for all subjects exposes many women to unnecessary morbidity. Less morbid techniques include sentinel node biopsy and node sampling alone or in combination. Both will incur a small failure rate compared with node clearance. The overall failure rate of sentinel node biopsy (failure to identify a sentinel node or a false negative sentinel node) is approximately 5–10%. The rate of regional recurrence after such procedures is likely to be lower than this, due to case selection, adjuvant therapy effect (approximately 20% odds reduction in local or regional recurrence) and the fact that approximately 50% of all node positive patients have only 1 node positive. It is now possible to avoid performing full axillary clearance for all women with node negative disease. Women with minimal nodal involvement (1 or 2 nodes positive) may also be treated with axillary radiotherapy rather than axillary clearance.

RADIOTHERAPY

Like surgery, radiotherapy is a local treatment. Intact breast radiotherapy is given routinely after breast-conserving surgery. Evidence suggests that women under age 40 also benefit from a radiotherapy boost to the site of excision. Methods of partial breast irradiation are currently being investigated in trials. These involve either interstitial wires, an inflatable device placed inside the excision cavity or intra-operative radiotherapy.

Radiotherapy is also given after mastectomy in women at high risk of local/chest wall recurrence. Definitions of high risk vary but having two of the following factors is a common protocol: high grade; vascular invasion and node positivity. Occasionally radiotherapy is used pre-operatively for cancers inoperable at presentation.

SYSTEMIC THERAPY

Systemic therapy is administered on the basis of likelihood of metastatic spread. The degree of risk to justify therapy varies and is a balance of morbidity versus benefit versus cost restraints. Informed patient choice is essential. In some countries evidence of a 1% absolute benefit is considered sufficient to justify therapy whereas in others, evidence of a larger percentage benefit is deemed to be necessary.

Options for systemic therapy include hormone therapy, chemotherapy and immunotherapy. Hormone therapy is only effective in ER positive disease; the optimum duration of treatment is currently believed to be five years and the benefit (approximately 30 % odds reduction of death from breast cancer) is maintained. In pre-menopausal women, hormone therapy involves ovarian ablation/suppression and Tamoxifen. In post-menopausal women aromatase inhibitors Tamoxifen is used. Prolongation of endocrine treatment by switching medication at 2–5 years may be appropriate in some high-risk women and is under investigation. Chemotherapy has a greater role in younger women, with a proportionate reduction in benefit with advancing age beyond the menopause. In young women chemotherapy is associated with a reduction in odds of death from breast cancer of approximately 20 %. A combination of drugs is more effective than a single agent but prolonged treatment beyond 4–6 months and high dose treatment has not been shown to be of benefit. Chemotherapy has a bigger role in ER negative disease and it is generally accepted that some of the effects in ER positive disease are due to an ovarian suppression effect. Therapy targetting the HER-2 receptor (Herceptin) has shown a large benefit (50 % odds reduction in breast cancer related deaths) in the small percentage of women that are HER-2 positive.

PROGNOSIS AFTER BREAST CANCER TREATMENT

The outcome after treatment is dependent upon the extent of disease at the time of diagnosis and the effectiveness of therapy. Essentially it is the likelihood that systemic metastatic disease is present that predicts overall survival. Local control of disease is also likely to have a very small effect on patient survival. Various models for predicting outcome are available. The most validated is the Nottingham Prognostic Index based upon size, grade and lymph node stage (see Chapter 20).

OUTCOME OF BREAST CANCER TREATMENT

Considerable improvements in overall survival after a diagnosis of breast cancer have been observed over the past 15–20 years, despite a rising incidence. This is attributed to various factors among which are greater breast cancer awareness, better and more organized methods of breast assessment and better local and adjuvant treatments. Mammographic screening for breast cancer after age 50 is associated with an absolute reduction in mortality from the disease of 20–30 %. Taking all women diagnosed with breast cancer, approximately 80 % can be expected to be alive at ten years after diagnosis. Importantly, breast cancer treatment is now associated with less morbidity.

SUGGESTED READING

Elston CW, Ellis IO. eds. The Breast Systemic Pathology Volume 13. Edinburgh: Churchill-Livingstone, 1998.

Harris JR, Lippman ME, Morrow M, Osbourne CK eds. Diseases of the Breast. Third edition. Lippincott, Williams and Wilkins, 2004.

Silverstein MJ, Recht A, Lagios MD eds. Ductal Carcinoma in situ of the Breast. Second edition. Lippincott, Williams and Wilkins, 2002.

5 Overview of Radiologic Aspects of Breast Disease

Andrew J Evans · Jonathan J James

INTRODUCTION

Imaging is crucial in the diagnosis of breast disease. It is used to screen for breast cancer, diagnose symptomatic breast problems and guide biopsies and marker localizations.

Mammography and ultrasound are still the most commonly used modalities for breast diagnosis. In recent years magnetic resonance imaging (MRI) has also emerged as a useful tool for the diagnosis and local staging of breast cancer.

MAMMOGRAPHY

Mammograms are radiograph images of the breast that are taken using low energy x-rays to enhance the contrast between fat, breast tissue and breast lesions, all of which have similar attenuation characteristics. Two views are normally taken of each breast: the medio-lateral oblique view and the cranio-caudal view (Figure 5-1).

The appearance of normal breast tissue varies greatly from woman to woman. Some women have very dense breast tissue (Figure 5-2A), while other women have almost completely involuted breasts where the entire breast is made up of fatty tissue (Figure 5-2B). There is a trend for younger women to have denser breasts and older women to have fatty breasts. Other factors known to influence mammographic background pattern are hormone replacement therapy (HRT) use and patient weight. The sensitivity of mammography for the detection of malignancy is reduced in women with a dense mammographic background pattern.

The main advantages of mammography as an imaging modality are that it is quick to perform and interpret, it images the whole of both breasts and has a high sensitivity for the detection of both ductal carcinoma *in situ* (DCIS) and invasive breast cancer. The disadvantages of mammography are that it uses ionizing radiation, the compression required can be uncomfortable, it requires highly trained radiographers and speci-

ficity is relatively low unless combined with ultrasound and biopsy.

In the last few years we have seen major advances in mammography technology with the development of digital mammography systems. Digital mammography allows each step of the imaging chain, from image acquisition to display, to be optimized, leading to an improvement in image quality. It is thus hoped that digital mammography will outperform conventional film mammography, leading to an increase in cancer detection rates.

MAMMOGRAPHIC ABNORMALITIES

MASSES

Mass lesions are commonly found on the mammograms of both symptomatic and asymptomatic women. Abnormalities such as cysts, fibroadenomas and lymph nodes account for the vast majority of the benign mass lesions. The most important feature to help distinguish benign from malignant mass lesions is the margin definition. Masses with a well-defined margin are almost always benign (Figure 5-3); approximately one-third of ill-defined masses and over 90% of spiculated masses are malignant (Figure 5-4). Mammographic spiculation is due to two processes. The desmoplastic reaction incited by low grade invasive carcinomas causes in-pulling of normal Cooper's ligaments into the lesion producing spiculation. Shorter spicules are sometimes caused by direct extension of tumor into breast parenchyma.

MALIGNANT MICROCALCIFICATIONS

Microcalcification is a common feature of both invasive and *in situ* malignancy. The features that suggest calcifications are malignant are clustering, pleomorphism (calcifications of different sizes, density and shapes), the presence of rod- and branching-shaped calcifications, and a ductal distribution (Figure 5-5). Approximately

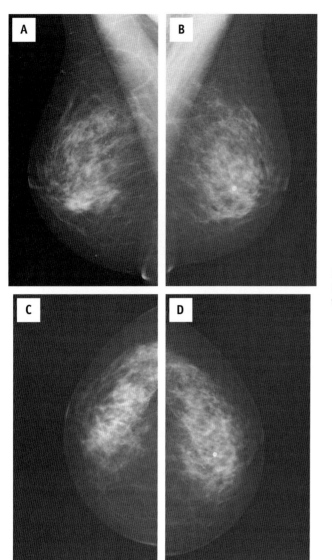

FIGURE 5-1

Mammography. A standard set of mammogram films consists of an oblique view (A,B) and a craniocaudal view (C,D) of each breast.

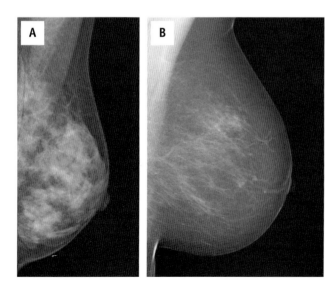

FIGURE 5-2

Breast density varies between women. The sensitivity of mammography for detecting malignancy is significantly reduced if the breast consists of a high proportion of fibro-glandular (dense) breast tissue (A) compared to a breast that is fatty (B).

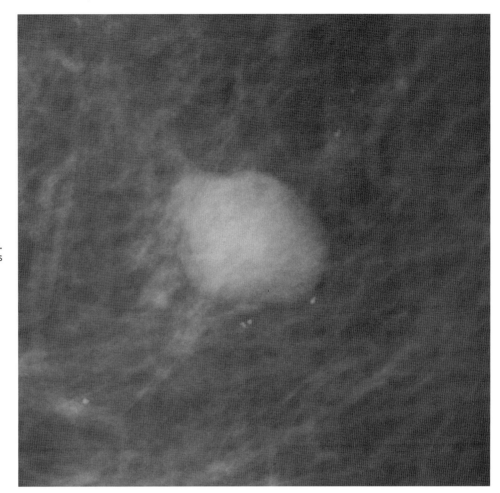

FIGURE 5-3

Mammographic abnormalities: masses. A well-defined benign looking mass which proved to be a simple cyst.

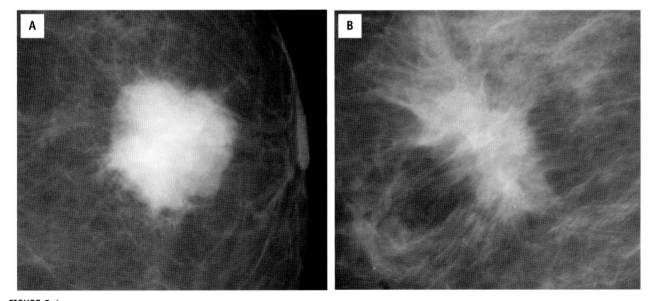

FIGURE 5-4

Mammographic abnormalities: masses. Ill-defined and spiculate masses are the typical mammographic features of carcinomas. (A) An ill-defined mass in the retroareolar region of the left breast. Biopsy showed a high grade ductal/no special type carcinoma. (B) A spiculate mass that proved to be a grade 2 ductal/no special type carcinoma.

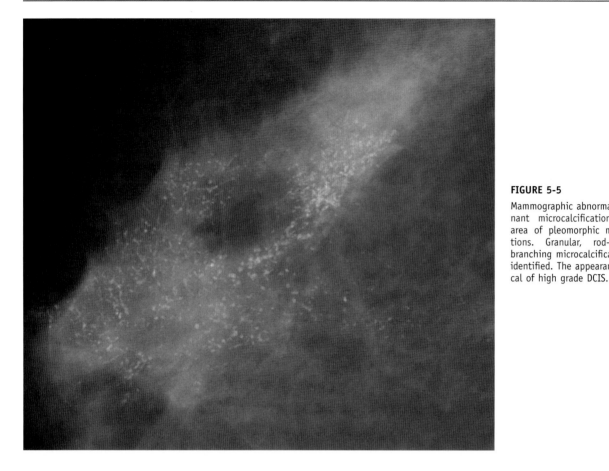

FIGURE 5-5

Mammographic abnormalities: malignant microcalcifications. Extensive area of pleomorphic microcalcifications. Granular, rod-shaped and branching microcalcifications can be identified. The appearances are typical of high grade DCIS.

one-third of malignant microcalcification clusters have an invasive focus within them at surgical excision. The presence of a mass associated with malignant microcalcification increases the chance of invasion being present. However, DCIS alone can occasionally cause a mammographic mass.

BENIGN MICROCALCIFICATIONS

The most common causes of benign mammographic microcalcification are fibrocystic change, vascular calcification, fibroadenomatoid hyperplasia, duct ectasia and sclerosing adenosis. Microcalcifications may be present in normal breast tissue such as calcification within atrophic lobules and calcification in normal stroma. Vascular microcalcifications do not normally cause diagnostic difficulty as the 'tramline' appearance caused by calcification in both sides of the vessel wall is normally evident (Figure 5-6).

Fibrocystic change is a common cause of mammographically indeterminate calcification. A proportion of cases do not need to undergo biopsy as, on a lateral magnification mammographic view, layering of calcific fluid within small cysts results in a 'tea-cup' appearance (Figure 5-7). Calcifications due to fibroadenomatoid

hyperplasia often have an indeterminate appearance, which is indistinguishable from DCIS. Calcifications due to sclerosing adenosis, atrophic lobules and benign stromal calcification often appear as clusters of irregular granular microcalcification. Percutaneous biopsy is frequently required to distinguish benign microcalcifications from DCIS (Figure 5-8).

Calcifications can be due to duct ectasia (Figure 5-9). Coarse rod and branching calcifications due to calcification of debris within dilated ducts are typical. These calcifications have been described as having a 'broken needle' appearance. Extrusion of debris from dilated ducts can lead to fat necrosis in a periductal distribution, in this situation 'lead pipe' calcifications may be seen. The calcifications of duct ectasia are normally coarser than those seen in DCIS. Usually duct ectasia can be diagnosed with confidence based on the mammographic appearance, but there may be diagnostic uncertainty on occasions, especially if the calcifications are unilateral and focal.

PARENCHYMAL DISTORTION

Parenchymal distortion is present when the Cooper's ligaments are seen to be drawn to one area of the breast,

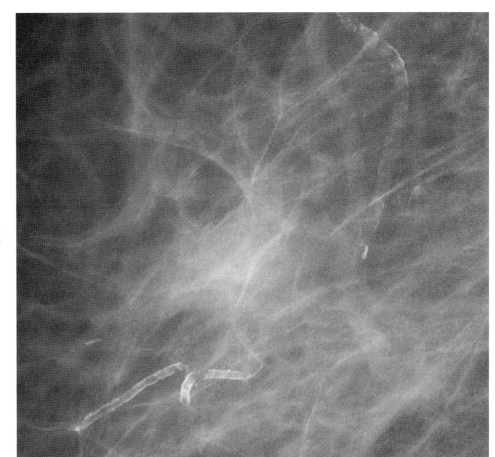

FIGURE 5-6

Mammographic abnormalities: benign microcalcifications. 'Tramline' vascular calcifications.

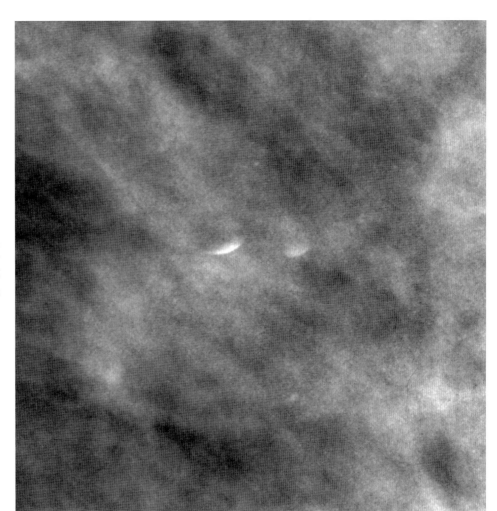

FIGURE 5-7

Mammographic abnormalities: benign microcalcifications. Lateral magnification view of an area of microcalcifications demonstrates 'tea-cup' appearances, indicating fibrocystic change

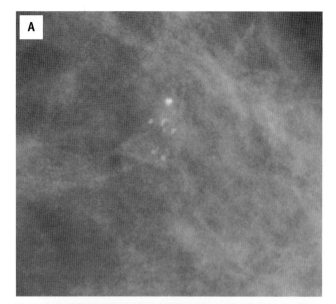

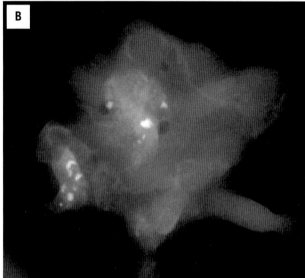

FIGURE 5-8

Mammographic abnormalities: benign microcalcifications. A tiny cluster of microcalcifications (A). They are difficult to characterize with variations in their size and shape. Vacuum assisted stereotactic biopsy was performed. The specimen radiographed confirms adequate sampling (B). Histology showed benign stromal calcifications.

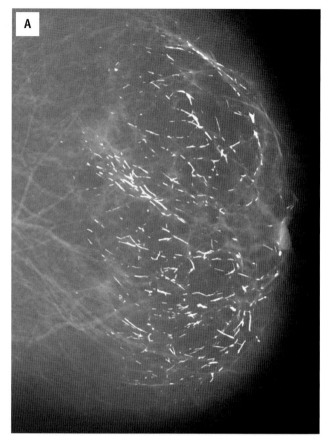

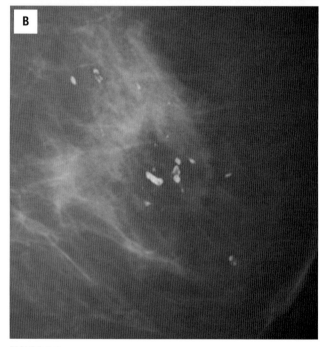

FIGURE 5-9

Mammographic abnormalities: benign microcalcifications. Coarse rod and branching shaped calcifications are typical of duct ectasia (A). These calcifications show a 'broken needle' appearance. Sometimes thicker more localized calcifications can be seen giving a 'lead pipe' appearance (B).

giving a stellate appearance without a central mass. The commonest malignant correlates of parenchymal distortion are small, low grade invasive cancers with tubular features.

The most common benign causes of architectural distortion are surgical scars (particularly if radiotherapy has been given) and complex sclerosing lesions (radial scars) (Figure 5-10). A proportion of complex sclerosing lesions have associated in situ or invasive malignancy. Consequently, it has been normal surgical practice to excise these lesions. There is now, however, a trend to offer percutaneous vacuum-assisted excision.

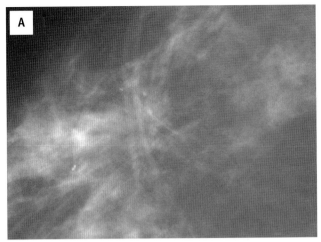

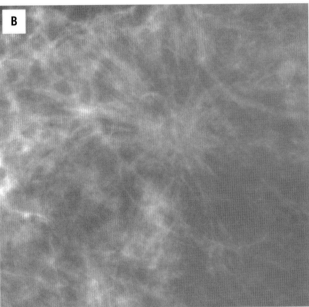

FIGURE 5-10
Mammographic abnormalities: parenchymal distortion. A stellate appearance with no central mass (A). It is not possible to differentiate reliably benign and malignant causes of parenchymal distortion on the basis of imaging alone. In this case stereotactic biopsy revealed a radial scar. Diagnostic excision was undertaken. Following surgery a parenchymal distortion persists, this time the result of a surgical scar (B).

ASYMMETRY

Asymmetry in the density of breast tissue on a mammogram is a normal feature in some women. The positive predictive value of an asymmetry as a sign of malignancy is less than 1%. Asymmetry can, however, be a useful sign at mammographic screening if the asymmetry is a new finding compared to previous films or the asymmetric density is in an unusual position, for example, in the inframammary fold.

SKIN CHANGES

Skin thickening is often accompanied by thickening of the Cooper's ligaments. Skin and Cooper's ligament thickening can be caused by tumor, inflammation or edema. Skin thickening is the mammographic correlate of the clinical sign 'peau d'orange' and may be seen in so called inflammatory breast cancer. Skin thickening is often seen associated with breast infections and when there is either venous or lymphatic obstruction within the axilla.

VARIATIONS IN THE MAMMOGRAPHIC APPEARANCES OF MALIGNANCY RELATED TO PATHOLOGIC FEATURES

High grade invasive ductal/no special type carcinomas normally present mammographically as an ill-defined mass, as the lack of a desmoplastic reaction histologically in many of these tumors means that spiculation is often not seen. Low grade invasive cancers more typically present either as a small spiculated mass or an architectural distortion. This is due to an associated desmoplastic reaction commonly present with these lesions.

Lobular cancers are often difficult to perceive mammographically because of this tumor's ability to diffusely infiltrate fat. Compared with ductal/no special type carcinoma, lobular cancers are more likely only to be seen on one mammographic view, are less likely to display microcalcification, and are more often seen as an ill-defined mass or newly developed asymmetry.

Tubular cancers and invasive cribriform carcinoma typically present as architectural distortion or small spiculated masses. Invasive papillary and mucinous cancers normally present as a new or enlarging multilobulated mass, sometimes part well defined and part ill defined.

High grade invasive ductal/no special type carcinomas are often associated with high grade DCIS. In this situation any associated microcalcifications are rod-shaped or branching and have a ductal distribution. These calcifications, also termed casting or comedo type, are the classical features of high grade DCIS on mammography. Calcification is a less common feature of low grade invasive breast cancer because any associated low grade DCIS may not calcify due to the lack of intraductal necrosis. If low grade DCIS does calcify, the microcalcifications are much less characteristic, tending to be small clusters of granular microcalcifications that vary in size, shape and density. Low grade DCIS can also present as a mass without microcalcification. In many cases where low grade DCIS is present, mammography is normal. Consequently, mammography is much better at predicting the size of high grade DCIS compared with low grade DCIS.

ULTRASOUND

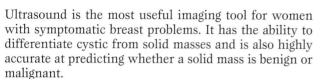

Ultrasound is the most useful imaging tool for women with symptomatic breast problems. It has the ability to differentiate cystic from solid masses and is also highly accurate at predicting whether a solid mass is benign or malignant.

Ultrasound is not, however, a suitable modality for breast cancer screening due to its limited sensitivity for small and *in situ* carcinomas. In the screening setting it is used for the assessment of lesions demonstrated on a mammogram and is the method of choice for image guided breast biopsy.

Breast ultrasound requires the use of high frequency ultrasound of at least 7.5 MHz. The higher the frequency the better the spatial and contrast resolution of the image. However, with increasing frequency the ability of the sound beam to penetrate deeper breast tissue decreases. Ultrasound is well tolerated by patients and is safe involving no ionising radiation.

ULTRASOUND ABNORMALITIES

CYSTIC LESIONS

Breast cysts can be definitively diagnosed with ultrasound (Figure 5-11). Simple cysts are well defined, exhibit no internal echoes (anechoic) and show posterior enhancement of the ultrasound beam. Some cysts are more complex, containing internal echoes reflecting debris within the cyst fluid. Lesions that do not exhibit all the characteristics of a simple cyst require further workup, with aspiration and core biopsy, if solid.

Filling defects may be seen within a cyst. Papillomas frequently have this appearance (Figure 5-12). However larger multi-lobulated filling defects within cysts can be due to malignancy, particularly papillary carcinoma. Filling defects seen in recently aspirated cysts may be due to blood clot.

Mucinous carcinomas can occasionally mimic complex cysts, due to their high water content. The high

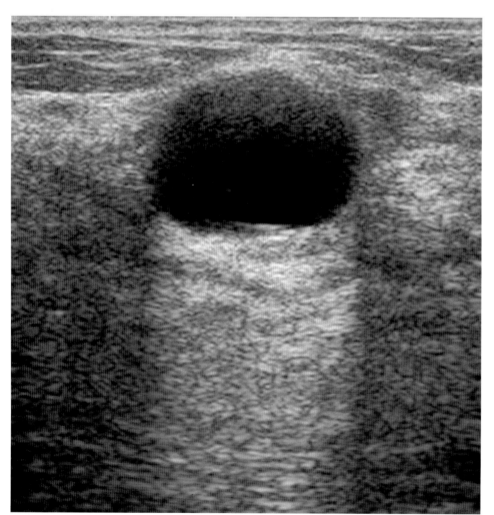

FIGURE 5-11

Ultrasound abnormalities: cystic lesions. The lack of any internal echoes and the posterior enhancement of the ultrasound beam confirm that this is a simple cyst.

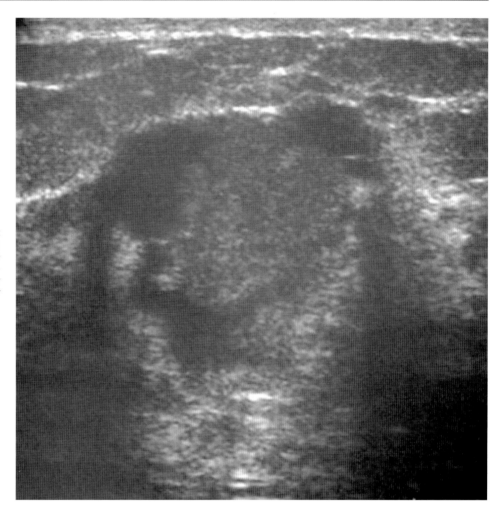

FIGURE 5-12

Ultrasound abnormalities: cystic lesions. The presence of a filling defect within this cystic structure suggests the diagnosis of a papilloma. Core biopsy showed a papillary lesion with no evidence of cellular atypia.

mucin content of the tumors means there is usually marked posterior enhancement behind the lesion.

BENIGN SOLID MASSES

Fibroadenomas are the most frequently encountered causes of a benign mass on ultrasound. They appear as an oval, solid mass with a homogenous internal echo pattern and smooth margins (Figure 5-13). There is often a well-defined echogenic capsule and edge attenuation. Fibroadenomas are usually wider than they are tall. The lesions are often compressible and many show macro-lobulation. Calcification and cystic changes are occasionally seen.

Lymph nodes are often demonstrated as a normal feature on ultrasound, most frequently within the upper outer quadrant of the breast and in the axilla (Figure 5-14). Normal lymph nodes can be quite large and the best differentiating features between normal/benign nodes and nodes bearing malignancy are the cortical thickness and shape. A lymph node with a cortical thickness of greater than 2 mm should be viewed as abnormal and image guided biopsy undertaken. Lymph nodes that are round rather than elongated are also suspicious.

There are other more unusual benign lesions that may be encountered. Phyllodes tumors may have a similar appearance to a fibroadenoma, but tend to be larger and sometimes echogenic. Leaf-like septations and cystic spaces can sometimes be seen. Hamartomas can sometimes be confidently diagnosed on ultrasound if interspersed fat is identified within the mass, but in many cases core biopsy will be required to make the diagnosis of a hamartoma.

MALIGNANT MASSES

Invasive breast cancer presents on ultrasound as an irregular mass with ill-defined margins and an inhomogeneous echo texture (Figure 5-15). Approximately 50% of invasive breast cancers are taller than they are wide. Malignant masses often display an ill-defined echogenic halo, distal shadowing and micro-lobulation.

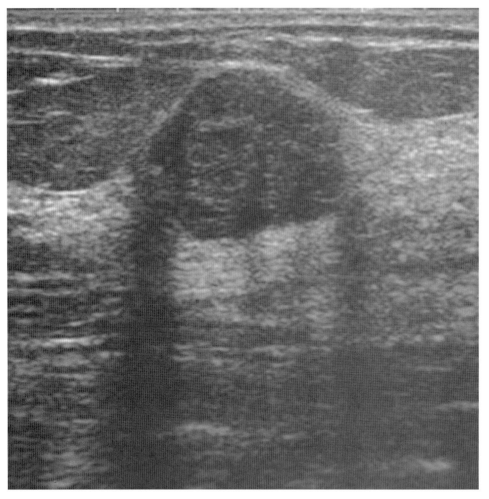

FIGURE 5-13
Ultrasound abnormalities: benign solid masses. This well-defined mass shows edge attenuation. The appearances are typical of a fibroadenoma. This was confirmed on ultrasound guided core biopsy.

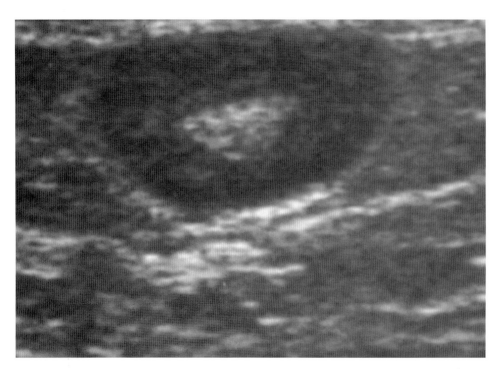

FIGURE 5-14
Ultrasound abnormalities: benign solid masses. Typical ultrasound appearances of a lymph node. Note the echogenic, fatty hilum and the hypoechoic cortex.

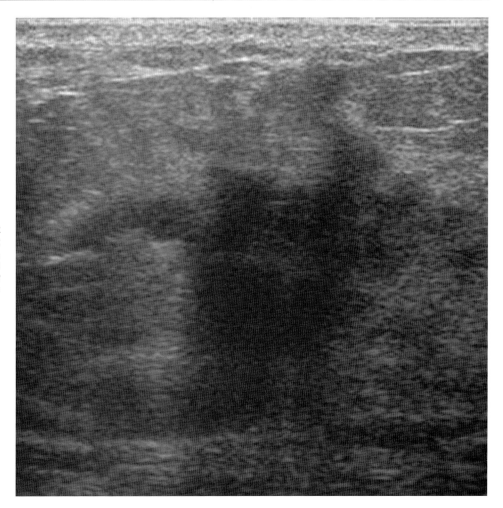

FIGURE 5-15

Ultrasound abnormalities: malignant lesions. An ill-defined hypoechoic mass with some posterior shadowing. Note the intraductal tumor extension on the left of the image. Core biopsy showed ductal/no special type carcinoma of histologic grade 2.

Breast cancers are non-compressible and they may show distortion of the adjacent breast tissue. Doppler examination of malignant masses shows neo-vascularity with irregular, centrally penetrating blood vessels. In contrast, doppler examination of benign lesions such as fibroadenomas typically shows displacement of normal blood vessels around the edge of the lesion with just the occasional penetrating blood vessel.

Ultrasound is particularly useful when estimating the size of invasive tumors. Ultrasound is a better predictor of tumor size than mammography. It will often pick up intraductal extension of tumor (Figure 5-15) and small satellite foci of invasive tumor that may not be visible on mammography.

There are, however, a number of benign lesions that can mimic the ultrasound appearances of carcinomas. The most common are radial scar/complex sclerosing lesion, surgical scar and fat necrosis. Rarer lesions that can appear malignant on ultrasound also include granulomatous mastitis and lymphocytic lobulitis. Focal areas of fibrocystic change can occasionally mimic lobular carcinoma.

ULTRASOUND OF DUCTAL CARCINOMA IN SITU

The sensitivity of ultrasound for the detection of DCIS is lower than that of mammography. This is one of the reasons why ultrasound is of limited value as a primary screening tool for breast cancer. However, ultrasound is often useful for assessment, when a malignant cluster of microcalcification has already been identified mammographically. Sometimes the calcifications can be seen within distended ducts allowing ultrasound guided biopsy.

There are a number of atypical presentations of DCIS that may be seen on ultrasound. Low grade DCIS may present as a solid mass lesion and intracystic DCIS is also recognized. DCIS can also be diagnosed after percutaneous biopsy associated with apparently benign lesions such as radial scars or papillomas.

VARIATIONS IN THE ULTRASOUND APPEARANCES OF MALIGNANCY RELATED TO PATHOLOGIC FEATURES

High grade invasive breast cancers often appear as fairly well defined masses without distal shadowing. Intraductal extension may be identified and calcifications may be seen on ultrasound when the tumor is associated with high grade DCIS. However, sometimes high grade tumors may appear identical to fibroadenomas on ultrasound. This shows the importance of performing core biopsy on any solid lesion to establish a diagnosis even when the ultrasound appearances are benign. Doppler examination of high grade lesions may demonstrate a highly vascular lesion representing the marked neo-angiogenesis present.

Low grade invasive breast cancers, including tubular carcinomas, may present as small, poorly defined hypoechoic masses with marked distal attenuation (Figure 5-16). This posterior shadowing may completely obscure the posterior border of the mass.

Invasive lobular cancers are more frequently occult at ultrasound examination than ductal/no special type carcinomas. Lobular carcinomas tend to diffusely infiltrate fat, producing rather vague abnormalities on ultrasound. Some lobular cancers may be partly echogenic in appearance. This appearance can be easily mistaken for an area of fibrocystic change. Ultrasound, like mammography, tends to underestimate the size of lobular carcinomas.

Ultrasound of inflammatory breast cancer usually shows markedly thickened skin and dilated lymphatics throughout the breast. An underlying mass lesion is only sometimes seen. Subtle areas of inflammation and skin thickening associated with invasive breast cancers are sometimes seen at ultrasound examination even when clinically unapparent.

MAGNETIC RESONANCE IMAGING

Magnetic resonance imaging (MRI) has emerged as a promising modality for imaging the breast due to its high sensitivity for detecting invasive breast carcinoma, which in some studies approaches 100%. There are, however, problems with specificity with some benign lesions and even normal tissue having a worrying appearance on MRI. The problems with specificity are compounded by the lack of availability of MR guided biopsy. In addition, although MRI is highly sensitive for invasive breast cancer, its sensitivity for DCIS is considerably less. Finally, MRI is both expensive and time consuming and can be poorly tolerated by some patients due to claustrophobia.

To carry out successful breast MRI examinations, a high field strength magnet (at least 1.5 Tesla) is required. A dedicated breast coil is also needed. The patient lies prone on the couch of the MR scanner, with the breasts hanging down into the coil.

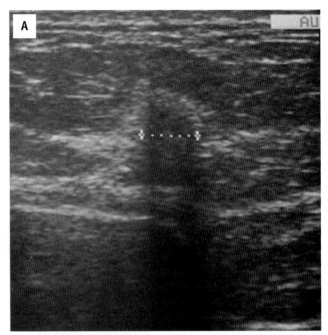

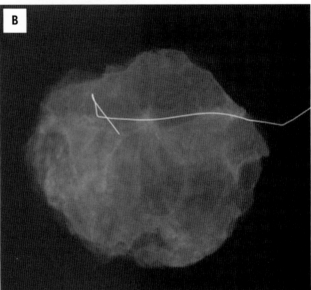

FIGURE 5-16

A small, poorly defined hypoechoic mass with marked acoustic shadowing was seen on ultrasound. The surgical specimen shows the corresponding mammographic appearance of a small spiculate mass (B). A wire localization was required as this screen detected cancer was impalpable. The imaging features suggest a low grade tumor and histology confirmed a tubular carcinoma.

There are specific indications where MRI is invaluable in the assessment of women with breast abnormalities. MRI is most frequently used for local staging of breast carcinomas prior to breast conserving surgery and is the most accurate modality at sizing invasive breast cancers. In an ideal world there would be an argument for breast MRI in all patients considering breast conserving surgery. However, due to expense and scarcity of resources, MRI is best reserved for patients where estimating size using conventional means is difficult. These include patients whose tumors have lobular features, patients with normal mammograms and patients where there is disparity between size estimations at mammography, ultrasound and clinical examination (Figure 5-17).

Another important role for MRI is identifying an occult primary tumor in women presenting with malignant axillary lymphadenopathy with normal mammography and ultrasound. MRI in this clinical setting is highly sensitive at demonstrating the presence of a primary lesion within the breast. MRI is also useful in the post-surgical breast, differentiating surgical scarring from recurrent tumor. Research is currently underway into the use of breast MRI in screening young women with a high familial risk of breast cancer as the sensitivity of mammography in these women is much reduced due to dense breast parenchyma. Other groups are also investigating using MRI to assess early response to treatment in women receiving neo-adjuvant chemotherapy for primary breast cancer.

All the above indications require contrast enhancement, as the increased vascularity of malignancy is the means by which these lesions are identified. Image inter-

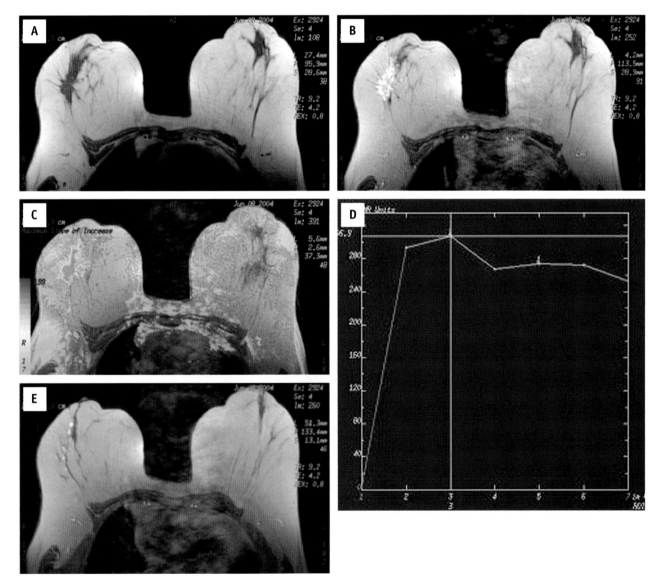

FIGURE 5-17

Magnetic resonance imaging. An MRI was performed for local staging of an invasive lobular carcinoma. The initial MR images suggest the presence of a spiculate mass in the right breast (A). Following injection of gadolinium contrast agent, a large area of enhancement measuring 40 mm can be seen corresponding with the tumor (B). A colour map shows the areas in red that exhibit the most intense contrast agent uptake and so are the areas that are most likely to be malignant (C). Measuring the enhancement pattern shows a rapid uptake of contrast agent followed by a wash out phase, which is typical of malignancy (D). Additional enhancing nodules are also demonstrated away from the primary tumor site indicating unsuspected multifocal disease. Consequently, this tumor was not suitable for breast conserving surgery. Histology confirmed a 43 mm lobular carcinoma with additional tumor foci behind the nipple.

pretation is based on the morphology of the abnormality as well as an assessment of how the lesion enhances following the injection of the MR contrast agent, gadolinium (Figure 5-17). Architectural features that indicate benign disease and malignancy are similar to those already described for mammography and ultrasound. Benign lesions tend to be well-defined with smooth margins whereas malignant lesions are poorly-defined and may show spiculation or parenchymal deformity.

Malignant lesions tend to enhance rapidly following the injection of the contrast agent and may well show ring enhancement. One of the strengths of MRI is that invasive carcinoma can be excluded with a high degree of certainty if no enhancement is seen. More detailed enhancement curves can be calculated to try and characterize lesions. Lesions that show rapid uptake of contrast agent followed by a washout phase (decrease of signal intensity after a peak has been reached) are highly likely to be malignant. Benign lesions tend to enhance more slowly, less avidly and do not tend to show washout during the time course of the examination.

MRI is the imaging modality of choice for assessing the integrity of breast implants. In this situation, contrast agent injection is not required unless associated malignancy is suspected. MRI is able to detect both intra-capsular and extra-capsular rupture with a high degree of certainty (Figure 5-18). It is also useful for diagnosing the complications of implant rupture such as free silicon, silicon granulomas and silicon in axillary lymph nodes. Extra-capsular rupture is diagnosed when silicon is demonstrated outside the fibrous implant capsule while intra-capsular rupture is diagnosed when silicon has escaped from the plastic implant shell, but is contained by the fibrous capsule.

SCINTIMAMMOGRAPHY

Scintimammography is a nuclear medicine technique. It has been developed following the observation that breast tumors often show uptake of the isotopes used in cardiac imaging. So far scintimammography has failed to establish a place in routine breast imaging due to its inability to accurately detect small invasive breast cancers and DCIS. Possible future indications would include the detection of local recurrence in women whose original tumor was mammographically occult.

BREAST CANCER SCREENING

Breast screening, using mammography, was introduced following a number of randomized control trials (RCT). The most modern and best RCTs of screening were undertaken in Sweden. The most recent overview of the results of the Swedish RCTs was performed in 2002 where the median trial time was 6.5 years and the median follow-up was 16 years. For all age groups there was a statistically significant 21% mortality reduction.

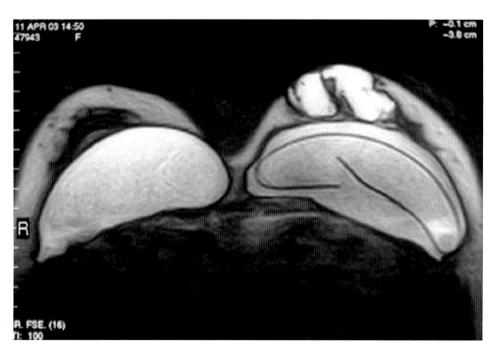

FIGURE 5-18

MRI images of a patient with bilateral breast implants. The implant on the left shows signs of intracapsular and extracapsular rupture with a clear hole in the shell of the implant and a siliconoma in the breast tissue adjacent to the implant.

This mortality reduction was largest in women aged 60–69 years who had a 33 % mortality reduction. There was also a statistically significant mortality reduction in women aged 55–64 years. The mortality benefit began to emerge at 4 years follow-up and continued to increase up until 10 years follow-up and this was then maintained.

RCTs are the best method of showing that a benefit is present, due to the exclusion of biases such as lead time bias (lead time is the period between early detection of disease and the time of its usual clinical presentation). RCTs tend, however, to underestimate the benefit for a woman attending for screening because the mortality reduction relates to women *invited* for screening and includes both those who do and do not attend. The Swedish RCTs also had significant contamination of the control groups who also received mammography. A recent paper by Laslo Tabar has suggested that regular attendance for mammographic screening results in a 63 % mortality reduction in breast cancer deaths.

The reduction in breast cancer mortality in many parts of the developed world appear to be due to a combination of factors including screening, better and more widely used systemic therapy, and increasing breast awareness in the female population.

WHO SHOULD BE SCREENED?

There is an established body of evidence supporting the regular mammographic screening of women aged 50–69 years. There is no randomized control evidence to support mammographic screening of women over the age of 70 years. Two RCTs have shown a statistically significant mortality benefit when screening women under the age of 50 years. These are the Malmo and the Gothenburg studies. The women in these studies, although randomized for screening under the age of 50, had a significant number of their screening episodes over the age of 50. Thus the mortality benefit seen in this age group remains controversial. Problems encountered when screening younger women include a lower breast cancer incidence and decreased specificity. The lead time of screening is also significantly shorter in younger women compared with older women, meaning the frequency of screening has to be increased.

HOW OFTEN SHOULD WOMEN BE SCREENED?

The frequency of the screening test is determined by lead time (period between earlier disease detection and time usual clinical presentation) achieved in that subpopulation and should not be affected by the cancer incidence. Even though breast cancer is less common in women in their 40s compared with older women, the shorter lead time of approximately 2.2 years in the younger group indicates that the maximum screening interval in this age group should be 18 months and the ideal 12 months. The lead time of screening of women over the age of 50 years is 3–4 years and the ideal screening interval for women of this age group is two years, although three years may be adequate.

THE SCREENING PROCESS

As an example, in the United Kingdom, breast screening is available to all women between the ages of 50 and 70 years of age. This is carried out every three years with two view mammography at each screening round. Approximately 80 % of women invited for screening attend. Screening mammography is carried out by trained female radiographers and women are sent their screening result within three weeks. Approximately 5 % of women are recalled for further assessment and the majority of these undergo further imaging, including extra mammographic views and ultrasound. When abnormalities are identified, percutaneous biopsy is crucial in making the diagnosis. Between 10 and 20 % of women recalled have breast cancer.

In the year 2002/2003, nearly 1.4 million women attended screening clinics in the UK. Nearly 10 000 breast cancers were detected, a rate of 7.3 per 1000 women screened. There was a small cancer (<15 mm) detection rate of 3.1 per 1000 women screened.

IMAGE GUIDED BREAST BIOPSY

The vast majority of breast lesions can be adequately diagnosed non-operatively, meaning that surgery is only performed to treat breast cancer or occasionally to excise lesions of uncertain malignant potential. The majority of breast cancers diagnosed at screening are impalpable, increasing the importance of image guided breast biopsy. Pre-operative diagnosis rates for screen detected invasive breast cancer are greater than 90 % in most institutions and greater than 80 % for DCIS in the UK. Lesions visible on ultrasound are biopsied under ultrasound guidance. Abnormalities such as microcalcifications frequently not visible on ultrasound are biopsied under stereotactic x-ray guidance.

Fine needle aspiration (FNA) is the method of percutaneous biopsy that has been around the longest. A fine needle (typically 21G) is passed into the lesion several times, and suction is applied with each needle pass. The aspirate can be smeared on to slides or injected into a preservative. The specimens are then sent for cytologic analysis.

Automated core biopsy devices for percutaneous breast biopsy became available in the mid 1990s (Figure 5-19). A cutting needle is fired into the lesion and a core of tissue obtained for histologic assessment. Typically

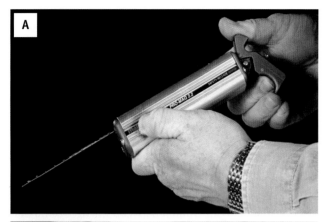

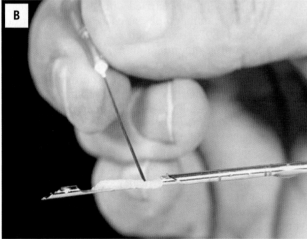

FIGURE 5-19

Image guided breast biopsy. Biopsy 'gun' used for core biopsies (A). A cutting needle is fired into the lesion; a small piece of tissue is contained within the sampling trough (B).

14G needles are used. Smaller needles result in less diagnostic tissue specimens.

Core biopsy has clear advantages over FNA. FNA is unable to differentiate between *in situ* and invasive breast cancer. In addition, FNA may precipitate more open surgical biopsies when indeterminate or suspicious cytology is encountered and it is also associated with a higher rate of inadequate samples. It has been shown that the absolute sensitivity of core biopsy for diagnosing malignancy in the breast is higher than FNA. This is particularly so if a stereotactic guided biopsy is performed. Stereo FNA has an absolute sensitivity of 62% compared with stereo core biopsy at 91%. Ultrasound guided core biopsy is also superior to ultrasound guided FNA, but the difference is less marked, with the absolute sensitivity of ultrasound FNA for diagnosing malignancy being 83% compared with ultrasound guided core biopsy at 97%. The reason for the difference is that stereotactic biopsy is required for the diagnosis of microcalcifications because most microcalcifications are not visible on ultrasound. Consequently it is now recommended that stereotactic FNA is not used for the biopsy of microcalcifications. In the United Kingdom there was a dramatic (50%) decline in the open surgical biopsy rate between 1996 and 1999, and at least part of this can be attributed to a move from FNA to core biopsy for both stereotactic and ultrasound guided breast biopsy.

Most microcalcifications can be adequately sampled using automated core biopsy, but in a small number of cases core biopsy may fail to provide a definitive diagnosis. This may be because some borderline pathologic conditions, such as radial scar, papillary lesions, atypical epithelial hyperplasias and low grade DCIS, require a larger volume of tissue to be sampled before a definitive histologic diagnosis is possible. In addition, small clusters of microcalcifications may be difficult to hit with a 14-G needle or the calcifications may be at a site which is difficult to target. Traditionally, in this situation, open surgical biopsy has been required. In recent years percutaneous vacuum-assisted biopsy devices have been developed capable of sampling much larger volumes of tissue.

Vacuum-assisted breast biopsy combines core biopsy with a vacuum system for acquiring and retrieving biopsy samples. The needle, which may be 14, 11 or 8-G, is positioned adjacent to the area to be sampled. Tissue is then sucked into the sampling aperture, a rotating blade spins forward cutting and capturing the specimen. In the most widely used commercial system the Mammotome™ (Ethicon Endosurgery), the tissue is transported to a tissue collection port, while the biopsy needle remains in the breast. The biopsy sample can then be removed. The biopsy needle can be rotated through 360° and the sampling procedure repeated as many times as required. Using this method the whole of an imaging abnormality can be removed if required.

Vacuum-assisted breast biopsy can be performed under ultrasound or stereotactic x-ray guidance (Figure 5-20). As already mentioned, stereotactic vacuum-assisted breast biopsy is ideal for sampling small clusters of microcalcifications and clusters in locations difficult to access with conventional core biopsy. Another important advantage of performing vacuum-assisted biopsy rather than conventional core biopsy when sampling calcifications is that understaging of disease tends to occur less frequently. In one study, conventional core biopsy underestimated the presence of invasive malignancy associated with DCIS in just over 20% of cases, while this occurred in only 11% of cases sampled by vacuum-assisted biopsy.

There are two methods for performing stereotactic breast biopsy, whether conventional automated core or vacuum-assisted. It can be performed with the patient in the prone position using a dedicated prone table system or in the upright position using an add-on device to a conventional mammography unit (Figure 5-20). The main advantage of the add-on unit over the prone table systems relates to cost. Add-on units are less expensive than prone table systems and the prone table systems can only be used to perform biopsies. In contrast, a mammography machine with an add-on device can be used to obtain standard mammography images

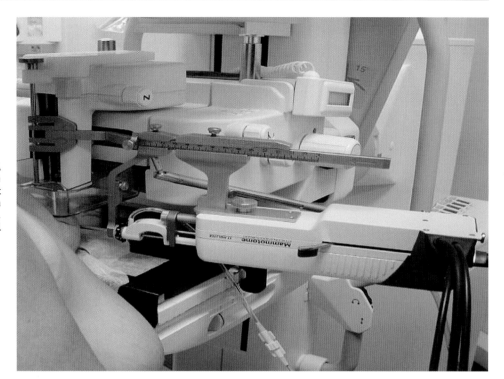

FIGURE 5-20

Image guided breast biopsy. A patient undergoing a vacuum assisted breast biopsy in the upright position using an add-on device to a conventional mammography unit. The biopsy device is held on a lateral arm support system.

when not employed for biopsy work. Prone tables are bulky items requiring a large room for installation. Consequently, upright add-on stereotactic biopsy systems remain the most frequent method of performing stereotactic biopsy in many Breast Units. The main disadvantage of the upright approach is that some patients may experience vaso-vagal symptoms leading to fainting. Patients in the prone position rarely faint.

The use of both methods is well established. In experienced hands, upright stereotactic biopsy with an add-on device is just as effective as using a dedicated prone table. Using modern digital add-on devices, around 95 % of microcalcifications can be successfully sampled using core needle biopsy. This rises to 98 % using an upright unit, vacuum-assisted biopsy and a lateral arm-support system. These results are in keeping with those obtained using the same needles and prone tables.

When performing stereotactic breast biopsy of microcalcifications it is vital to perform a specimen radiograph to ensure that representative calcifications have been obtained, confirming the abnormality has been adequately sampled (Figure 5-21). A minimum of five cores is required when sampling microcalcifications. There is a trend for increasing accuracy with increasing numbers of cores. Absolute and complete sensitivity are increased when six or more cores are taken compared to five. Another approach to deciding if microcalcifications have been adequately sampled is to count the number of calcifications present in the sample on the specimen radiograph. The number of flecks of calcification retrieved and the number of cores containing

calcifications is related to biopsy sensitivity. In one study, 100 % complete sensitivity was obtained once three individual flecks of calcifications were obtained, but for 100 % absolute sensitivity five or more flecks were required on the specimen radiograph. In addition, for 100 % complete sensitivity, two of the cores should show at least one fleck of calcifications and for 100 % absolute sensitivity, three separate cores should contain at least one fleck of calcification. Consequently, when performing stereotactic biopsy for calcifications, if only one or two flecks of calcifications are identified on the specimen radiograph more samples are required.

In general, percutaneous breast biopsy by whatever method is well tolerated by patients. There is no difference in the pain produced by core biopsy, cyst aspiration or FNA. Vacuum-assisted biopsy using larger bore needles is equally well tolerated, with many patients finding stereotactic vacuum-assisted biopsy preferable to multiple automated core biopsies when sampling microcalcifications.

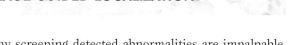

IMAGE GUIDED LOCALIZATION

Many screening detected abnormalities are impalpable, so methods are required to mark their position prior to

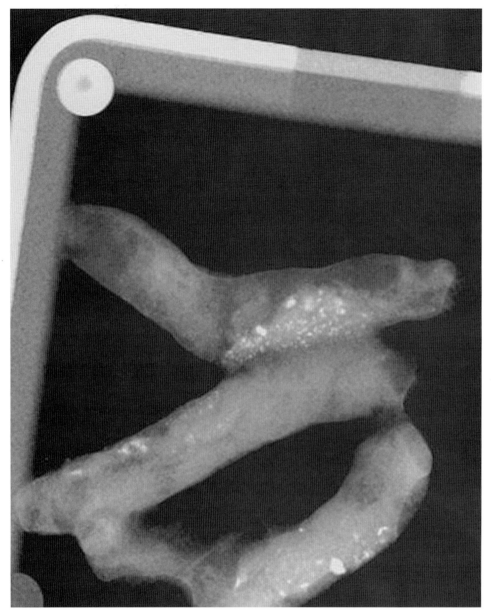

FIGURE 5-21
Image guided breast biopsy. Specimens from a vacuum-assisted stereotactic breast biopsy. Specimen radiography is crucial to confirm the lesion has been adequately sampled. Histology showed benign calcifications within an area of columnar cell change.

surgery. Impalpable breast lesions have traditionally been localized using hook wires placed under either ultrasound or stereotactic guidance. Alternatives to wire localization are skin marking, carbon granules and radio isotope localization. Radioisotope localization involves injecting Technetium labelled colloid into the lesion. The surgeon then uses a hand held gamma probe to localize the lesion while in the operating room.

Specimen radiographs should be performed on diagnostic excisions to assess the presence of the mammographic abnormality. They are also valuable on therapeutic excisions where the adequacy of the excision can be determined (Figure 5-22). The surgeon can thus view the specimen radiograph prior to completing the procedure. An assessment of the surgical margins can be made and, if necessary, a further excision can be taken prior to closing the wound. Specimen radiographs should be orientated to direct further surgery and allow more informed pathologic examination.

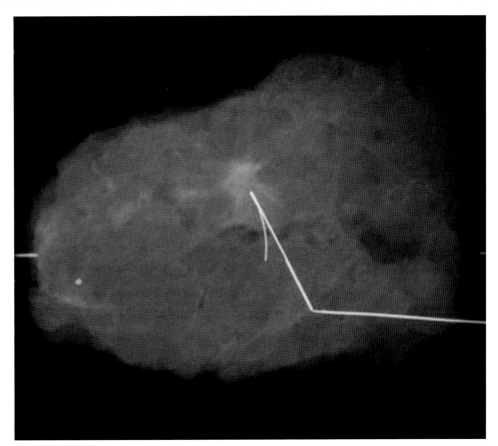

FIGURE 5-22

Image guided localization. A Hawkins wire has been used to mark a small screen detected carcinoma. Specimen radiographs can be used by the surgeon to estimate the adequacy of the resection whilst the patient is still in the operating theater. Final histology revealed complete excision of this 8 mm grade 2 lobular carcinoma.

SUGGESTED READING

Mammography

Burrell HC, Pinder SE, Wilson ARM, et al. The positive predictive value of mammographic signs: a review of 425 Non-palpable breast lesions. Clinical Radiology 1996: 51;277–281.

De Nunzio MC, Evans AJ, Pinder SE, et al. Correlations between the mammographic features of prevalent round screen detected invasive breast cancer and pathological prognostic factors. The Breast 1997;6:146–149.

Sala E, Warren R, McCann J, et al. Mammographic parenchymal patterns and mode of detection: implications for the breast screening programme. J Med Screen 1998;5:207–212.

Ultrasonography

Lister D, Evans AJ, Burrell HC, et al. The accuracy of breast ultrasound in the evaluation of clinically benign discrete, symptomatic breast lumps Clin Radiol 1998;53:490–492.

Stavros AT, Thickman D, Rapp CL, et al. Solid breast nodules: use of sonography to distinguish between benign and malignant lesions. Radiology 1995;196:123–134.

MRI

Boetes C, Mus RD, Holland R, et al. Breast tumours: comparative accuracy of MR imaging relative to mammography and ultrasound for demonstrating extent. Radiology 1995;197:743–747.

Tofani A, Sciuto R, Semprebene A, et al. ^{99}Tcm-MIBI scintimammography in 300 consecutive patients: factors that may affect accuracy. Nuc Med Com 1999;20:1113–1121.

Breast Screening

Nystrom L, Andersson I, Bjurstam, et al. Long term effects of mammographic screening: overview of the Swedish randomised trials. Lancet 2002;359:909–919.

Tabar L, Vitak B, Chen HH, et al. Beyond randomised controlled trials: organised mammographic screening substantially reduces breast cancer mortality. Cancer 2001;91:1724–1731.

Biopsy Techniques

Britton PD. Fine needle aspiration or core biopsy Breast 1999;8:1–4.

Evans A, Pinder S. Fine needle aspiration cytology and core biopsy of mammographic microcalcifications. In: Evans A, Pinder S, Wilson R, Ellis I, eds Breast Calcification: A Diagnostic Manual. London UK: Greenwich Medical Media, 2002;74–75.

Litherland J, Evans A, Wilson A, et al. The impact of core biopsy on preoperative diagnosis rate of screen detected breast cancer. Clin Radiol 1996;51;562–565.

Rich PM, Michell MJ, Humphreys S, et al. Stereotactic 14-G core biopsy of non-palpable breast cancer: what is the relationship between the number of core samples taken and the sensitivity for detection of malignancy? Clin Radiol 1999;54:384–389.

Normal Breast

James J Going

SURFACE AND MACROSCOPIC ANATOMY

In the adult woman, the breasts extend between, approximately, the second rib above, the sixth rib below, lateral border of the sternum medially and the mid-axillary line laterally, with a variable axillary tail extending towards the axilla (Figure 6-1). Anteriorly, the breast is bounded by the skin, from which it is derived, while posteriorly lie pectoralis major, serratus anterior and the superior rectus sheath. Loose connective tissue in the retromammary space allows significant mobility of the breast on the chest wall.

In males and females alike each breast possesses a central, erectile nipple or papilla with a circular or ovoid areola of darker skin. The degree of pigmentation is proportionate to overall skin color; the areolae in nulliparous fair-skinned women are pink but become brown with pregnancy / lactation. Smooth muscle fibres in circular and longitudinal bundles erect the nipple and contract the areola in response to thermal, tactile and psychological stimuli. On the areola low elevations (Montgomery's tubercles) indicate the presence of modified sebaceous glands.

The breasts vary markedly in form from person to person. The contours of the breast are normally smooth, and irregularities of their outline can be a consequence of benign or malignant breast disease.

Internally, the resting (non-pregnant, non-lactating) breasts are composed of a relatively small volume fraction of ducts radiating from the nipple and glandular parenchymal tissue ('lobules') embedded in a stroma of fibrous connective tissue (Figure 6-2) and fat in proportions that vary widely between individuals and with age; the volume fraction of collagen-rich fibrous tissue is greater in younger adult women prior to the menopause, and appears to be responsible for the greater mammographic density of the pre-menopausal breast. Varying proportions of fat, fibrous and parenchymal tissue also appear to account for this difference. The radiolucent pattern (N1 Wolfe pattern), seen in mammographic images has been associated with the lowest breast cancer risk and the dense pattern (D4 Wolfe pattern) with the greatest risk. This may reflect a possible association between parenchymal mass and cancer risk, but there is no definite relationship between overall breast volume and cancer risk, possibly because large breasts do not necessarily contain more parenchyma.

Collagenous bands tether the fibrous tissue of the breast to the overlying skin; these so-called 'suspensory ligaments' of Astley Cooper lack the dense bundles of long parallel collagen fibres characteristic of true ligaments. It is said that they are more numerous in the upper portion of the breast and increasing laxity with time may contribute to breast ptosis.

The ductal-glandular tissue of the breast is organized into ducts and lobules. Unlike most glandular organs, the breast has multiple central ducts and they converge on the nipple to form a bundle of parallel ducts in the papilla running forwards to the skin surface on the apex of the nipple (Figures 6-3 and 6-4). The number of nipple ducts is usually given as 15–20 or sometimes 20–25. In a mastectomy series of 72 breasts with cancer there was a slightly larger median of 27 ducts. Whether all of these ducts open onto the surface of the nipple is open to question; the number of ducts from which milk can be expressed in lactating women, and the number of nipple ducts which can typically be cannulated, are substantially smaller (typically 6–10). Possible explanations for this discrepancy include duct branching in the nipple itself but it is also possible that not all of the ducts present in the nipple open directly on to the nipple surface. Those that do, open into a funnel-shaped vestibule lined by stratified squamous epithelium and plugged by keratin. There is an abrupt transition between the bilayered duct epitheium and squamous epithelium (Figure 6-5), which appears to form a barrier to the extension of intraductal carcinoma onto the surface of the nipple except for those epitheliotropic tumors associated with Paget's disease of the nipple. A population of benign epidermal clear cells, known as Toker cells, are present in about 10 % of normal nipples and it has been proposed that some examples of Paget's disease of the nipple arise from these cells. Immediately deep to this point, the duct in the nipple adopts a characteristically convoluted outline (Figure 6-6) for a variable distance before opening out into a smooth-profiled lactiferous sinus just deep to the nipple.

'LOBAR' ORGANIZATION IN HUMAN BREAST

Many images of breast parenchymal anatomy published in books or on the internet imply that individual ducts contribute equally to the breast volume and suggest a relatively regular architecture of approximately equal 'lobes' possessing radial symmetry arranged around the nipple like segments of an orange. Such an arrangement, while possible, is not supported by any considerable body of evidence; indeed, there is limited evidence for much greater variation in the configuration of individual duct systems (for which the term 'lobes' could usefully be retained: Figures 6-7 and 6-8). Such variation is not easily studied because the lobar architecture cannot be inferred merely by inspection of breast tissue, as the thin-walled ducts and their branching pattern can barely be discerned, and injection studies *in vivo* (ductography) or using surgical or autopsy tissues are technically challenging. Improved knowledge of this 'lobar' anatomy would be helpful for understanding normal breast development and possible pathways for the spread of preinvasive neoplastic cell populations (e.g, ductal and lobular carcinomas in situ) in the breast. A specific unresolved question is whether or not anastomotic peripheral connections exist between different duct systems. Such anastomoses might allow in situ carcinoma to spread widely within a breast.

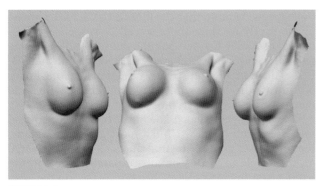

FIGURE 6-1
Three views of a 3-D digital surface model of the anterior thorax and breasts of a normal volunteer. The model was created by high-resolution close-range digital photogrammetry with unstructured illumination. (Image courtesy of Colin Urquhart (Virtual Clones Ltd, Glasgow, Scotland), Arup Ray and Helga Hensler (Canniesburn Plastic Surgery Unit, Glasgow Royal Infirmary) and the volunteer subject.)

BLOOD SUPPLY

The blood supply of the breast derives medially from the internal thoracic (mammary) artery from which perforating branches run forward in the second to the fourth intercostal spaces, and laterally from branches of the axillary artery including the lateral thoracic and acromiothoracic arteries. Posterior intercostal arteries also supply the breast with some blood. Venous drainage is principally via tributaries of the axillary vein but blood also drains via posterior intercostal veins in the second to sixth intercostal spaces and also to the internal thoracic vein from medial parts of the breast. Varia-

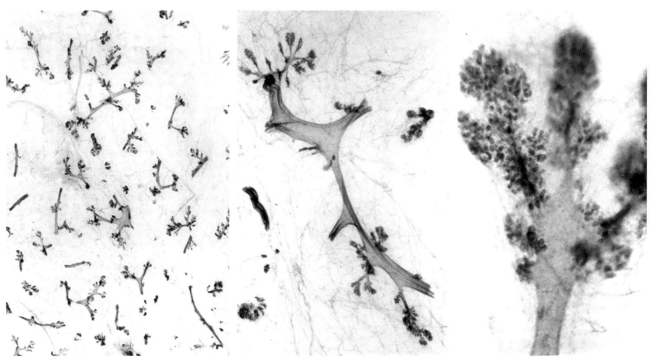

FIGURE 6-2
Appearance of breast parenchyma (ducts and lobules) in normal breast tissue at low, medium and high power. A 2 mm thick section of breast tissue was stained with hematoxylin and cleared in methyl salicylate. The low-power view shows numerous branching ducts. One of these is shown in the medium-power middle view and the high power view (right) shows one medium-sized duct dividing into three terminal ducts and forming lobules.

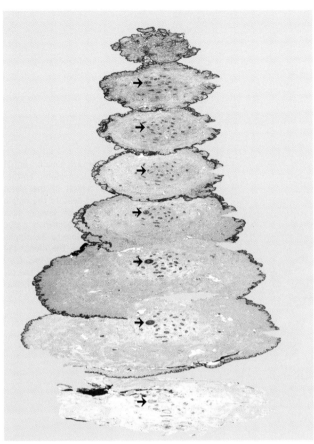

FIGURE 6-3

Ducts in the nipple. Eight parallel histologic sections each separated by approximately 2 mm have been taken at right angles to the duct bundle in a mastectomy nipple. These stacked digital images of the hematoxylin and eosin stained sections show the ducts converging on the apex of the papilla of the nipple. In this case, one of the ducts (indicated in each section by an arrowhead) was expanded by high grade ductal carcinoma in situ.

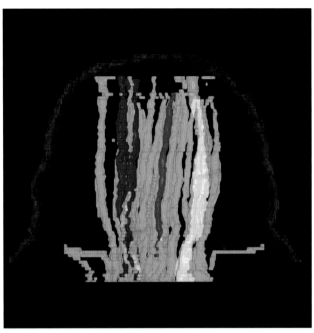

FIGURE 6-4

A 3-D reconstruction of the major ducts in a nipple from a mastectomy, viewed from the side. The reconstruction was made from 68 100 micron sections. Outline of the nipple skin is shown in red. Five ducts have been allocated different colors to emphasize the unbranching, independent courses of the ducts in the nipple. Notice that while a minority of ducts expand in caliber towards the skin surface on the apex of the nipple, the majority taper down and appear to terminate about 1 mm beneath the skin surface.

FIGURE 6-5

The mammary squamo-columnar junction, where the epithelial-myoepithelial bilayer lining the breast ducts meets the squamous epithelium of the nipple skin. This junction appears to offer a barrier to the further extension of ductal carcinoma in situ, except in cases which progress to Paget's disease of the nipple. (Hematoxylin and eosin).

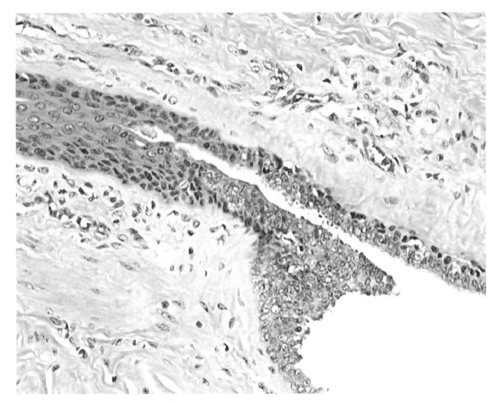

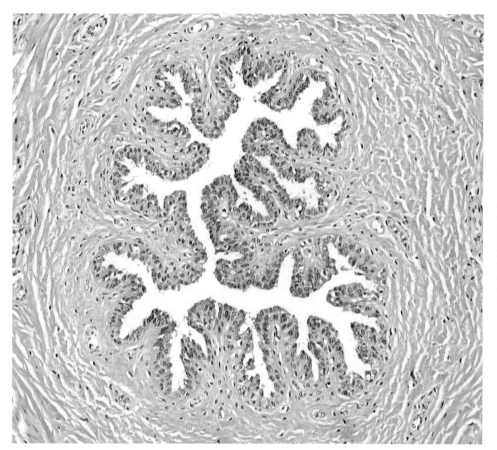

FIGURE 6-6

Cross-section through a major central breast duct. The convoluted epithelial profile is typical of the major ducts in and just deep to the nipple and the presence of several such ducts in a biopsy specimen is a clue to an origin from close to the nipple. Slightly further from the nipple the ducts may open out into a smoother, ovoid profile characteristic of the so-called 'lactiferous sinuses'. (Hematoxylin and eosin).

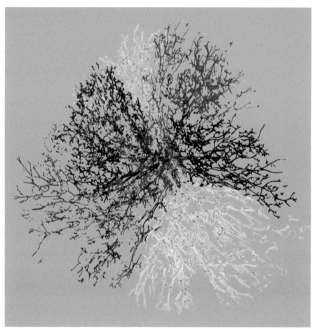

FIGURE 6-7

'Lobar' anatomy of a normal human breast. Individual duct systems were reconstructed by tracing their branches from slice to slice in a stack of 2 mm 'subgross' serial sections in the coronal plane. Different colors indicate individual systems, each draining to the nipple via a single central duct. Great variation in the extent of individual duct systems is a feature of the lobar anatomy. (Reproduced with permission from Going JJ and Moffat DF. Escaping from flatland: clinical and biological aspects of human breast duct anatomy in three dimensions. Journal of Pathology, 2004:202:538–544. © 2004, Pathological Society of Great Britain and Ireland).

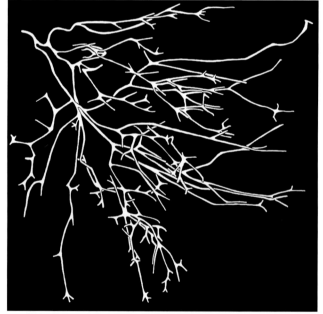

FIGURE 6-8

The duct 'skeleton' of a complete single duct system in an autopsy breast. Terminal ducts and lobules are not shown. Reconstructed from serial subgross sections. This particular system accounted for about 25% of the whole breast illustrated in Figure 6-7. Theoretically, mammary intraepithelial neoplasia could colonize an entire duct system such as this.

tions in both the arterial and the venous systems of the breasts can be seen between individuals.

LYMPHATIC DRAINAGE

The lymphatic drainage of the breasts has been studied for many years, and such an important route for the spread of breast cancer is more significant than ever with the advent of sentinel node biopsy in breast cancer.

Two main destinations for lymph draining from the breasts have been recognized for over 200 years: nodes in the axilla, and nodes along the internal mammary blood vessels. Quantitative studies in the 1950s indicated that about 75 % of breast lymph passes to ipsilateral axillary nodes, and confirmed significant lymphatic drainage to the internal mammary nodes from lateral as well as medial parts of the breast. Direct drainage to supraclavicular nodes, to contralateral internal mammary nodes behind the sternum and to posterior intercostal nodes are less common. Anomalous drainage to the contralateral axilla or retrograde flow in the internal mammary chain towards the liver have been associated with lymphatic blockage by tumor cells.

The course of lymph flow from the breast has been, and to some extent still remains, a subject of controversy. Sappey's belief that lymph drained to the axilla via the subareolar lymphatic plexus was supported by other pioneers but was challenged by Turner-Warwick and other more recent workers using methods including lymphoscintigraphy, which usually indicates a small number of lymphatics following more or less direct paths to a sentinel node or nodes in the axilla, or to an internal mammary node, without involving the subareolar lymphatic plexus.

Methods of sentinel lymph node identification have been influenced by these anatomical considerations. Intradermal and subcutaneous injection of tracers appear to be less likely to identify internal mammary sentinel nodes than peritumoral injection for deeply located tumors, when such nodes may be identified in up to one-third of cases. Occasionally, supraclavicular, intra-pectoral or intramammary sentinel nodes may be identified and such nodes appear more likely to be identified by deep rather than intradermal or subcutaneous injection of tracer.

INNERVATION AND SENSATION

Innervation of the breast is via branches of the intercostal nerves. The lateral part of the breast is innervated by lateral cutaneous branches of intercostal nerves II–VII arising in the mid-axillary line, which pierce serratus anterior and give off branches which run forward into the breast over pectoralis major. Anterior cutaneous branches of the intercostal nerves I–VI enter the medial breast just lateral to the sternum. Innervation of the nipple–areola complex is rather consistently from the anterior and lateral branches of the intercostal nerve IV with lesser contributions from III and V. The nipple–areola area is well supplied with tactile receptors such as Meissner's corpuscles. Cutaneous sensitivity of the breast varies between women and at different times in the menstrual cycle but nipple stimulation initiates the afferent limb of the milk ejection reflex via cutaneous nerves, relayed via the spinothalamic tracts to oxytocin-containing cells in the supraoptic and paraventricular nuclei of the hypothalamus. These cells have axons ending in the posterior pituitary where they release oxytocin and its carrier neurophysin into the blood, constituting the efferent limb of this important neuroendocrine reflex.

NORMAL DEVELOPMENT AND INVOLUTION

The earliest sign of the developing breast is the appearance, during the fourth week of gestation, of the curvilinear ectodermal thickenings known as the 'milk lines' extending from the axilla down to the medial thigh. Subsequent regression occurs except in the fourth intercostal space where the breast will subsequently develop. Here the primary mammary bud begins to grow down into the subjacent dermis, at about the seventh week of intrauterine life, and forms branches over the following weeks which subsequently become canalized and form glandular tissue under the influence of maternal hormones and important paracrine/juxtacrine interactions between the ectoderm of the milk line and the subjacent mesoderm. Under the influence of maternal hormones, the mammary glands of both male and female neonates may secrete 'witch's milk' for a while. At birth, the nipple is represented by a shallow pit into which the central ducts open, but proliferation of the surrounding mesoderm soon gives the nipple its characteristically everted form in most cases.

The relatively small, and not very complex, gland established *in utero* is quiescent until puberty. Although breast growth is a characteristic event in females with the onset of puberty, about two-thirds of males will also experience some mammary gland enlargement (gynecomastia) at this time, and may require reassurance that this is unlikely to persist. In the rare X-linked androgen insensitivity syndrome, there is a loss-of-function androgen receptor gene mutation. In these individuals peripheral conversion of testosterone to estradiol stimulates a female pattern of breast development despite the XY genotype.

In females, thelarche initiates a sustained period of mammary gland growth during which the deposition of fat and periductal connective tissue occur *pari passu* with the elongation and further branching of the duct systems and the formation of terminal duct – lobular units, although these are not functionally secretory at this stage. This contrasts with rodent mammary gland development in which the formation of secretory (glandular) tissue is largely deferred until pregnancy.

Tanner described five characteristic stages of mammary gland development in adolescent girls:
- Stage 1: small elevated nipple, no palpable breast tissue.
- Stage 2: pale areola begins to enlarge, small mound forms over breast bud.
- Stage 3: areola less pale, continuing breast enlargement.
- Stage 4: nipple and areola form a separate elevation on the breast mound.
- Stage 5: mature breast. Areola no longer elevated above surrounding breast (but this elevation may persist in some women).

Full, functional development of the mammary gland is only achieved as a consequence of hormonal changes associated with pregnancy and lactation. During pregnancy breast growth occurs and there is a reduction in the proportion of the breast composed of fibrous and fatty connective tissue and a concomitant increase in the proportion of glandular tissue. Following parturition, lactation may become established if the infant suckles regularly, and in response to the stimulation of the nipple by the suckling infant, oxytocin release causes contraction of the myoepithelial cells around the glandular alveoli, thereby increasing the supply of milk for the infant on the breast ('let-down'). With weaning the production of milk is inhibited as a consequence, inter alia, of its non-withdrawal and systemic hormonal effects. In both mice and humans the end of lactation initiates a dramatic phase of glandular involution characterized by a profound wave of cell death and tissue remodelling which eventually returns the gland to something like its pre-pregnancy condition.

With the onset of the menopause, the epithelial elements of the breast enter a further phase of gradual involution which will establish the characteristically stroma-predominant post-menopausal breast in which fatty tissue predominates with relatively little fibrous connective tissue and rather attenuated ducts leading to small, withered lobules composed of small, loose aggregates of ductuli in a stroma which tends to be more collagenous than myxoid. Eventually, lobular elements may disappear almost completely.

VARIATIONS IN MAMMARY DEVELOPMENT

Complete bilateral or unilateral absence of mammary development is very unusual. Small hypoplastic breasts are more often encountered and may be associated with Poland's syndrome (pectoral dysplasia – dysdactyly), in which unilateral absence of pectoralis major, pectoralis minor and abnormal development of the chest wall (including breast), arm and hand may occur in varying degrees. Nipple and breast agenesis or hypoplasia occur

in the rare autosomal dominant Finlay-Marks scalp-ear-nipple syndrome, along with cataracts and renal abnormalities. In the, also rare, autosomal dominant Pallister-Schinzel ulnar-mammary syndrome limb defects and abnormal apocrine gland and mammary development are caused by mutation of the TBX3 gene which encodes a T-box transcription factor. Mammary hypoplasia may also be a component in hypohydrotic/anhydrotic ectodermal dysplasia syndromes.

Minor degrees of asymmetry in breast development are so common that they can hardly be regarded as truly abnormal. More marked differences are less common and may include a small, hypoplastic breast with normal contralateral development, or a normal breast on one side with an unusual degree of enlargement of the other breast (juvenile hypertrophy, usually beginning with puberty). Juvenile hypertrophy is more commonly bilateral, and may lead to back problems and body image difficulties for young women so affected.

That trauma to the breast bud prior to thelarche may cause failure of subsequent breast development was known to those classical writers who claimed that the 'Amazons' seared the rudimentary right breast during infancy to prevent its later development. Asynchronous thelarche is not uncommon and inappropriate surgery on the unilaterally enlarging breast under the misapprehension that a pathologic process is present may severely disrupt its subsequent growth, and require ultimate cosmetic correction. Premature thelarche may be unilateral or bilateral, usually regresses eventually, and only a small minority go on to develop true precocious puberty. Subsequent development is usually normal.

The commonest actual aberrations of mammary development are supernumerary nipples, with or without associated breast tissue. These occur most frequently along the 'milk line' from axilla to groin, but may occur in other locations as well. They are not always recognized for what they are, but may enlarge during pregnancy and produce milk during lactation. Accessory breast tissue can be identified in about 1–3 % of males and twice as many females, at more than one site in about one-third of cases. Most examples occur on the thoraco-abdominal milk lines with a left sided preponderance. Almost any combination of nipple, areolar and breast tissue can be found. Polythelia (extra nipples) are most frequent, and usually infra-mammary. Accessory breast tissue may develop any of the disease processes to which normally located breasts are susceptible.

HISTOLOGIC ORGANIZATION

The parenchymal tree from the central ducts out to the lobules is lined by cuboidal or low columnar epithelial cells which form the interior layer of the epithelial lining of the ducts and are surrounded by a more or less continuous layer of outer myoepithelial cells.

The lobules are found attached to the parenchymal trees via the terminal ducts and are composed of a compact, rounded or ovoid clump of individual ductules or acini embedded in a specialized myxoid connective tissue stroma, within which a scattering of lymphoid or plasma cells are often present (Figure 6-9). This is in contrast to the appearance of the fully differentiated lobule during lactation (Figure 6-10). The size of lobules varies, with most in the range 0.5–2 mm in the resting adult breast. Lobular development is minimal in pre-pubertal female and male breasts. Their density varies greatly from sparse to very numerous between

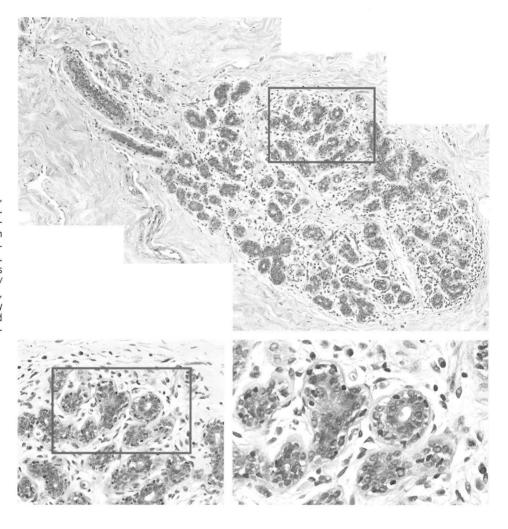

FIGURE 6-9

'Resting' human breast lobule, stained with hematoxylin and eosin. Top: low power view showing terminal duct (upper left) entering an individual lobule composed of individual ductules or glandular acini. Intermediate and high power views show the two-layered epithelial/myoepithelial lining of the acini, the myxoid stroma in which they are embedded, and the associated plasma cells, stromal and intraepithelial lymphocytes.

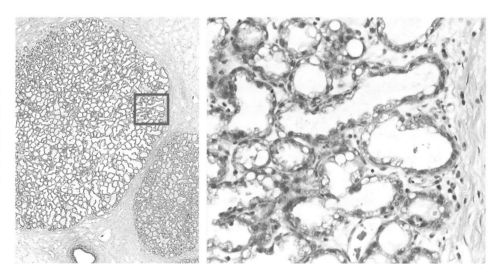

FIGURE 6-10

Lactational change in breast lobules: low and high power (left and right). The volume fraction of the lobule occupied by the intralobular stroma is reduced, with an increase in the proportion of the lobule occupied by glandular acini. The cells of the lobular epithelium contain numerous lipid vacuoles and have a characteristic 'hobnail' appearance.

individuals, and even between different areas within one breast. To the naked eye lobules may be a little more transparent than the surrounding collagenous breast tissue. Neither ducts nor lobules can usually be discerned on a plain mammogram.

TURNOVER OF CELLS

Although the term 'resting' breast is often applied to the non-pregnant and non-lactating breast, this term is misleading in that the breast is not quiescent, and there is significant proliferative activity of lobular and ductal epithelium, with a cycle of proliferation and apoptosis in pre-menopausal women. Proliferation is maximal in the second half (secretory phase) of the menstrual cycle, unlike the endometrium and oral contraceptive use is not associated with any significant reduction in proliferative activity of breast epithelium. Breast epithelial proliferation is maximal in young women and decreases gradually in the 30s and 40s, and further beyond the menopause.

STEM CELLS AND PATHWAYS OF DIFFERENTIATION

There has been a great deal of attention devoted in recent years to defining mammary stem cells and pathways of differentiation in the mammary epithelium. Not surprisingly, more is known about the situation in experimental animals (mainly rodents) but there is also some human data. Striking facts from the world of animal mammary gland biology include the fact that an entire mouse mammary gland can be reconstituted from a single mammary gland cell, and the even more striking fact that in the case of 'Dolly' the famous Finn Dorset sheep, it was possible to create a complete organism from a nucleus derived from a stem cell of adult mammary gland origin.

Pathways of cellular differentiation in the mammary gland are generally considered in the light of differentiation towards luminal and basal (or myoepithelial) cellular phenotypes (Figure 6-11). These pathways are characterized in the case of luminal epithelial cells by specific cytokeratins especially 8/18 and 19, whereas the basal lineage is more typically characterized by cytokeratins 5 and 14 (Figure 6-12) (which, like 8 and 18, are also partners in the Moll catalog of cytokeratins) and other markers of smooth muscle differentiation including smooth muscle actin, CALLA (CD10), S100 protein and p63. Figure 6-13 illustrates the expression of six different markers in a normal pre-menopausal breast lobule. Expression studies of lineage-specific markers

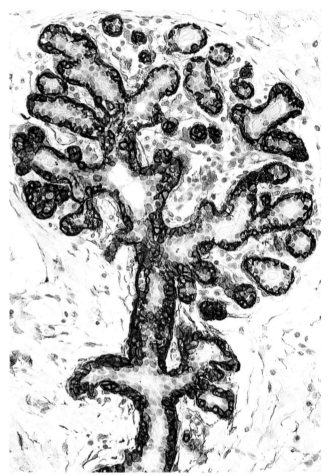

FIGURE 6-11

The architecture of a normal 'resting' human breast lobule. Immunohistochemistry with the basal/myoepithelial marker CALLA (CD10) shows the epithelial bilayer of the terminal duct and the branching ductules within the lobule with great clarity, as expression of this marker is almost dichotomous between the negative luminal and the strongly positive basal cells.

suggest that in normal breast small numbers of CK5/6 positive epithelial cells which express neither luminal (CK 8/18/19) nor basal lineage markers (smooth muscle actin) are present and may represent precursor cells uncommitted to either lineage. Subsequent expression of markers appropriate to one or other of the major mammary epithelial lineages appear and fully mature cells may lose CK5/6 positivity. These lineage-specific markers may be helpful in discriminating between hyperplasia of usual type (HUT) in which a mixture of immature epithelial and myoepithelial phenotypes is characteristic, from ADH and DCIS in which mature luminal phenotypes characteristic of the neoplastic cells generally are seen.

Identification of very early stem cells remains a significant challenge but certain signalling molecules of the Notch family (e.g., the Notch-4 receptor) and biochemical activities such as the exclusion of certain vital dyes by viable cells (so called 'side' populations) which may

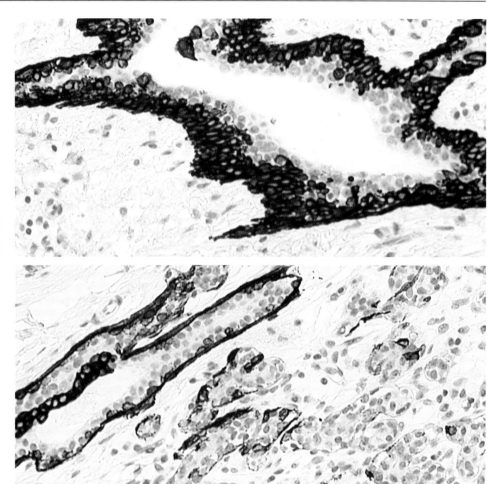

FIGURE 6-12

Variability of the immunophenotype of myoepithelial cells in a large duct (above), terminal duct and lobule (below). In the large duct and the terminal duct, the basal myoepithelial cells are strongly positive for cytokeratin 14, which is lost in the intralobular ductules and acini. Contrast this variability with the uniform expression of CD10 in Figure 6-11.

be characteristic of stem cell populations are beginning to be identified in the mammary gland.

HORMONE RECEPTOR EXPRESSION

Expression of estrogen and progesterone receptors (ER and PR, respectively) are, as one might expect for a sex hormone responsive tissue, invariably found in normal breast tissue, but the pattern of expression is distinctive in that normal breast epithelium never shows 100% positivity (Figure 6-14) and a striking feature of normal breast epithelium is that the proliferating cell population shows very little overlap with the ER and PR positive cells. This pattern strongly suggests that in normal breast epithelium the proliferative stimulus of steroids is indirectly acting, presumably via paracrine or juxtacrine signalling between the receptor-positive cells

and the receptor negative but proliferating cells. This is in distinction to neoplastic epithelial populations in which co-expression of steroid receptors and proliferation markers in the same cells is frequently found.

ULTRASTRUCTURAL FEATURES

Electron microscopy is not used very often in the clinical investigation of breast tissue but has been used extensively to characterize breast tissue in terms of cellular differentiation and, for instance, in looking for candidate stem cells and possible maturational pathways. The cuboidal to columnar epithelial (luminal) cells lining the ducts and ductules within the lobules usually show surface specialization with microvilli on the luminal surface and may contain secretory droplets towards the luminal pole. They may rest basally on

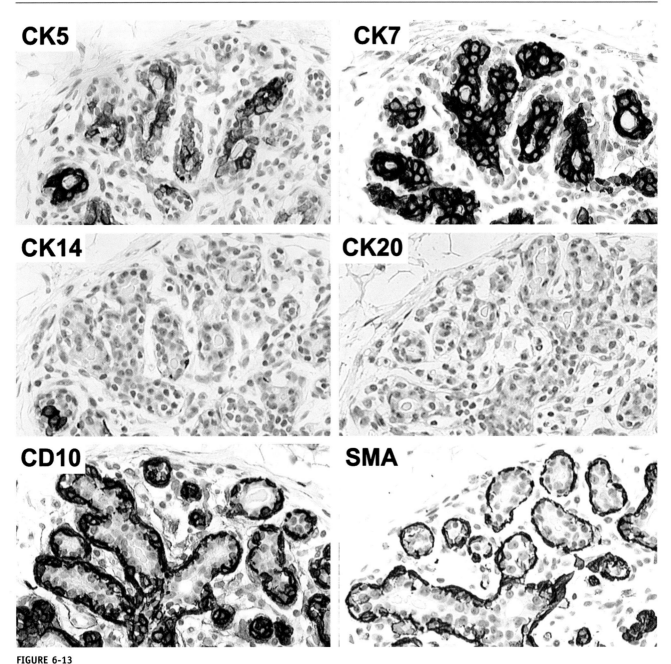

FIGURE 6-13

Expression of a variety of lineage markers in adjacent sections of the same normal breast lobule. The basal markers CD10 and smooth muscle actin (SMA) are pretty strictly confined to the basal cell population whilst CK7 is purely luminal. There is no expression of CK20 and limited expression of CK14. CK5 expression is heterogeneous and not confined to basal cells in this particular lobule

either the basement membrane or on cells of the discontinuous layer of myoepithelial cells, which tend to be orientated at right angles to the epithelial cells. Both cell types contain mitochondria. A Golgi apparatus is present in the epithelial cells while the smaller myoepithelial cells are characterized by their contractile actin filaments. Cytoplasmic density varies and both 'light' and 'dark' variants of epithelial and myoepithelial cells are probably related to different stages in the differentiation of these cells from their stem cell precursors. Lymphoid cells are observed quite frequently and tend to occupy a niche between the epithelial and myoepithelial cells. Elongated fibroblastic cells characteristically invest the glandular acini.

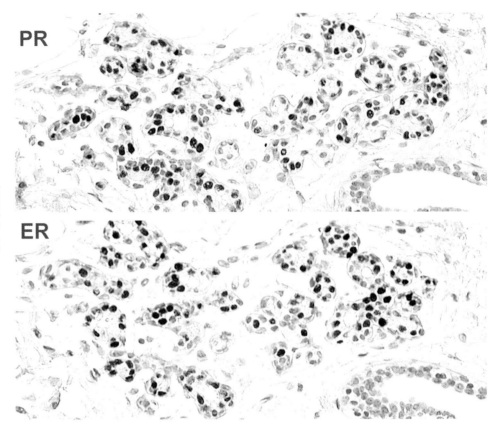

FIGURE 6-14

Expression of progesterone receptor (PR) and estrogen receptor (ER) in adjacent sections of the same normal breast lobule. Although there are many steroid-receptor positive cells, there are also many cells in which no receptor expression is detectable.

SUGGESTED READING

Anderson TJ, Battersby S, King RJB, et al. Oral contraceptive use influences resting breast proliferation. Hum Pathol 1989;20:1139–1144.

Boecker W, Buerger H. Evidence of progenitor cells of glandular and myoepithelial cell lineages in the human adult female breast epithelium: a new progenitor (adult stem) cell concept. Cell Prolif 2003;36(Suppl. 1):73–84.

Dontu G, El-Ashry D, Wicha MS. Breast cancer, stem/progenitor cells and the estrogen receptor. Trends Endocrinol Metabol 2004;15:193–197.

Gilbert SF. Multiple hormone interactions in mammary gland development. In: Developmental Biology, 4e. Sunderland, MA Sinauer Associates, Sunderland, Massachusetts, 1994.

Going JJ, Moffat DF. Escaping from Flatland: clinical and biological aspects of human mammary duct anatomy in three dimensions. J Path 2004;203:538–544.

Jaspars JJP, Posma AN, van Immerseel AAH, Gittenberger-de Groot AC. The cutaneous innervation of the female breast and nipple-areola complex: implications for surgery. Br J Plast Surg 1997;50:249–259.

Ohtake T, Kimijima I, Fukushima T, et al. Computer-assisted complete three-dimensional reconstruction of the mammary ductal/lobular systems. Cancer 2001;91:2263–2272.

Rosen PP. Anatomy and physiologic morphology: In: Rosen's Breast Pathology. New York, Lippincott Williams & Wilkins, 2001 p 1–21.

Smith GH, Boulanger CA. Mammary epithelial stem cells: transplantation and self-renewal analysis. Cell Prolif 2003; 36(Suppl.1):3–15.

Tanis PJ, Niewg OE, Olmos RAV, Kroon BBR. Anatomy and physiology of lymphatic drainage of the breast from the perspective of sentinel node biopsy. J Am Coll Surg 2001;192:399–409.

Tavassoli FA. Normal development and anomalies. In: Pathology of the Breast. Norwalk, CT Appleton and Lange, 1992m p 1–24.

7 Inflammatory Lesions, Infections and Silicone Granulomas

Andrew HS Lee

This chapter focuses on the common inflammatory conditions affecting the breast. Less common conditions are mentioned briefly.

DUCT ECTASIA

Duct ectasia is a common disorder affecting the larger ducts and characterized by duct dilatation with periductal inflammation and fibrosis.

CLINICAL FEATURES

Duct ectasia is most common in women between the ages of 30 and 70 years, although it can rarely occur in men and children. Mild forms of duct ectasia may be asymptomatic. The high frequency of duct ectasia at post mortem examination suggests that only a small proportion is symptomatic. Common symptoms include nipple discharge, which may be serous, creamy or blood stained, a mass, nipple retraction and pain. The features may mimic carcinoma. Duct ectasia may have acute inflammatory episodes, which may be self limiting or result in abscess or fistula formation. Infection appears to be important in the acute inflammatory complications of duct ectasia, but not in duct ectasia itself.

Clinical features of pain and a mass and histologic periductal inflammation are seen more in younger women; the label periductal mastitis may be applied to this group. By contrast, duct dilatation and nipple retraction are seen more in older women; some authors restrict the term duct ectasia to this group. Using these definitions, cigarette smoking is associated with periductal mastitis, but not with duct ectasia. It is uncertain whether periductal mastitis can progress to duct ectasia or whether they should be regarded as two separate conditions. Acute inflammatory complications appear to be particularly associated with periductal mastitis.

RADIOLOGIC FEATURES

The dilated ducts may be seen on mammography and ultrasound. Mammography may show calcification.

PATHOLOGIC FEATURES

DUCT ECTASIA – FACT SHEET

Definition
▶ Dilatation of larger ducts with periductal inflammation and fibrosis.

Incidence
▶ Common

Gender and Age Distribution
▶ Most common in women aged 30 to 70 years

Clinical Features
▶ Nipple discharge, mass, pain or nipple retraction.

Radiologic Features
▶ The dilated ducts may be seen on mammography and ultrasound
▶ Mammography may show calcification

Prognosis and Treatment
▶ Benign condition
▶ May be complicated by abscess formation

DUCT ECTASIA – PATHOLOGIC FEATURES

Gross Findings
▶ Dilated subareolar ducts containing cheesy or brown material.

Microscopic Features
▶ Dilated ducts with luminal amorphous material and macrophages.
▶ Periductal inflammation (predominantly chronic) and fibrosis.

Fine Needle Aspiration Cytology Features
▶ Debris, foamy macrophages, lymphocytes and plasma cells.
▶ Epithelium is scanty, but may appear mildly atypical.

Pathologic Differential Diagnosis
▶ Cysts

GROSS FINDINGS

The characteristic appearance is dilated subareolar ducts containing soft creamy or brown material. Occasionally more peripheral ducts are affected.

MICROSCOPIC FINDINGS

The lumina of the dilated ducts typically contain eosinophilic amorphous debris and foamy macrophages (Figure 7-1). Crystalline material is occasionally present. The epithelium lining the ducts is often thinned and may contain inflammatory cells, particularly macrophages (Figure 7-2). Epithelial hyperplasia is not a feature of duct ectasia. The adjacent tissues contain chronic inflammation composed of macrophages, lymphocytes and plasma cells (Figure 7-1). Granulomatous inflammation, including giant cells, may be present. Acute inflammation is occasionally seen. Periductal fibrosis is another common feature and explains nipple retraction. Occasionally obliteration of ducts secondary to the fibrosis may occur. Calcification is another uncommon feature.

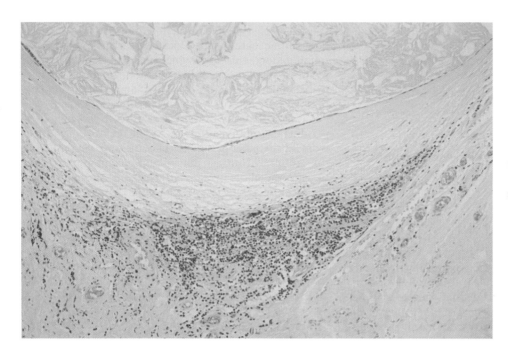

FIGURE 7-1
Duct ectasia. Dilated duct with fibrosis and chronic inflammation.

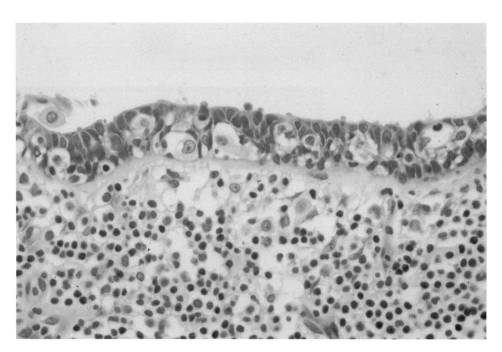

FIGURE 7-2
Duct ectasia. Note the macrophages in the epithelium.

FINE NEEDLE ASPIRATION CYTOLOGY

There is debris, foamy macrophages, lymphocytes and plasma cells. Epithelium is scanty, but may appear mildly atypical.

DIFFERENTIAL DIAGNOSIS

The diagnosis of duct ectasia is usually straightforward. Potential confusion with cysts may occur. Duct ectasia involves central ducts with luminal debris and macrophages and surrounding inflammation and fibrosis with elastic tissue in the wall. Cysts are rounded and usually lack luminal debris, inflammatory changes and fibrosis, and do not have elastic tissue in the wall.

PROGNOSIS AND THERAPY

Duct ectasia is a benign condition with no increased risk of malignancy. Antibiotics do not appear to be helpful in uncomplicated duct ectasia. Duct excision is not indicated for uncomplicated duct ectasia, except perhaps for persistent troublesome discharge. The complications of duct ectasia are discussed below. Stopping smoking may be helpful in periductal mastitis.

INFECTIONS

Bacterial infections related to pregnancy or duct ectasia are not uncommon. Tuberculous mastitis is briefly discussed below. Fungal and parasitic infections are rare and are not described in detail here.

ABSCESS

An abscess is an acute inflammatory mass that yields pus on incision. Mammography may show an ill-defined mass, with thickening of adjacent trabeculae and skin. Ultrasound shows an ill-defined fluid collection with surrounding edema. There are two common patterns of abscess related either to lactation or to duct ectasia:

- Acute mastitis during lactation is common. It is often due to staphylococcal or streptococcal infection. Stasis of milk or cracks in the skin of the nipple may allow entry of bacteria. It may progress to abscess formation. *Staphylococcus aureus* is the most frequently isolated organism in puerperal abscesses.
- Non-puerperal abscesses are frequently subareolar and associated with duct ectasia. *S. aureus* or anaerobic organisms are commonly grown.

Histology shows a central area of acute inflammation with surrounding granulation tissue and chronic inflammation, and fibrosis at the edge (Figures 7-3 and

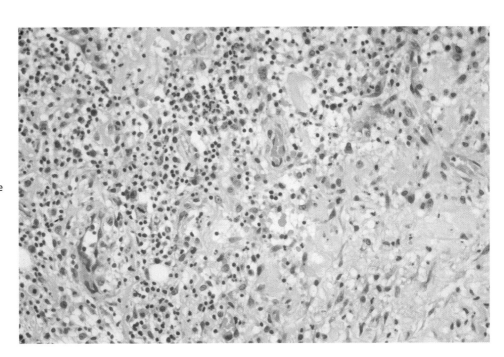

FIGURE 7-3

Abscess. At the center there is acute inflammation.

7-4). Lactational changes or duct ectasia may be seen depending on the etiology. Cytology shows polymorphs, macrophages and debris. Reactive epithelial atypia may be present. If the woman is lactating, lactational changes may also be present.

An abscess is usually treated successfully by aspiration and antibiotics or occasionally by incision to allow drainage. Surgery is rarely needed.

MAMMARY FISTULA

This is a fistula of lactiferous ducts. The commonest clinical association is with a preceding breast abscess, usually secondary to duct ectasia. Often the abscess will have been previously incised, but spontaneous fistula formation from an abscess can also occur. Some authorities advocate excision of the fistula with packing of the wound. Recurrence may occur following excision and primary closure; antibiotics may be important in reducing the risk of recurrence. Histology shows a track lined by granulation tissue and sometimes also by squamous epithelium (Figure 7-5). *S. aureus* and enterococcus are commonly grown.

MAMMARY TUBERCULOSIS

Tuberculosis of the breast is rare in western countries, but is more common in developing countries. The

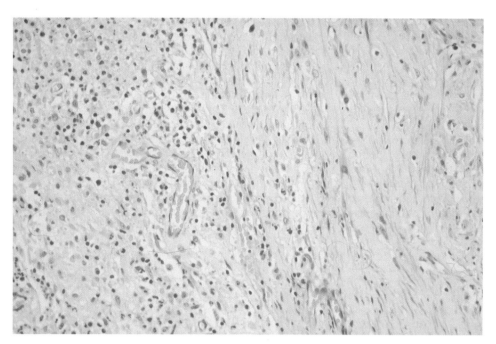

FIGURE 7-4

Abscess. At the edge there is granulation tissue and fibrosis.

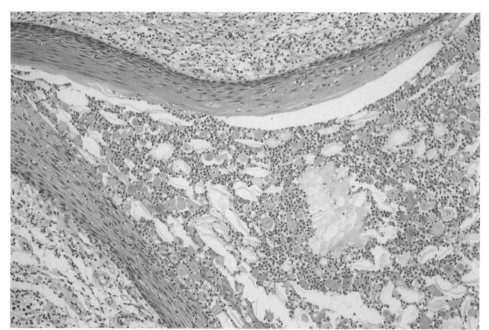

FIGURE 7-5

Fistula. The track is lined by squamous epithelium.

commonest presentations are with a mass, a sinus or a combination of the two. The clinical appearance may mimic carcinoma. Women are much more frequently affected than men, with most being between 20 and 50 years old. The typical histologic appearance is like tuberculosis in other organs: granulomas with epithelioid macrophages, Langhan's giant cells and caseous necrosis. The typical cytologic appearance shows epithelioid granulomas, Langhan's giant cells, lymphocytes and polymorphs. Necrosis is often present. For a definitive diagnosis tubercle bacilli should be both demonstrated on Ziehl-Neelsen (ZN) stain and grown on culture. Most cases reported in the literature have neither positive ZN stain nor positive culture. In Western countries a typical histologic picture or evidence of tuberculosis elsewhere may be sufficient for starting anti-tuberculous therapy. It is important to exclude other infections with similar histologic features including syphilis, fungal infections and parasitic infestations. Less stringent criteria are reasonable in areas with a high incidence of tuberculosis. If a diagnosis is made without positive ZN stain or positive culture and the patient fails to respond to anti-tuberculous therapy, then the diagnosis should be reconsidered.

SARCOIDOSIS

Sarcoidosis rarely involves the breast. Usually there is involvement of other organs; indeed the diagnosis is difficult without such evidence. Presentation is with single or multiple breast masses. The radiologic features are not specific. The pattern of the inflammation is the same as in other organs: non-caseating granulomas with epithelioid macrophages and Langhan's giant cells. Associated lymphocytes and fibrosis are often present. The inflammation may be centered on lobules. The diagnosis requires exclusion of other causes of granulomatous inflammation and clinical evidence of disease elsewhere. In particular tuberculosis must be excluded. If there is no extra-mammary disease then idiopathic granulomatous mastitis must be considered. Inflammation resembling sarcoidosis may rarely be seen in association with carcinoma.

IDIOPATHIC GRANULOMATOUS MASTITIS

Histology of idiopathic granulomatous mastitis shows lobulocentric granulomatous inflammation. Other causes of granulomatous inflammation need to be excluded before the diagnosis of idiopathic granulomatous mastitis can be made.

IDIOPATHIC GRANULOMATOUS MASTITIS – FACT SHEET

Definition
▶ Idiopathic granulomatous mastitis shows lobulocentric granulomatous inflammation
▶ It is a diagnosis of exclusion

Incidence
▶ Uncommon

Gender and Age Distribution
▶ Most often affects women between the ages of 20 and 40 years

Clinical Features
▶ Frequently associated with a recent pregnancy
▶ Palpable mass which is often tender

Radiologic Features
▶ Mammography may show an ill-defined mass or an asymmetric density
▶ Ultrasound typically shows multiple clustered hypoechoic masses

Prognosis and Treatment
▶ Benign, but disease may persist for several years
▶ Possible role for steroid treatment
▶ Some cases require surgery

CLINICAL FEATURES

This condition typically occurs in young women between the ages of 20 and 40 years and is frequently associated with a recent pregnancy. The usual presentation is with a palpable mass which is often, but not always, tender. The disease is bilateral in about one-quarter of patients. In up to half of cases the clinical impression is of carcinoma. Some reports emphasize the extra-areolar position of the mass, but the mass may be retroareolar. Axillary lymphadenopathy may be present. Persistent and recurrent disease may occur. Patients with idiopathic granulomatous mastitis do not have granulomatous disease at extra-mammary sites, in contrast to other granulomatous disorders.

RADIOLOGIC FEATURES

Mammography may show an ill-defined mass or an asymmetric density. Ultrasound typically shows multiple clustered hypo-echoic masses, which are often contiguous.

PATHOLOGIC FEATURES

IDIOPATHIC GRANULOMATOUS MASTITIS – PATHOLOGIC FEATURES

Gross Findings
▸ Ill-defined mass

Microscopic Features
▸ Non-caseating granulomas centered around lobules
▸ May be neutrophil polymorphs and microabscess formation
▸ No foreign material is present
▸ Special stains for organisms are all negative

Fine Needle Aspiration Cytology Features
▸ Epithelioid macrophages, giant cells and neutrophils

Pathologic Differential Diagnosis
▸ Tuberculosis
▸ Fungal infection
▸ Sarcoidosis
▸ Wegener's granulomatosis
▸ Granulomatous inflammation in association with duct ectasia

GROSS FINDINGS

The macroscopic features are not distinctive. An ill-defined mass up to 8 cm may be seen.

MICROSCOPIC FINDINGS

The characteristic histologic appearance is of non-caseating granulomas centered on lobules (Figure 7-6).

The inflammation sometimes extends into interlobular tissue. There are epithelioid macrophages and Langhan's multinucleated giant cells (Figures 7-6 and 7-7). Neutrophil polymorphs are often present and microabscess formation may occur (Figure 7-8). Lymphocytes, plasma cells and eosinophils are also present in varying numbers. Clear spaces, probably representing lipid, may occasionally be seen, sometimes within granulomata. Foamy macrophages may be prominent. Necrosis is occasionally present, but there is no caseation. Fat necrosis is described. Vasculitis is not seen. No foreign material is present and special stains for organisms (ZN, periodic acid Schiff and Gram stain) are all negative. Duct dilatation occurs in a small proportion of cases. Ulceration of the ductular epithelium with luminal polymorphs is described. One hypothesis is that granulomatous mastitis represents a reaction to luminal secretions leaked into the perilobular connective tissue secondary to epithelial damage.

ANCILLARY STUDIES

FINE NEEDLE ASPIRATION CYTOLOGY

Epithelioid macrophages, giant cells and neutrophils are commonly seen in cytologic specimens. Necrosis is not present. However specific features are absent, making definite cytologic diagnosis difficult. Because idiopathic granulomatous mastitis is a diagnosis of exclusion, reliable diagnosis requires histology, clinical details and exclusion of infection.

MICROBIOLOGY

Almost all studies have not demonstrated organisms either with special stains in histologic sections or by

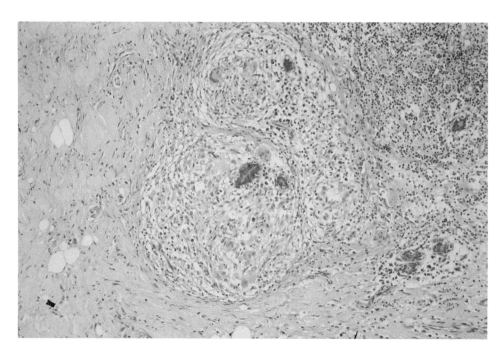

FIGURE 7-6

Granulomatous mastitis. Lobulocentric granulomatous inflammation.

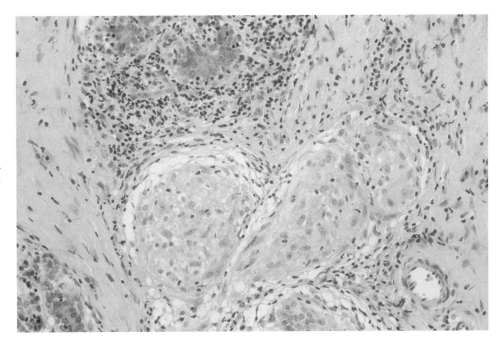

FIGURE 7-7

Granulomatous mastitis. High power showing the granulomatous inflammation.

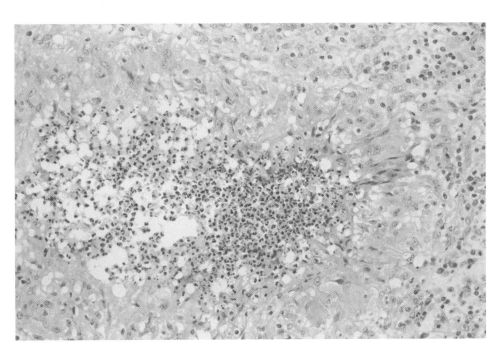

FIGURE 7-8

Granulomatous mastitis. Granulomatous inflammation with central microabscess.

culture. One recent large study from New Zealand found evidence in some patients of *Corynebacteria* on histology or by culture.

DIFFERENTIAL DIAGNOSIS

Idiopathic granulomatous mastitis is a diagnosis of exclusion. Infective causes should be excluded by undertaking special stains for tuberculosis and fungi. When possible, culture of tissue for tuberculosis should be performed. Sarcoidosis is histologically similar and clinical evidence of disease elsewhere should be sought. In Wegener's granulomatosis a vasculitis may be identified and respiratory tract and renal disease should be sought. Granulomatous inflammation may also be seen in association with duct ectasia, however the inflammation is centred on ducts and not lobules and there is prominent duct dilatation. Very occasionally a granulomatous reaction to carcinoma is present and a biopsy may be taken from this area, missing the malignant lesion.

PROGNOSIS AND THERAPY

Persistent disease lasting for several years is well recognized. An apparent response to steroid treatment is described, but there are limited data. Some cases require surgery, but there is a risk of recurrent disease, which may clinically mimic wound infection.

SCLEROSING LYMPHOCYTIC LOBULITIS

Sclerosing lymphocytic lobulitis is characterized by perilobular and perivascular lymphocytic infiltrate. It is thought be of autoimmune etiology. It is also known as lymphocytic mastopathy. Older descriptions of fibrous mastopathy or fibrous disease often had associated lymphocytic infiltrate suggesting that it is, at least in some cases, the same disease.

CLINICAL FEATURES

Most patients present with a breast mass. Usually the mass is interpreted as benign on clinical examination, but sometimes the appearances may mimic carcinoma.

A minority of patients also complain of pain; occasionally the mass is tender. The masses are sometimes bilateral and recurrences can occur. It is seen most commonly in women between the ages of 25 and 60 years; occasionally men are affected.

Sclerosing lymphocytic lobulitis is thought to have an autoimmune etiology. There is an association with other autoimmune diseases, especially longstanding insulin dependent diabetes mellitus and Hashimoto's thyroiditis. It has been suggested that sclerosing lymphocytic lobulitis is associated with certain human leukocyte antigen types. However a controlled study showed that the increased frequency of HLA-DR4 is a reflection of the association of this genotype with insulin dependent diabetes mellitus. The pattern of inflammation resembles that seen in other autoimmune disorders including Hashimoto's thyroiditis, myoepithelial sialadenitis and insulin dependent diabetes mellitus.

RADIOLOGIC FEATURES

Mammography often shows a dense parenchymal pattern with no discrete mass. Sometimes there is an asymmetric density and occasionally a circumscribed mass. Mammography may, however, be normal. Ultrasound often shows a hypoechoic mass, sometimes with associated acoustic shadowing.

PATHOLOGIC FEATURES

SCLEROSING LYMPHOCYTIC LOBULITIS– FACT SHEET

Definition
▸ Inflammatory disorder of the breast characterized by perilobular and perivascular lymphocytic infiltrate
▸ Thought to be of autoimmune etiology

Incidence
▸ Uncommon

Gender and Age Distribution
▸ Most common in women aged 25 to 60 years
▸ Occasionally seen in men

Clinical Features
▸ Usually presents with a mass
▸ Association with autoimmune diseases especially longstanding insulin dependent diabetes mellitus

Radiologic Features
▸ Mammography usually shows no specific features
▸ Ultrasound often shows a hypoechoic mass with acoustic shadow

Prognosis and Treatment
▸ Benign disorder
▸ Recognition of the diagnosis prevents unnecessary surgery

SCLEROSING LYMPHOCYTIC LOBULITIS – PATHOLOGIC FEATURES

Gross Findings
▸ Cut section shows ill-defined rubbery or firm, gray white tissue

Microscopic Features
▸ Circumscribed perilobular and perivascular aggregates of small lymphocytes
▸ Lobular atrophy and fibrosis
▸ Stromal fibrosis with epithelioid fibroblasts

Fine Needle Aspiration Cytology Features
▸ Often inadequate/insufficient

Immunohistochemical Features
▸ The infiltrate is predominantly composed of B lymphoid cells with a smaller proportion of T cells

Pathologic Differential Diagnosis
▸ Duct ectasia
▸ Granulomatous mastitis
▸ Carcinoma with associated periductal and perivascular inflammation

GROSS FINDINGS

Cut section shows ill-defined rubbery or firm gray white tissue up to 6 cm.

MICROSCOPIC FINDINGS

The characteristic histologic feature is circumscribed aggregates of small lymphocytes around lobules, ducts and vessels (Figures 7-9 and 7-10). Typically there are small numbers of plasma cells and germinal centers are sometimes present. There may be small numbers of intraepithelial lymphocytes. The vessels, in both the perivascular and perilobular lymphoid aggregates, often have plump endothelium resembling high endothelial venules (Figure 7-10). Affected lobules may show atrophy and fibrosis. There is also fibrosis of the interlobular stroma with plump epithelioid fibroblasts frequently present (Figure 7-11). Some authors have suggested that epithelioid fibroblasts are only seen in patients with associated diabetes mellitus and the term diabetic mastopathy has been used. However, epithelioid fibroblasts are also present in patients without diabetes mellitus and a pathologic term such as sclerosing lymphocytic lobulitis or lymphocytic mastopathy is preferable. Patients with a sequential series of biopsies

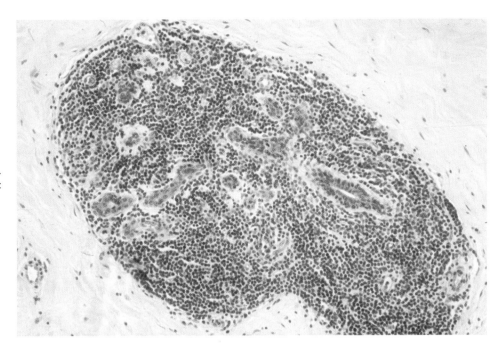

FIGURE 7-9

Sclerosing lymphocytic lobulitis. Circumscribed perilobular lymphocytic infiltrate.

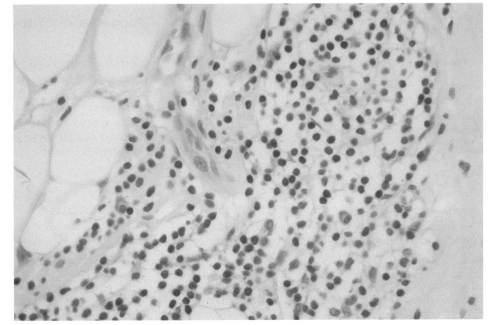

FIGURE 7-10

Sclerosing lymphocytic lobulitis. Perivascular lymphocytic infiltrate around vessel resembling a high endothelial venule.

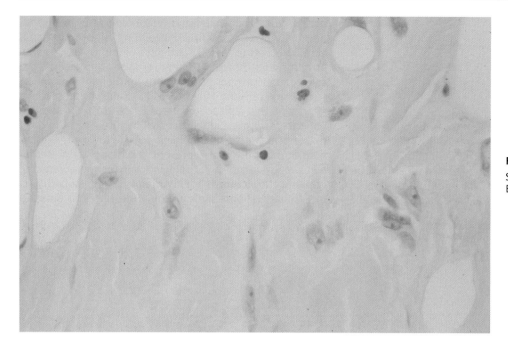

FIGURE 7-11
Sclerosing lymphocytic lobulitis. Epithelioid fibroblasts in the stroma.

often show a progression from prominent inflammation to increasing lobular atrophy and fibrosis with less inflammation. The features in the later fibrotic phase are not specific and histologic diagnosis is then difficult. Diagnosis can be made on core biopsy if the typical pattern of inflammation is present.

ANCILLARY STUDIES

IMMUNOHISTOCHEMISTRY

The lymphoid infiltrate is predominantly composed of B cells and to a lesser extent T cells. The B cells are polyclonal. There is increased expression of class II MHC by the epithelium. This pattern of changes is similar to other autoimmune diseases.

FINE NEEDLE ASPIRATION CYTOLOGY

Cytology may show benign epithelial cells, lymphocytes, connective tissue and epithelioid fibroblasts, but aspirates are often inadequate and specific diagnosis is difficult if not impossible.

DIFFERENTIAL DIAGNOSIS

The distinction from other disorders with periductal or perilobular inflammation is usually straightforward. Important features in the diagnosis of sclerosing lymphocytic lobulitis are the circumscription of the perilobular and perivascular aggregates and the lymphocytic nature of the infiltrate. In duct ectasia the inflammation is centered on ducts and is usually poorly circumscribed. In idiopathic granulomatous mastitis the inflammation is centered on lobules but is granulomatous rather than lymphocytic. The histologic features of the later, more fibrotic, stages of sclerosing lymphocytic lobulitis are not specific and a definite diagnosis is often not possible. A pattern of inflammation resembling sclerosing lymphocytic lobulitis can also be seen associated with carcinoma of the breast, particularly invasive lobular carcinoma (Figure 7-12). If the inflammation is marked, care must be taken to avoid missing a small carcinoma. The main pattern of inflammation associated with ductal carcinoma *in situ* is perivascular aggregates of B and T cells, but perilobular inflammation is not a feature.

PROGNOSIS AND THERAPY

Sclerosing lymphocytic lobulitis is a benign condition. An important reason to make the diagnosis is to avoid unnecessary surgery. An association with lymphoma with some features of extranodal marginal zone (mucosa associated lymphoid tissue) lymphoma was described in a Japanese series, but was not seen in European studies.

FAT NECROSIS

CLINICAL FEATURES

Fat necrosis of the breast most commonly presents as a mass. The mass is often firm and there may be

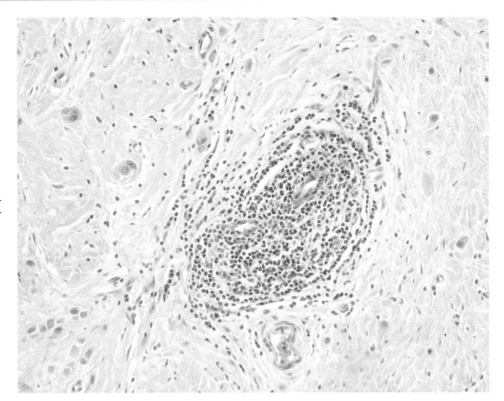

FIGURE 7-12
Invasive lobular carcinoma. Perivascular inflammation mimicking sclerosing lymphocytic lobulitis.

FAT NECROSIS – FACT SHEET

Definition
▶ Reaction of adipose tissue to injury

Incidence
▶ Common, particularly after surgery

Clinical Features
▶ Most commonly presents as a firm mass
▶ May be skin retraction, thickening or tethering
▶ May clinically mimic carcinoma
▶ History of trauma in some patients
▶ May occur after surgery or radiotherapy

Radiologic Features
▶ Mammographic appearance is very variable
▶ Ultrasound shows hyperechogenicity in the acute phase and later usually shows a mass

Prognosis and Treatment
▶ Benign
▶ Important to establish diagnosis as clinically can mimic carcinoma

---

skin retraction, thickening or tethering. Thus the clinical features may resemble carcinoma. It may occur anywhere in the breast. There is a history of trauma in some patients. Symptomatic fat necrosis may occur after surgery (including wide local excision, reduction mammoplasty and breast reconstruction) or following radiotherapy including irridium implants. Asymptomatic fat necrosis may be detected by mammography.

RADIOLOGIC FEATURES

The characteristic ultrasound appearance of acute fat necrosis is an area of hyperechogenicity, which may have a central decrease in echogenicity. Ultrasound of more longstanding fat necrosis usually shows a mass, which may be circumscribed or ill defined and may show posterior acoustic shadowing or enhancement. The mammographic appearance of fat necrosis is very variable from normal to suspicious of malignancy. Lipid cysts on mammography are diagnostic of fat necrosis. There may be calcification or a spiculated mass that is indistinguishable from carcinoma.

PATHOLOGIC FEATURES

GROSS FINDINGS

The typical appearance is a yellow discoloration of the fat. There is often associated fibrosis. Cyst formation and calcification may be present.

MICROSCOPIC FINDINGS

The typical histologic appearance of fat necrosis is an infiltrate of foamy macrophages adjacent to adipose

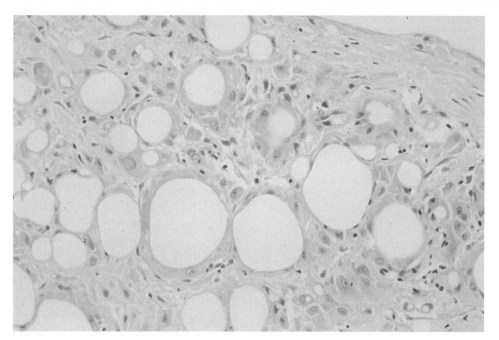

FIGURE 7-13
Fat necrosis. Typical appearance of foamy macrophages.

FAT NECROSIS – PATHOLOGIC FEATURES

Gross Findings
▸ Yellow discoloration of the fat, often with associated fibrosis

Microscopic Features
▸ Foamy macrophages adjacent to adipose tissue.
▸ Multinucleate giant cells, lymphocytes and plasma cells are often present
▸ Later changes include fibrosis and calcification

Fine Needle Aspiration Cytology Features
▸ Foamy macrophages, multinucleate giant cells and background of acellular debris

Pathologic Differential Diagnosis
▸ Occasionally invasive lobular carcinoma may mimic fat necrosis

ANCILLARY STUDIES

IMMUNOHISTOCHEMISTRY

Usually the histologic diagnosis is straightforward on hematoxylin and eosin sections. Occasionally immunohistochemistry is useful when the macrophages are atypical (Figure 7-15) and raise the possibility of malignancy. The macrophages express CD68 and are negative for cytokeratins.

FINE NEEDLE ASPIRATION CYTOLOGY

Typical features are foamy macrophages, multinucleated giant cells and a background of acellular debris. There are usually few or no epithelial groups. Sometimes the macrophages appear atypical and may mimic carcinoma cells.

DIFFERENTIAL DIAGNOSIS

The diagnosis of fat necrosis is usually straightforward. Occasionally invasive lobular carcinoma of the breast may infiltrate adipose tissue with minimal fibrosis and mimic fat necrosis (Figure 7-16). This is usually only a problem on core biopsy.

PROGNOSIS AND THERAPY

Fat necrosis is a benign condition. It is important to establish the diagnosis, particularly when the clinical or

tissue (Figure 7-13). Multinucleated giant cells, lymphocytes and plasma cells are often present, but polymorphs are uncommon. Initially there is associated hemorrhage, then hemosiderin-laden macrophages and occasionally cholesterol clefts (Figure 7-14). Later changes include fibrosis and calcification. Sometimes there are oil cysts: cystic spaces lined by eosinophilic material. The changes may persist for months or years. If the fat necrosis is secondary to radiation therapy, then epithelial atypia and vascular changes secondary to the radiation may also be present.

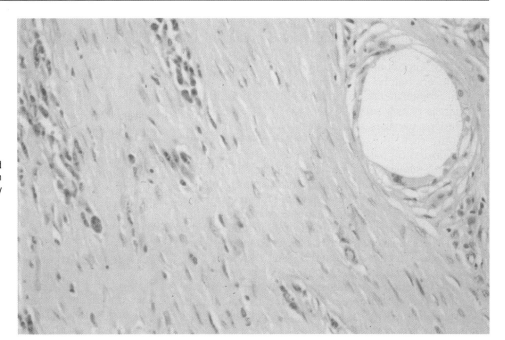

FIGURE 7-14

Fat necrosis. Fibrosis and hemosiderin-laden macrophages in addition to the small area of foamy macrophages.

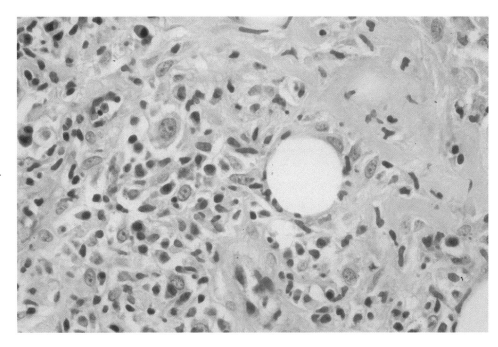

FIGURE 7-15

Fat necrosis. Some of the macrophages show atypia.

radiologic features suggest carcinoma. Core biopsy and fine needle aspiration cytology are useful in establishing the diagnosis. Caution is necessary as occasionally both fat necrosis and carcinoma may be present: follow-up or excision biopsy may be needed.

INFARCTION OF THE BREAST

Spontaneous infarction of the breast is rare. Localized infarction is seen most frequently in the third trimester of pregnancy or early puerperium and clinically presents as a mass that is sometimes painful. Such infarction is often noted to occur in lactational adenomas or fibroadenomas. Histology shows a circumscribed area of coagulative necrosis with granulation tissue and fibrosis at the periphery. It has been suggested that infarction is due to 'relative vascular insufficiency' because of the increased metabolic demands placed on the breast in pregnancy and lactation. Vessels with organizing thrombi have been described, but are not always present.

Localized infarction not associated with pregnancy is well recognized in benign lesions including fibroadenomas and papillomas. Procedures such as core biopsy or fine needle aspiration cytology can contribute to the infarction. Recognition of the underlying lesion may be difficult or impossible. Connective tissue stains, such as reticulin, are helpful in showing the underlying structure. Squamous metaplasia may be present. Infarction of carcinomas is very rare.

Extensive necrosis of the breast is very rare. It is most commonly seen in association with warfarin therapy. The majority of patients are being treated for deep venous thrombosis or pulmonary embolism. The typical presentation is with discoloration of the skin progressing to necrosis within several days of starting warfarin treatment. About half the patients require surgical treatment. Inflammation is often seen in and around vessels. Thrombosis of small vessels, particularly veins, is described. This has prompted the suggestion that the mammary infarction represents part of a generalized tendency to venous thrombosis. However, the association of mammary infarction with warfarin treatment suggests that the drug has a role. Abnormalities of coagulation may also contribute.

TISSUE REACTION TO BREAST IMPLANTS

In the past, liquid silicone was injected directly into the breast to achieve augmentation of the breasts. This causes a foreign body type reaction. Nowadays, breast implants contain silicone gel or saline in a bag made of silicone elastomer or polyurethane. A fibrous capsule develops around breast implants. There may also be pseudosynovial changes on the surface of the capsule. Silicone may leak from intact implants or there may be rupture of the implant.

CLINICAL FEATURES

Injection of liquid silicone, as undertaken historically, may present as a firm breast mass. There may be fixation to skin, skin retraction and nipple inversion. Occasionally associated enlargement of axillary lymph nodes may be noted. Silicone may also migrate to the chest wall and other sites. Similar clinical signs may be seen with implant rupture, but the changes are usually less marked. The reaction to silicone may mask carcinoma, making clinical and radiologic diagnosis difficult.

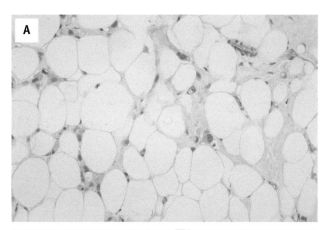

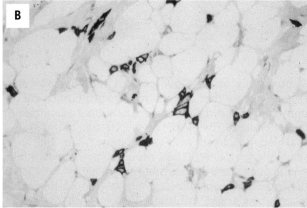

FIGURE 7-16

Invasive lobular carcinoma. (A). The appearances mimic fat necrosis. (B) The diagnosis of carcinoma is confirmed by cytokeratin immunohistochemistry (CAM5.2).

TISSUE REACTION TO BREAST IMPLANTS – FACT SHEET

Definition
▸ Reaction to implants may consist of macrophages and giant cells, fibrosis and pseudosynovium

Incidence
▸ Common in those with implants

Clinical Features
▸ May present as firm breast mass
▸ May be fixation to skin, skin retraction, nipple inversion
▸ The reaction to silicone may mask carcinoma

Radiologic Features
▸ Mammography may show formation of a fibrous capsule, calcification and rupture
▸ Ultrasound of silicone granulomas shows a snowstorm appearance
▸ Magnetic resonance imaging is valuable for detecting implant rupture

Prognosis and Treatment
▸ Reaction may require removal of the implant
▸ Implants do not appear to increase the risk of carcinoma of the breast or of connective tissue diseases

RADIOLOGIC FEATURES

Mammographic examination of breast prostheses frequently shows formation of a fibrous capsule. Rupture may be seen as high-density masses. Calcification may also be present. Ultrasound of silicone granulomas shows a snowstorm appearance. Magnetic resonance imaging is valuable for detecting both intracapsular and extracapsular implant rupture.

PATHOLOGIC FEATURES

GROSS FINDINGS

Cut section shows firm tissue. Calcification or spaces containing liquid material may be apparent.

MICROSCOPIC FINDINGS

Leakage or injection of liquid silicone causes a foreign body giant cell reaction. The reaction to breast implants varies according to the nature of the implant. Textured implants have knob-like projections on the surface. Most implants develop a surrounding capsule composed of a band of paucicellular fibrous tissue with scattered chronic inflammatory cells. Silicone that has leaked from the implant is seen as clear spaces, typically of variable size, with macrophages, foreign body giant cells and lymphocytes (Figure 7-17). Occasional plasma cells and polymorphs may be present. Prominent acute inflammation suggests infection. Most of the silicone is dissolved in tissue processing, but sometimes the sections show visible material in the clear spaces that is often refractile, but not usually birefringent (Figure

7-18). Silicone gel can also migrate to sites far from the implant. Polyurethane is seen as brown-yellow or blue-gray geometric crystalline structures that are refractile and sometimes polarize, with an associated inflammatory reaction of macrophages, giant cells and lymphocytes. Talcum powder may also be seen. Calcification may occur within the fibrous capsule.

There may be amorphous material on the surface adjacent to the implant (Figure 7-19). The surface of the capsule adjacent to the implant may bear a layer of

---

TISSUE REACTION TO BREAST IMPLANTS – PATHOLOGIC FEATURES

Gross Findings
▶ Cut section shows firm tissue.
▶ May be calcification or spaces containing liquid material

Microscopic Features
▶ Foreign body giant cell reaction
▶ Silicone is seen as clear spaces, typically of variable size
▶ Fibrosis
▶ Pseudosynovial reaction at the surface of the implant

Ultrastructural Features
▶ Silicone appears as intracellular and extracellular amorphous material
▶ Polyurethane inclusions have a geometric shape and electron-dense outer rim

Pathologic Differential Diagnosis
▶ Usually a straightforward diagnosis
▶ Fat necrosis
▶ Could be mistaken for liposarcoma

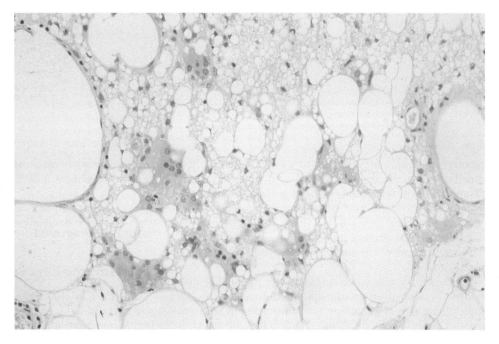

FIGURE 7-17

Breast implants. Reaction to silicone: clear spaces of variable size with adjacent macrophages and giant cells.

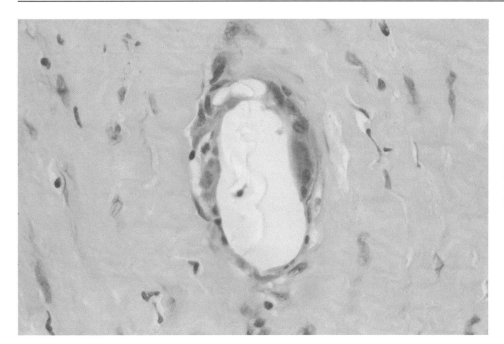

FIGURE 7-18

Breast implants. Clear space with refractile material, adjacent macrophages and surrounding fibrosis.

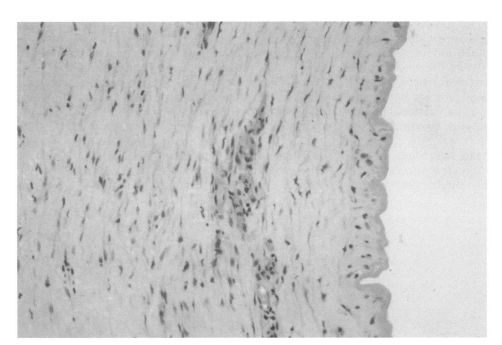

FIGURE 7-19

Breast implants. Lining of the capsule by amorphous material with fibrosis and chronic inflammation in the wall.

macrophages; this may consist of a single layer of flattened cells or a thicker layer either with no organization (Figure 7-20) or with cells arranged perpendicular to the surface with basally located nuclei. There is no basement membrane beneath the layer of macrophages. Occasionally the surface may have a papillary structure. The architecture of the surface macrophage layer resembles synovium.

Silicone may also cause a reaction in regional lymph nodes. This is often an incidental finding in patients undergoing surgery for another reason. Some patients present with lymphadenopathy which may be painful.

Histology shows clear spaces of variable size with adjacent macrophages and foreign body giant cells.

ANCILLARY STUDIES

ULTRASTRUCTURAL FEATURES

Electron microscopy shows silicone as intracellular and extracellular amorphous material. Polyurethane inclusions have a geometric shape and electron-dense

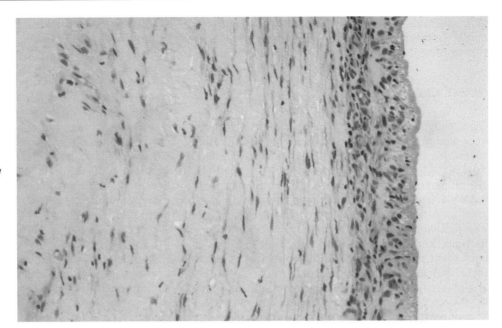

FIGURE 7-20

Breast implants. Capsule lined by pseudosynovium.

outer rim. Scanning electron microscopy and energy-dispersive X-ray microanalysis can identify the elements, such as silicone, present in the fibrous capsule. Other techniques, like Raman spectroscopy are needed to identify the molecules present.

IMMUNOHISTOCHEMISTRY

Immunohistochemistry shows that the pseudosynovium is composed of macrophages and that the inflammatory cells in the capsule are predominantly macrophages and T cells.

DIFFERENTIAL DIAGNOSIS

A characteristic feature of the reaction to silicone granulomas is vacuoles of variable size. This feature is useful in making the distinction from fat necrosis. The reaction to silicone has been misinterpreted as liposarcoma.

PROGNOSIS AND THERAPY

Although carcinomas and connective tissue disorders associated with breast prostheses are described, there does not appear to be an increase in the risk of either disorder with breast prostheses. The reaction to silicone may, however, mask carcinoma, so careful follow up is needed.

VASCULITIS OF THE BREAST

Vasculitis of the breast is rare. Only about 40 cases have been described in the medical literature. It may affect the breast alone or can be part of a systemic disease and should be distinguished from vasculitis affecting the skin or subcutaneous adipose tissue overlying the breast. The breast is one of the more common sites in which vasculitis may present as a tumor-like mass and thus clinically often mimics carcinoma. Both clinical and pathologic features are important in making a specific diagnosis. Three types of vasculitis affecting the breast parenchyma are described: polyarteritis nodosa, giant cell arteritis and Wegener's granulomatosis.

POLYARTERITIS NODOSA

Polyarteritis nodosa rarely involves the breast. It presents as a firm tender breast mass in women between 45 and 80 years. Bilateral involvement is seen in half of cases. Approximately half of the reported patients have had constitutional symptoms including headache, tiredness, pyrexia, myalgia and arthralgia. Raised erythrocyte sedimentation rate (ESR), mild anemia and raised peripheral white cell count may be present. In the majority of patients the vasculitis is confined to the breast, but occasionally there is involvement of the skin or systemic disease. Histology shows vasculitis affecting small and medium sized arteries with fibrinoid necrosis and infiltrates of lymphocytes, neutrophils and eosinophils. In most patients corticosteroids or surgical excision of the mass have produced resolution of symptoms.

GIANT CELL ARTERITIS

Giant cell arteritis of the breast usually presents with a firm tender breast mass in women between 50 and 80 years. In about half of patients there are bilateral masses. Skin fixation may occur. Some women have symptoms suggestive of polymyalgia rheumatica, including malaise, fever, anorexia, weight loss, arthralgia and myalgia. Mild anemia and a raised ESR may be present. The pathologic features are as seen in temporal arteritis. Small and medium sized arteries show inflammation with giant cells, macrophages, lymphocytes and sometimes polymorphs with destruction of the internal elastic lamina. In most patients the vasculitis appears to be restricted to the breast; the temporal artery is affected in a minority, but few patients have had a biopsy performed at the time of diagnosis of the breast lesion. Most patients have an uneventful postoperative course with either improvement of symptoms with corticosteroids or spontaneous resolution with no treatment other than excisional biopsy.

WEGENER'S GRANULOMATOSIS

Wegener's granulomatosis is a necrotizing granulomatous vasculitis of both arteries and veins that typically involves the upper and lower respiratory tract and kidneys. Involvement of the breast is rare. Almost all the patients with breast disease also have systemic involvement, although this may appear at a later time. Serum anti-neutrophil cytoplasmic antibodies are present in most patients with systemic or localized disease, but the value of this test in patients with disease restricted to the breast is uncertain. Patients present with a breast mass, which is usually tender and sometimes bilateral. The women are typically younger than the patients with the above two vasculitides (40 to 60 years). Histology typically shows acute and chronic inflammation of the vessels with necrosis. Inflammation, including granulomas, is also present in adjacent fat and parenchyma. Infarction or fat necrosis may obscure the vasculitis and in some cases the necrotizing vasculitis and granulomatous inflammation are limited or absent, making pathologic diagnosis difficult. This emphasizes the importance of clinical features and clinicopathologic correlation in making the diagnosis. The majority of patients respond to the standard treatment of prednisolone and cyclophosphamide.

MONDOR'S DISEASE

Superficial thrombophlebitis of the chest or Mondor's disease is an uncommon condition that predominantly affects women between the ages of 30 and 50 years. An association with trauma, including surgical procedures, is described. There is a possible association with breast cancer.

The typical presentation is with pain or a mass. Examination shows a subcutaneous linear cord-like swelling that is usually tender and often associated with a groove in the skin. The lateral thoracic and thoraco-epigastric veins are commonly affected. The diagnosis is usually made clinically. Mammography shows a superficially located tubular density corresponding to the clinical abnormality. Ultrasound shows a tubular structure with no flow. Histology shows a vein with luminal thrombus. In later lesions there may be organization or recanalization of the thrombus and fibroblastic proliferation in the wall of the vein. The pain usually resolves spontaneously within 10 weeks and the palpable cord disappears within a few months. Symptomatic treatment is given.

INFLAMMATORY DISEASES NOT SPECIFIC TO BREAST

There are numerous inflammatory diseases that can affect the skin and subcutaneous adipose tissue of the breast, but are not specific to the breast. Examples include eczema of the nipple, psoriasis, candida infection and lupus panniculitis.

SUGGESTED READINGS

Banik S, Bishop PW, Ormerod LP, O'Brien TEB. Sarcoidosis of the breast. J Clin Pathol 1986;39:446–448.

Catania S, Zurrida S, Veronesi P, et al. Mondor's disease and breast cancer. Cancer 1992;69:2267–2270.

Dixon JM, Ravisekar O, Chetty U, Anderson T. Periductal mastitis and duct ectasia: different conditions with different aetiologies. Br J Surg 1996;83:820–822.

Girling AC, Hanby AM, Millis RR. Radiation and other pathological changes in breast tissue after conservation treatment for carcinoma. J Clin Pathol 1990;43:152–156.

Janowsky EC, Kupper LL, Hulka BS. Meta-analyses of the relation between silicone breast implants and the risk of connective-tissue diseases. N Engl J Med 2000;342:781–790.

Lee AHS, Bateman AC, Turner SJ, et al. HLA class II DRB1 and DQB1 allelic polymorphism and sclerosing lymphocytic lobulitis of the breast. J Clin Pathol 1999;52:445–449.

Scholefield JH, Duncan JL, Rogers K. Review of a hospital experience of breast abscesses. Br J Surg 1987;74:469–470.

Shinde SR, Chandawarkar RY, Deshmukh SP. Tuberculosis of the breast masquerading as carcinoma: a study of 100 patients. World J Surg 1995;19:379–381.

Taylor GB, Paviour SD, Musaad S, et al. A clinicopathological review of 34 cases of inflammatory breast disease showing an association between corynebacteria infection and granulomatous mastitis. Pathology 2003; 35:109–119.

Whitaker-Worth DL, Carlone V, Susser WS, et al. Dermatologic diseases of the breast and nipple. J Am Acad Dermatol 2000;43:733–751.

8 Sclerosing Lesions: Sclerosing Adenosis, Radial Scar/Complex Sclerosing Lesion

Timothy W Jacobs

Sclerosing adenosis and radial scar are two entities included in the category of benign sclerosing lesions of the breast. Like other sclerosing lesions, both may mimic invasive carcinoma clinically, radiologically and on gross or microscopic pathologic examination. Recent data suggest that radial scars represent independent markers of a generalized increased risk for subsequent breast cancer.

SCLEROSING ADENOSIS

Sclerosing adenosis is a benign proliferative lesion composed of distorted epithelial, myoepithelial and stromal elements. Because of the sclerotic pattern, these lesions may be confused with invasive carcinomas (particularly low grade infiltrating ductal and tubular carcinoma).

CLINICAL FEATURES

Sclerosing adenosis is often an incidental microscopic finding in breast specimens removed for other indications and therefore the true incidence in the general population is not exactly known. These lesions may present at any age, but may be larger in pre- or perimenopausal patients. However, because these lesions are sclerotic and often contain calcifications, they may present mammographically as architectural distortion and/or microcalcifications. Lesions may be solitary or multiple. In addition, sclerosing adenosis may less commonly present as a mass lesion on palpation or by imaging.

RADIOLOGIC FEATURES

On mammography, sclerosing adenosis may present as an area of architectural distortion, microcalcifications (often clustered), and/or a mass.

SCLEROSING ADENOSIS – FACT SHEET

Definition
▶ A benign sclerosing lesion arising in association with the terminal duct lobular unit, composed of distorted epithelial elements surrounded by myoepithelial cells in a fibrotic stroma.

Incidence and Location
▶ Most asymptomatic, therefore true incidence in general population is not accurately known
▶ May be solitary or multiple, any location in breast

Gender, Race and Age Distribution
▶ Occur at any age, but may be larger in pre- or perimenopausal women

Clinical Features
▶ Usually asymptomatic and found as incidental lesion
▶ Increasingly detected by mammography
▶ May present as mass lesion, mimicking carcinoma

Radiologic Features
▶ May present as microcalcifications, area of architectural distortion or a mass lesion

Prognosis and Treatment
▶ Benign lesion, categorized as proliferative without atypia
▶ If found on CNB and there is good correlation with imaging, does not require surgical excision
▶ No further treatment necessary if found on surgical excision

---

PATHOLOGIC FEATURES

GROSS FINDINGS

Although sclerosing adenosis is usually imperceptible on gross examination, an area of fibrosis, distortion or even a mass lesion suspicious for carcinoma may be seen, in keeping with the clinical and imaging features.

MICROSCOPIC FINDINGS

Sclerosing adenosis arises in association with the terminal duct lobular unit. This 'lobulocentric' pattern is key to the correct diagnosis of sclerosing adenosis and its variants and in the histologic distinction of this lesion from invasive carcinoma and is best appreciated at low microscopic power. Higher power examination reveals sclerosing adenosis to be composed of distorted, elongated and/or obliterated glands and tubules. These epithelial structures are surrounded by myoepithelial cells, within a fibrotic or sclerotic stroma (Figure 8-1). In some cases, the epithelial element may be less prominent or even appear to be absent, with mostly myoepithelial cells and sclerotic stroma present (Figure 8-2). The epithelium in sclerosing adenosis may undergo apocrine metaplasia (Figure 8-3). This may be confused with infiltrating carcinoma if the low power lobulocentric pattern and myoepithelial cells are not appreciated, and especially if the apocrine metaplasia is cytologically atypical. Sclerosing adenosis may also be involved by atypical lobular hyperplasia (ALH)/lobular carcinoma *in situ* (LCIS) (Figure 8-4), atypical ductal hyperplasia (ADH), or ductal carcinoma *in situ* (DCIS) (Figure 8-5), resulting in confusion with invasive carcinoma. Perineural 'pseudoinvasion' may be present in approximately 2% of sclerosing adenosis cases and should not be misinterpreted as invasive carcinoma (Figure 8-6). Sclerosing adenosis may also present as a mass lesion (also known as nodular adenosis or adenosis tumor). These lesions are composed of aggregates of well circumscribed nodules in which the characteristic

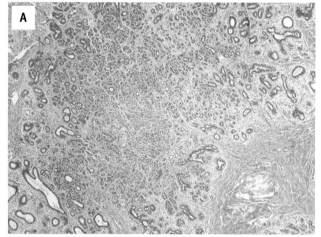

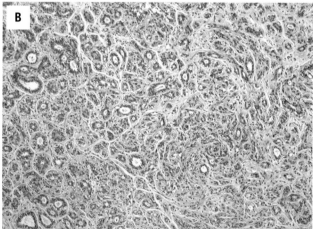

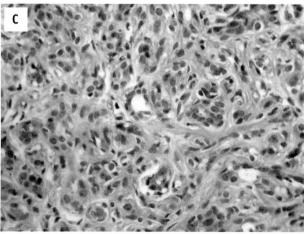

FIGURE 8-1

Sclerosing adenosis. (A) The characteristic 'lobulocentric' pattern best appreciated at low power; (B) distorted, elongated glands and tubules in a fibrotic stroma at intermediate power; and (C) high power demonstrating the epithelial structures surrounded by myoepithelial cells.

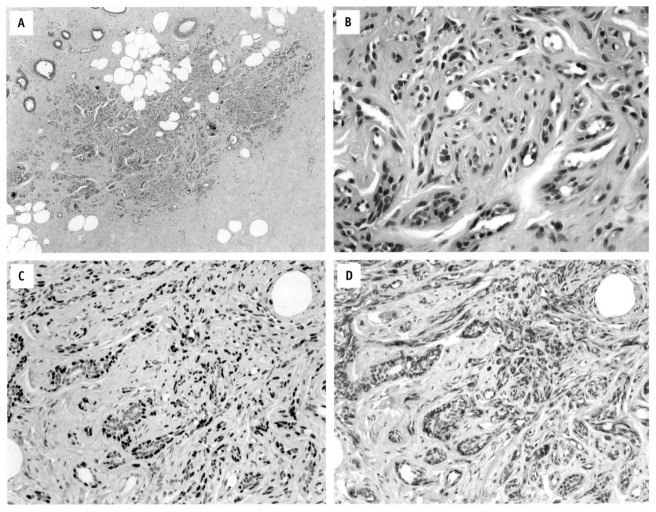

FIGURE 8-2

Sclerosing adenosis with inconspicuous epithelial cells. (A) Low power scerotic appearance in a lobulocentric pattern (note calcifications). (B) Higher power showing predominantly myoepithelial cells. (C) Immunostains for p63 and (D) smooth muscle myosin heavy chain, highlighting the myoepithelial cells.

lobulocentric configuration is easily appreciated at low power microscopic examination. At higher power, the arrangement of epithelial and myoepithelial cells, typical of sclerosing adenosis, is found (Figure 8-7).

ANCILLARY STUDIES

Immunohistochemistry to highlight the presence of myoepithelial cells is often useful in cases of sclerosing adenosis that are difficult to distinguish from invasive carcinoma on routine histology. Involvement by atypical hyperplasia or *in situ* carcinoma may be especially problematic, particularly when the lobulocentric pattern is not evident, in distorted specimens or those where tissue is limited. The most specific and useful markers are p63 (a nuclear antigen) and smooth muscle myosin – heavy chain (cytoplasmic). Use of both stains is often complementary (see Figures 8-2 and 8-5). Calponin is

more sensitive but less specific as myofibroblasts may be non-specifically immunostained. Immunohistochemical markers that may be useful in this setting are further discussed in Chapter 25.

DIFFERENTIAL DIAGNOSIS

Because of its sclerotic pattern, sclerosing adenosis may be confused with invasive carcinomas (in particular low grade infiltrating ductal carcinoma or tubular carcinoma, see Figure 8-8). However, there are several distinguishing histologic features (Table 8-1). The key feature of sclerosing adenosis is the 'lobulocentric' pattern (best appreciated at low magnification) which contrasts with that of tubular carcinoma which is infiltrative in nature and does not conform to the normal ductal and lobular architecture. In contrast to the distorted, elongated and often obliterated glands of

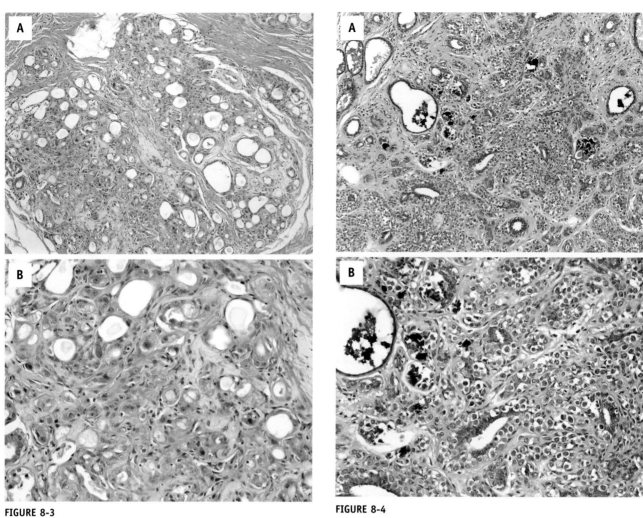

FIGURE 8-3

Sclerosing adenosis with apocrine metaplasia. (A) The lobulocentric configuration is appreciated at low power while at (B) high power apocrine epithelium is seen and may be mistaken for carcinoma particularly if cytologically atypical appearing.

FIGURE 8-4

Involvement of sclerosing adenosis by lobular carcinoma *in situ* (LCIS) with associated calcifications. (A) Low power demonstrating the typical architecture of sclerosing adenosis and (B) higher power showing the lobular neoplastic cells involving the lesion in a pagetoid fashion.

TABLE 8-1
Histologic Features of Sclerosing Adenosis Compared to Those of Tubular Carcinoma

Sclerosing adenosis	Tubular carcinoma
Present in association with the terminal duct lobular unit, i.e., 'lobulocentric', best appreciated at low power	Infiltrative appearance with haphazard arrangement of tubules at low power
Stroma is fibrotic	Stroma is desmoplastic (more cellular)
Distorted, compressed, and/or elongated tubules, often with obliterated lumens	Angulated tubules with open lumens
Myoepithelial cells always present surrounding distorted/compressed tubules (at least in part)	Absent myoepithelial cells

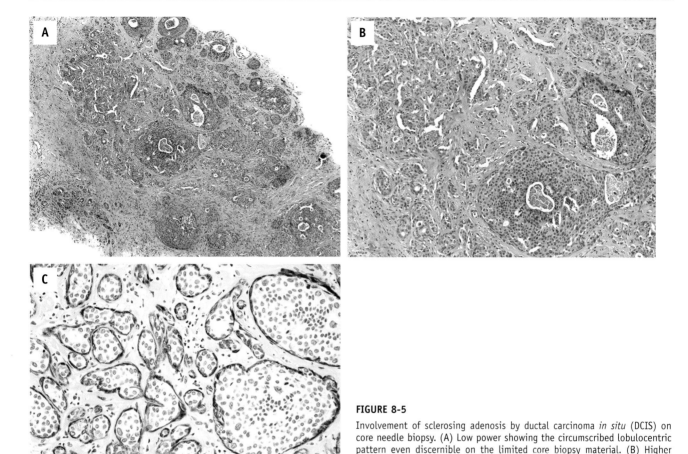

FIGURE 8-5

Involvement of sclerosing adenosis by ductal carcinoma *in situ* (DCIS) on core needle biopsy. (A) Low power showing the circumscribed lobulocentric pattern even discernible on the limited core biopsy material. (B) Higher power demonstrating the atypical glands in a sclerotic background. Myoepithelial cells can be seen surrounding most epithelial nests. (C) Smooth muscle myosin heavy chain immunostaining of myoepithelial cells around all epithelial nests confirming the absence of invasive carcinoma.

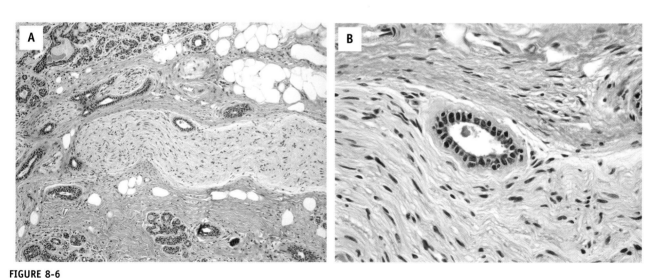

FIGURE 8-6

Sclerosing adenosis with 'pseudoinvasion' of a nerve. (A) Low power and (B) high power showing the myoepithelial cells surrounding the benign gland in the nerve.

sclerosing adenosis, tubular carcinoma is composed of angulated tubules with open lumens. Furthermore, the fibrotic (or sclerotic) stroma of sclerosing adenosis differs from the more cellular desmoplastic stroma of tubular carcinoma. Sclerosing adenosis contains epi-thelial cells with associated myoepithelial cells whereas these are absent in tubular carcinoma. Although the presence of apocrine metaplasia, atypical hyperplasia or carcinoma *in situ* involving sclerosing adenosis may be confused with invasive carcinoma, the lobulocentric

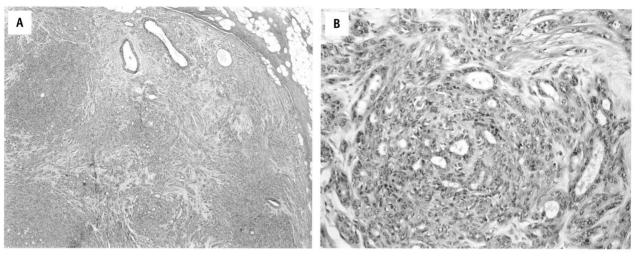

FIGURE 8-7

Nodular sclerosing adenosis. (A) Low power showing the well circumscribed configuration with the characteristic lobulocentric nodular pattern and (B) higher power showing the arrangement of epithelial and myoepithelial cells typical of sclerosing adenosis.

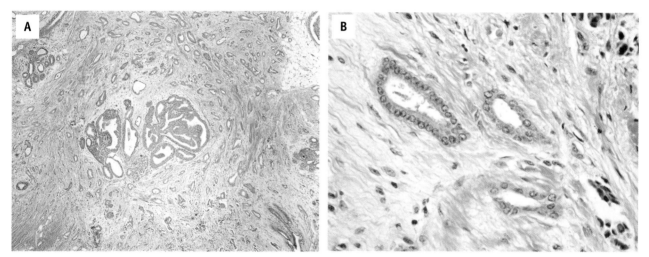

FIGURE 8-8

Tubular carcinoma. (A) Low power showing the haphazard 'sprinkling' of glands in a desmoplastic stroma throughout the lesion; note the low grade DCIS. (B) High power of an angulated tubule with an open lumen, with one epithelial layer with basally oriented nuclei, opposed directly to the underlying desmoplastic stroma without intervening myoepithelial cells. Several epithelial cells have characteristic apical snouts.

pattern and presence of myoepithelial cells are keys to the correct diagnosis.

THERAPEUTIC CONSIDERATIONS

Sclerosing adenosis is not a direct or obligate precursor of breast carcinoma and is rather grouped in the risk category of 'proliferative lesions without atypia,' such as florid ductal hyperplasia. The diagnosis of sclerosing adenosis is usually straightforward on core needle biopsy, with the lobulocentric pattern easily identifiable on low power in most cases. Therefore, patients with a diagnosis of sclerosing adenosis on core needle biopsy

can be safely managed by observation alone without surgical excision, provided the imaging studies are concordant with that diagnosis (e.g., corresponding calcifications) and another lesion requiring excision is not present (such as atypical ductal hyperplasia or DCIS).

RADIAL SCAR

Radial scars were first recognized by Semb in 1928. Although several names have been used for these lesions, the term 'radial scar' is the most widely used.

RADIAL SCAR – FACT SHEET

Definition

▶ A benign sclerosing breast lesion characterized by a central fibroelastotic core with radiating ducts and lobules exhibiting various proliferative changes and cysts.

▶ Term complex sclerosing lesion used if larger than 1 cm or composed of several closely contiguous fibroelastotic areas

Incidence and Location

▶ Usually incidental microscopic finding in breast tissue removed for other reasons, with incidence ranging from 4–28% depending on series (e.g., autopsy versus surgical excision).

▶ May occur anywhere in breast, may be multiple (up to 67%) and bilateral (up to 43%)

Gender, Race and Age Distribution

▶ May occur at any age

Clinical Features

▶ Usually incidental microscopic findings; rarely large enough to form a palpable mass mimicking carcinoma

Radiologic Features

▶ If large enough to be seen on mammography, characteristically stellate or 'spiculated' lesions, often with a radiolucent central area corresponding to the fibroelastotic core.

Prognosis and Treatment

▶ Considered generalized risk factors for subsequent breast cancer; risk is independent of other concurrent benign histologic risk lesions (twofold higher); risk increased with multiple or larger lesions

▶ If present on CNB, prudent to excise if clinically feasible due to the increased incidence of carcinoma associated with lesions which are large enough to be detected by imaging; carcinoma is more likely to be peripherally located.

▶ If found on surgical excision specimen, radial scar (by itself) does not require re-excision.

RADIAL SCAR – PATHOLOGIC FEATURES

Gross Findings

▶ If large enough to be detected grossly, appear as a stellate mass on cut surface, usually indistinguishable from invasive carcinoma

▶ Occasionally dilated cysts may be seen at the periphery of larger lesions

Microscopic Findings

▶ Central zone of fibroelastosis from which ducts and lobules radiate, exhibiting various benign alterations

▶ Radiating ducts and lobules appear to 'expand' or enlarge centrifugally

▶ Entrapped smaller ducts present withing central fibroelastotic stroma; lined by one or more layers of epithelium with an outer myoepithelial cell layer

▶ May be involved by atypical hyperplasia (ductal or lobular), LCIS, DCIS; rarely carcinoma (usually peripherally)

Immunohistochemical Features

▶ Myoepithelial markers (e.g., p63 or smooth muscle myosin-heavy chain) are useful adjunct in histologically challenging cases

Pathologic Differential Diagnosis

▶ Invasive carcinoma

▶ Other sclerosing lesions

Initially proposed by Linell, Ljungberg and Anderson in 1980, it translated from the German 'strahlige narben' introduced in 1975 by Hamperl. The term 'complex sclerosing lesion' is sometimes used for similar lesions which are larger than one centimeter in size or for those lesions with several fibroelastotic areas in close contiguity.

CLINICAL FEATURES

Radial scars are most often incidental microscopic findings in breast biopsies performed for other indications, however, some are large enough to be detected mammographically. The reported incidence of radial scars varies from 4% to 28%, and in a recent large nested case–control study, radial scars were identified in 7% of benign breast biopsies reviewed. Several studies have found radial scars to be bilateral and multicentric, with these frequencies reported to be as high as 43% and 67%, respectively.

RADIOLOGIC FEATURES

If large enough to be seen on mammography, radial scars are characteristically stellate or 'spiculated' lesions, often with a radiolucent central area (Figure 8-9). However, as alluded to above, distinction from a spiculated-appearing invasive carcinoma is often not possible.

PATHOLOGIC FEATURES

GROSS FINDINGS

If large enough to be detected grossly, radial scar appears as a stellate mass on cut surface, usually indistinguishable from invasive carcinoma (Figure 8-10). Occasionally dilated cysts may be seen at the periphery of larger lesions

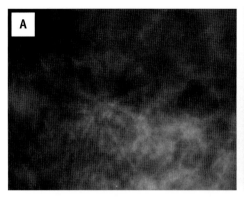

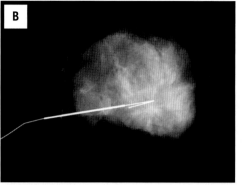

FIGURE 8-9

Mammography of radial scar demonstrating the characteristic spiculated lesion with a radiolucent central area corresponding to the fibroelastotic core. (A) Mammogram magnification view; (B) needle localization specimen radiograph.

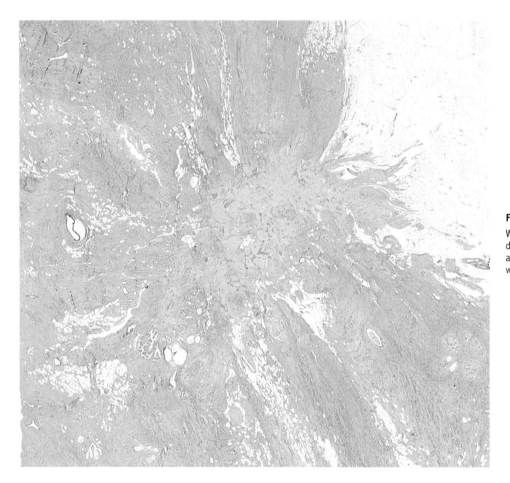

FIGURE 8-10

Whole mount view of a radial scar, demonstrating the stellate, sclerotic appearance which could be confused with carcinoma grossly.

MICROSCOPIC FINDINGS

On microscopic examination, radial scars are characterized by a central zone of fibroelastosis from which ducts and lobules radiate, exhibiting various benign alterations such as microcysts, apocrine metaplasia and proliferative changes (e.g. florid hyperplasia and papillomas). The 'radiating' ducts and lobules usually appear to expand or enlarge from the central fibroelastotic area in a 'centrifugal' manner. Within the central area of fibroelastostotic stroma, smaller entrapped ducts are present, which are often distorted or angular in appearance. These ducts are lined by one or more layers of epithelium with an outer myoepithelial cell layer (Figure 8-11). Often, epithelium of the entrapped glands appears to be retracted from the dense fibroelastotic stroma due to vacuolation of the interposed myoepithelial cells, with only the pyknotic appearing nuclei of the latter evident (Figure 8-12). As with sclerosing adenosis, radial scars may be involved by atypical hyperplasia (either ductal or lobular), LCIS (Figure 8-13) or DCIS (Figure 8-14). Rarely invasive carcinoma

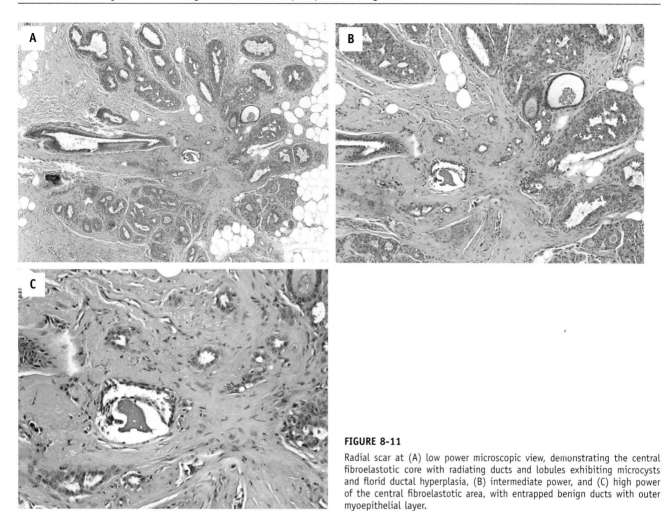

FIGURE 8-11

Radial scar at (A) low power microscopic view, demonstrating the central fibroelastotic core with radiating ducts and lobules exhibiting microcysts and florid ductal hyperplasia, (B) intermediate power, and (C) high power of the central fibroelastotic area, with entrapped benign ducts with outer myoepithelial layer.

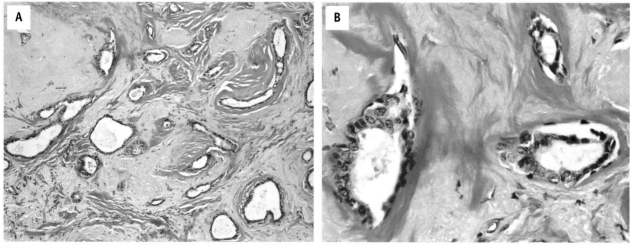

FIGURE 8-12

The central fibroelastotic core of another radial scar. (A) Intermediate power showing the entrapped glands within the fibroelastotic stroma. (B) High power showing the entrapped glands with the small pyknotic-appearing nuclei of the outer myoepithelial cells with the stroma appearing to retract. Note the myoepithelial cells are not present completely surrounding the entrapped glands, in part due to plane of sectioning.

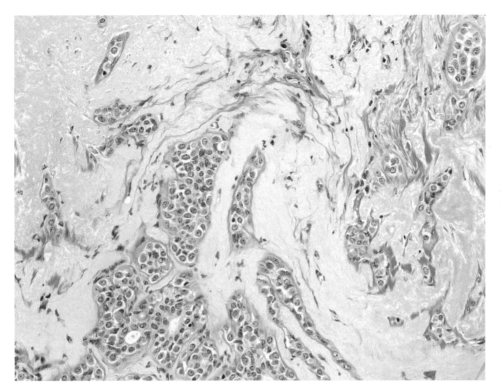

FIGURE 8-13

Lobular carcinoma *in situ* (LCIS) involving a radial scar. Entrapped and distorted ducts distended by lobular neoplastic cells are surrounded by myoepithelial cells.

may involve a radial scar, and when present, is usually at the periphery rather than in the central fibroelastotic area. Of note, atypical hyperplasia and carcinoma are more common in larger lesions and in radial scars in women greater than 50 years of age.

ANCILLARY STUDIES

If not readily apparent by routine hematoxylin and eosin staining, myoepithelial cells surrounding the entrapped glands within the central fibroelastotic area may be highlighted by immunohistochemistry (Figure 8-15). As with sclerosing adenosis, the most specific and useful markers are p63 and smooth muscle myosin – heavy chain, with use of both stains complementary. Of note, in many radial scars (even those which are histologically unambiguous) immunostains may only detect focal myoepithelial cells associated with individual entrapped glands and not be present completely circumferentially. In addition, some entrapped glands may appear not to have any surrounding myoepithelial cells, in part due to plain of sectioning. Therefore it is important not to over-interpret these perceived 'gaps' or 'absences' of myoepithelial cells as evidence of carcinoma, but to rather view the whole case in the appropriate histologic context.

DIFFERENTIAL DIAGNOSIS

As alluded to above, radial scars may mimic invasive carcinoma (particularly low grade invasive ductal and tubular carcinoma clinically, on imaging studies and on pathologic examination (Table 8-2 and contrast Figures 8-8, 8-11 and 8-12)). Both radial scars and invasive carcinomas may have a spiculated appearance on imaging, corresponding to stellate lesions on gross pathologic examination. In particular, tubular carcinoma may be confused with radial scars microscopically for several reasons. On low power examination, both radial scars and tubular carcinomas may exhibit stellate configurations. At higher magnification, the entrapped, distorted glands within the fibroelastotic center of a radial scar may be confused with invasive carcinoma. However, the entrapped glands within the fibroelastotic core of radial scar are surrounded at least in part by myoepithelial cells which are absent in tubular carcinoma. The stroma of radial scars is characteristically 'fibroelastotic' (i.e., composed of hyalinized collagen and elastic tissue), and is present only in the center of the lesion. In contrast, the stroma of tubular carcinoma tends to be more cellular ('desmoplastic') and is usually present throughout the lesion. In addition, cysts and/or proliferative changes tend to increase in magnitude peripherally in a radial fashion from the central fibroelastotic core in a radial scar. This configuration is usually not present in

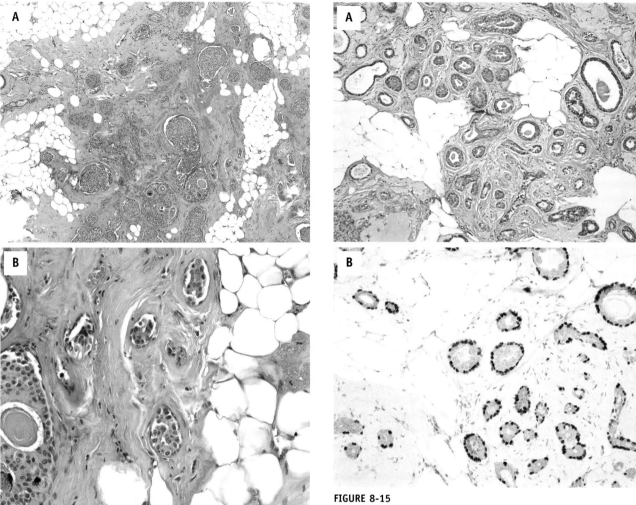

FIGURE 8-14

Ductal carcinoma *in situ* (DCIS) involving a complex sclerosing lesion. (A) Low power and (B) high power, showing the entrapped neoplastic cells, surrounded by myoepithelial cells consistent with their *in situ* nature.

FIGURE 8-15

Complex sclerosing lesion with several closely contiguous fibroelastotic areas amongst adipose tissue. This pattern may mimic invasive carcinoma on hematoxylin and eosin staining (A), with immunohistochemistry for myoepithelial markers, such as p63 helpful. (B) Note that even though this lesion is benign, the nuclear staining for p63 is not present completely surrounding all nests.

TABLE 8-2

Histologic Features of Radial Scar Compared to Those of Tubular Carcinoma

Radial scar	Tubular carcinoma
Low power stellate appearance; radiating ducts/proliferations increase in size centrifugally from central core	Low power infiltrative appearance with haphazard arrangement of tubules (but may be stellate)
Stroma is fibroelastotic, present centrally	Stroma is desmoplastic, present throughout lesion
Entrapped glands central; confined to fibroelastotic stroma	Tubules may be central and/or peripheral
Entrapped glands are distorted	Tubules are angulated, usually with open lumens
Myoepithelial cells surround the entrapped glands (at least in part)	No myoepithelial cells surrounding tubules
Glandular epithelium not usually polarized; no apical snouts	Glandular epithelium polarized, often with apical snouts
In situ carcinoma may be present, but rarer; most have benign epithelial proliferations and/or cysts	Low grade DCIS and/or ADH common

tubular carcinoma, with the cancerous, small angulated glands present haphazardly 'sprinkled' throughout the lesion (Table 8-2). It should be noted that the presence of a fibroelastotic stroma alone does not automatically equate with a diagnosis of radial scar and that invasive carcinomas may have similar elastotic stroma (Figure 8-16).

Furthermore, invasive carcinoma may occur in association with a radial scar, often peripherally. The presence of DCIS or LCIS within a radial scar may be particularly diagnostically challenging because the entrapped and distorted ducts involved by in situ carcinoma may simulate invasive carcinoma (Figures 8-13 and 8-14). However, the areas most worrisome for invasion are usually located within the central fibroelastotic core of the radial scar where entrapped ducts are most often situated, rather than at the periphery of the lesion where carcinoma is more apt to be. In addition, in contrast to true microscopic invasion, a cellular, desmoplastic stroma is not present around the worrisome cell nests. As with all radial scars, the entrapped glands with *in situ* carcinoma are surrounded by myoepithelial cells, which may be highlighted by immunohistochemistry if necessary.

The distinction between radial scar and invasive carcinoma may be especially problematic with core needle biopsy specimens due to the limited sample afforded by this technique. A histologic diagnosis of radial scar can be made when the characteristic central area of fibroelastosis is found with at least part of the radiating surrounding ducts and lobules present. However, the diagnosis may be particularly challenging when just the central fibroelastotic area of the radial scar is sampled by the needle. In this situation, only the entrapped distorted ducts within a fibroelastotic stroma may be present, without the typical radiating ducts and lobules containing proliferative and cystic changes. In these cases, immunohistochemical stains to demonstrate myoepithelial cells may be particularly helpful. However, even if carcinoma is not found in a core biopsy specimen that shows features of a radial scar, an excisional biopsy may still be advisable to exclude the possibility of concomitant carcinoma.

PROGNOSIS AND THERAPY

The observation that the entrapped epithelial elements within the central zone of fibroelastosis in radial scars may mimic tubular carcinoma has led several authors to postulate that radial scars represent an early phase in the development of some breast cancers. However, until recently, most reports had been observational and not validated by clinical follow-up studies. We recently reported the results of a large case–control study nested within the Nurses' Health Study which is a cohort of US women with prospectively collected data on risk factors for breast carcinoma. We found that women with a radial scar had a two-fold increase in breast cancer risk, independent of the histologic category of benign breast disease. In addition, the presence of a radial scar

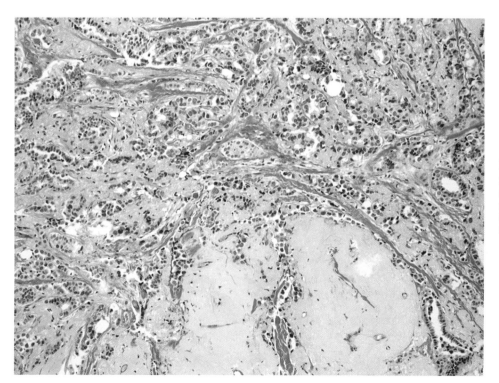

FIGURE 8-16

Invasive carcinoma, with haphazard arrangement of malignant glands; note the associated fibroelastotic stroma, particularly in the lower half of the field.

further increased the breast cancer risk among women with proliferative disease without atypia (e.g, florid ductal hyperplasia, sclerosing adenosis, fibroadenoma and papilloma) and among those with atypical hyperplasia. In addition, the breast cancer risk increased with larger and with multiple radial scars.

There was no significant difference between the number of women who developed cancer in the breast contralateral or ipsilateral to that of their original benign biopsy containing a radial scar and therefore, radial scars are probably best considered markers of generalized increased breast cancer risk. However, given that *in situ* and invasive carcinomas appear to be more common in larger than smaller radial scars, the possibility that at least some radial scars represent direct cancer precursors must also be considered. Based on our recent data, we believe that pathologists should note the presence of radial scars in benign breast biopsies and also indicate the size of the largest radial scar and number of lesions present. As alluded to above, patients in whom a radial scar is detected on a core biopsy of a lesion large enough to be detected by imaging should probably undergo excisional biopsy of the lesion due to the increased chance of carcinoma occurring in larger radial scars (and particularly at the periphery of these lesions). Furthermore, women who have breast biopsies that reveal radial scars should undergo regular clinical and mammographic follow-up, as for other patients with benign breast lesions that impart a moderately increased, bilateral breast cancer risk.

Radial scars present management issues when diagnosed on CNB. These lesions are not commonly encountered in CNB specimens, perhaps in part because at many institutions patients in whom such lesions are suspected mammographically are preferentially referred for surgical excision. As a consequence, only a few retrospective studies with very limited case numbers exist concerning the surgical outcome of radial scars without atypia diagnosed on core biopsy. Nonetheless, a proportion of cases with radial scar on CNB have had carcinoma at excision. Based on the results of studies showing an increased likelihood of finding carcinoma in larger radial scars, and having very limited objective data available from the CNB follow-up studies to date, it is prudent for all patients with radial scars diagnosed on CNB to undergo surgical excision if clinically feasible to exclude the possibility of concomitant carcinoma.

SUGGESTED READING

Sclerosing Adenosis

Eusebi V, Collina G, Bussolati G. Carcinoma in situ in sclerosing adenosis of the breast: an immunocytochemical study. Semin Diagn Pathol 1989;6:146–152.

Fechner RE. Carcinoma in situ involving sclerosing adenosis. Histopathology 1996;28:570.

Fechner RE. Lobular carcinoma in situ in sclerosing adenosis. A potential source of confusion with invasive carcinoma. Am J Surg Pathol 1981;5:233–239.

Gill HK, Ioffe OB, Berg WA. When is a diagnosis of sclerosing adenosis acceptable at core biopsy? Radiology 2003;228:50–57.

Gobbi H, Jensen RA, Simpson JF, et al. Atypical ductal hyperplasia and ductal carcinoma in situ of the breast associated with perineural invasion. Hum Pathol 2001;32:785–790.

Jensen RA, Page DL, Dupont WD, et al. Invasive breast cancer risk in women with sclerosing adenosis. Cancer 1989;64:1977–1983.

O'Malley FP, Bane AL. The spectrum of apocrine lesions of the breast. Adv Anat Pathol 2004;11:1–9.

Seidman JD, Ashton M, Lefkowitz M. Atypical apocrine adenosis of the breast: a clinicopathologic study of 37 patients with 8.7-year follow-up. Cancer 1996;77:2529–2537.

Spencer NJ, Evans AJ, Galea M, et al. Pathological-radiological correlations in benign lesions excised during a breast screening programme. Clin Radiol 1994;49:853–856.

Werling RW, Hwang H, Yaziji H, et al. Immunohistochemical distinction of invasive from noninvasive breast lesions: a comparative study of p63 versus calponin and smooth muscle myosin heavy chain. Am J Surg Pathol 2003;27:82–90.

Radial Scar

Adler DD, Helvie MA, Oberman HA, et al. Radial sclerosing lesion of the breast: mammographic features. Radiology 1990;176:737–740.

Anderson TJ, Battersby S. Radial scars of benign and malignant breasts: comparative features and significance. J Pathol 1985;147:23–32.

Douglas-Jones AG, Pace DP. Pathology of R4 spiculated lesions in the breast screening programme. Histopathology 1997;30:214–220.

Frouge C, Tristant H, Guinebretiere JM, et al. Mammographic lesions suggestive of radial scars: microscopic findings in 40 cases. Radiology 1995;195:623–625.

Jacobs TW, Byrne C, Colditz G, et al. Radial scars in benign breast-biopsy specimens and the risk of breast cancer. N Engl J Med 1999;340:430–436.

Jacobs TW, Connolly JL, Schnitt SJ. Nonmalignant lesions in breast core needle biopsies: to excise or not to excise? Am J Surg Pathol 2002;26:1095–1110.

Jacobs TW, Schnitt SJ, Tan X, et al. Radial scars of the breast and breast carcinomas have similar alterations in expression of factors involved in vascular stroma formation. Hum Pathol 2002;33:29–38.

Nielsen M, Christensen L, Andersen J. Radial scars in women with breast cancer. Cancer 1987;59:1019–1025.

Sloane JP, Mayers MM. Carcinoma and atypical hyperplasia in radial scars and complex sclerosing lesions: importance of lesion size and patient age. Histopathology 1993;23:225–231.

Wellings SR, Alpers CE. Subgross pathologic features and incidence of radial scars in the breast. Hum Pathol 1984;15:475–479.

9 Papillomas and Related Lesions

Beverley A Carter · Jean F Simpson

INTRODUCTION

Papillomas and related lesions of the breast are lesions of true ducts and encompass papillomas (both solitary and multiple), papillomas with atypical hyperplasia, papillomas with focal involvement by ductal carcinoma *in situ* (DCIS), ductal adenomas, nipple adenomas and encysted non-invasive papillary carcinomas. A papilloma or related lesion is diagnosed when a breast duct contains a lesion with fibrovascular stroma covered by epithelium. On multiple histologic sectioning, the attachment to the duct wall may be identified. Papillomas, particularly when solitary, may attain several centimeters in size, causing them to appear encysted with an apparent constant continuity with an often subtle encysting fibrous tissue representing the remnants of the duct wall.

PAPILLOMA

CLINICAL FEATURES

Papillomas of the breast are the most common focal mass lesion of the breast after fibroadenoma. Solitary papillomas are usually located beneath the areola, while multiple papillomas are often peripherally located. Usually multiple papillomas are clustered or at least regional and are continuous with hyperplasic alterations within adjacent lobular units, as shown in 3-D reconstruction studies. Either of these two locations may result in the clinical presentation of nipple discharge that may be bloody or clear.

RADIOLOGIC FEATURES

Women with a single papilloma often have normal mammograms, or a smooth walled well-defined mass may be seen. Multiple peripheral papillomas may have multiple nodular masses by mammography. Galactography identifies a filling defect.

Ultrasound is usually abnormal in patients with a papilloma and shows a well-defined hypoechoic mass or a solid and cystic lesion with a smooth wall. Adjacent ducts are often dilated.

PATHOLOGIC FINDINGS: GROSS AND MICROSCOPIC

These lesions range from less than 3–5 mm to up to several centimeters in size. They vary from soft to firm

PAPILLOMA AND RELATED LESIONS – PATHOLOGIC FEATURES

Gross Findings

▶ 3 mm–several centimeters
▶ Vary from soft to firm with dense sclerosis
▶ Focal hemorrhage and necrosis common

Microscopic Findings

▶ Multiple branching papillae lined by varying epithelium, may have usual or atypical ductal hyperplasia, apocrine or squamous metaplasia
▶ Surrounding stroma may be sclerotic with pseudoinvasive foci

Ultrastructural Features

▶ N/A

Fine Needle Aspiration Biopsy Findings

▶ 3-D clusters with fibrovascular cores
▶ Increased cellularity

Immunohistochemical Features

▶ Immunohistochemical stains for myoepithelial cells may aid in diagnosing pseudoinvasion

Differential Diagnosis

▶ Infiltrating mammary carcinoma

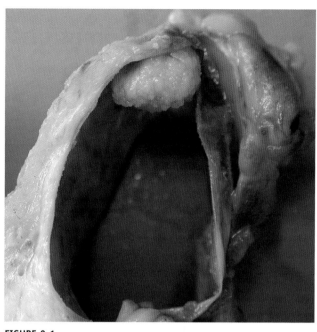

FIGURE 9-1

Papilloma. Gross image of a papilloma showing a cystically dilated, smooth-walled duct, with a focal solid papillary excrescence.

with dense sclerotic foci. Focal areas of hemorrhage and necrosis can be seen especially in larger lesions. Careful gross examination may show the lesion as lying within dilated ducts (Figure 9-1).

Microscopic examination of classic examples shows multiple branching papillae lined by two cell layers (Figure 9-2). The luminal epithelium is usually, but not always, cuboidal. The basal or myoepithelial layer may be round or spindled and is occasionally patchily present (Figure 9-3). Apocrine change is a relatively frequent change in papillomas and related lesions (Figure 9-4), while hypersecretory change and squamous metaplasia are relatively uncommon. Squamous metaplastic changes are often present in areas of infarction. When infarction occurs, this may cause compression and entrapment of epithelium, mimicking invasive carcinoma.

The luminal epithelium is subject to the same proliferative changes that occur elsewhere in the breast, most commonly florid usual hyperplasia and atypical ductal hyperplasia. These entities are diagnosed using criteria similar to those for usual and atypical hyperplasia elsewhere in the breast.

Usual hyperplasia involving a papilloma is diagnosed when the luminal cells, lacking cytologic uniformity, pile up, often forming irregular slit-like spaces (Figure 9-5). Atypical ductal hyperplasia (ADH) involving a papilloma is diagnosed if the histologic patterns and cytologic features of the hyperplastic epithelium approach, but do not fulfill standard diagnostic criteria for low grade ductal carcinoma *in situ*. As always, extent

is a defining feature of ADH. Often ADH only partially involves an otherwise ordinary papilloma, and the pathologist must measure the extent of involvement and not estimate percentage of the involvement. Any area consisting of uniform histology and cytology consistent with low grade DCIS that extends over an area less than 3 mm in greatest contiguous dimension qualifies as ADH involving a papilloma (Figure 9-6). Larger lesions merit a diagnosis of DCIS.

Multiple peripheral papillomas are much more likely to be associated with ADH or ductal carcinoma; up to 60% of these lesions in some series.

Adjacent breast tissue, especially in extensive lesions, may show atypical hyperplasia and/or ductal carcinoma *in situ*.

Other lesions bearing clinical and pathologic resemblance to papillomas include nipple adenoma (florid papillomatosis of the nipple) and ductal adenoma/sclerosed papilloma.

Nipple adenoma is a term used to describe a variety of benign proliferative lesions that are found in the area of the nipple (also see Chapter 12). They can be seen at any age, but are most common around the menopause. As with papillomas they may present with nipple discharge. Some cases present as a slightly red crusty nipple overlying a small firm palpable mass. They are usually less than 1 cm in size at time of diagnosis.

The histologic features are a mixture of papilloma, usual hyperplasia and adenosis, enveloped by fibrosis (Figure 9-7). Gynecomastoid hyperplasia of the

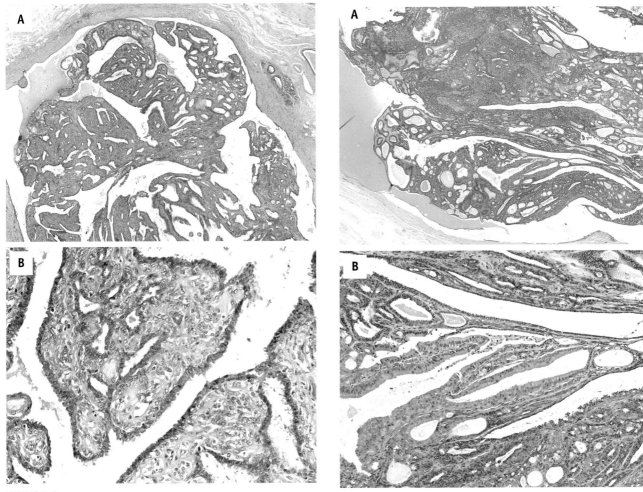

FIGURE 9-2

Papilloma. Low power view (A) showing a cystically dilated duct containing multiple branching papillae composed of fibrovascular stromal cores; (B) high power view showing fibrovascular cores lined by myoepithelial and epithelial cells.

FIGURE 9-4

Apocrine change within a papilloma. (A) Low power and (B) medium power view of a benign papilloma which contains a focal area of apocrine metaplasia.

FIGURE 9-3

Papilloma. High power view showing a dual cell layer lining the papillae. The luminal epithelial cells seen here are columnar and overlie a rather prominent layer of myoepithelial cells that contain abundant clear cytoplasm.

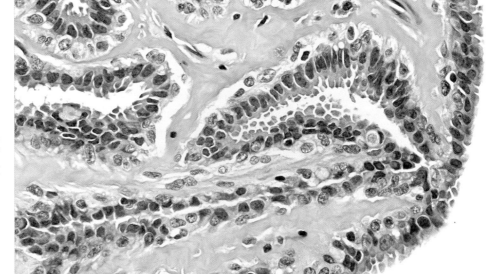

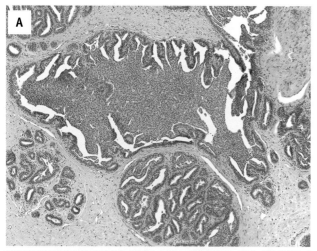

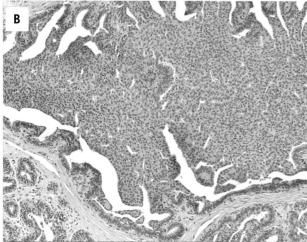

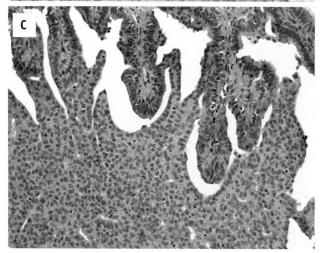

FIGURE 9-5

Florid epithelial hyperplasia of usual type in a papilloma. (A) Low power view of a papilloma showing florid epithelial hyperplasia of usual type. (B) The luminal cells pile up, forming irregular slit-like spaces, lacking the punched-out spaces often seen in ADH/DCIS. (C) The cells show slight nuclear irregularity typical of usual hyperplasia and the pattern is that of overlapping and streaming of the constituent cells.

glandular epithelium is especially common. The epithelium may display nuclear hyperchromasia and a high nuclear to cytoplasmic ratio that can look worrisome. Complex patterns of epithelial hyperplasia enveloped by fibrosis may lead to the mistaken diagnosis of malignancy. Careful histologic sampling and complete excision are important, because foci of carcinoma have rarely been described in such lesions.

Sclerosed papilloma and ductal adenoma are similar terms for an uncommon but important group of lesions closely related to papillomas. They are usually solitary lesions, but can be multiple and extensive in the breast. They are associated with larger ducts. Most occur in older women or in the perimenopausal era. The lesions are solitary, pale brown and firm on gross examination. They are usually thick walled. A duct lumen or site of attachment may be seen in larger lesions, but it is often obliterated. Histologically these are papillomas with unusual patterns of sclerosis and adenosis (Figure 9-8). Because these lesions are characteristically surrounded by dense fibrous tissue within which epithelial cells are pseudo invasive, they may be over diagnosed as malignancy by the unwary.

ANCILLARY STUDIES

Fine needle aspiration biopsy of papillomas gives 3-D papillary clusters with fibrovascular cores. Marked cellularity with cellular dissociation is usually seen. Monotony of the cellular population raises the possibility of a papilloma involved by DCIS or an encysted non-invasive papillary carcinoma (discussed in the next section).

If there is doubt about pseudoinvasion (Figure 9-9) of the surrounding duct wall, immunohistochemical stains for myoepithelial cells may be of some value.

DIFFERENTIAL DIAGNOSIS

The most important entity in the differential diagnosis of papilloma and related lesions is infiltrating carcinoma. Mammographically detected lesions, including papillomas, are increasingly evaluated by stereotactic core biopsy. Occasionally this can result in the displacement of epithelium into the surrounding tissue. The entrapped epithelium from a papilloma mimics an invasive process. This is less of a problem when the papilloma is not involved by atypia, but if the entrapped epithelium is dislodged from an area of DCIS within a papilloma (or even an encysted, non-invasive papillary carcinoma), misinterpretation can occur. Many sclerosed papillomas mimic other breast adenomas because there is no apparent space between the fibrovascular cores. Foci of sclerosis are quite common, by definition, in such lesions both within the substance

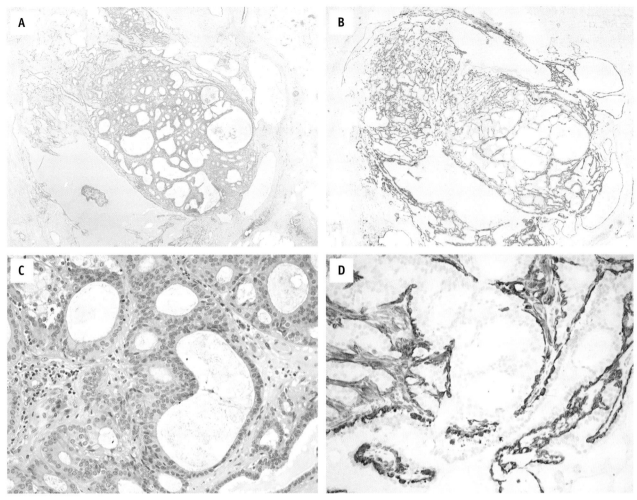

FIGURE 9-6

Atypical ductal hyperplasia occurring within a papilloma. (A) At the lower, cental aspect of the lesion, a focus of ADH is seen, with the formation of rigid lumina and a monotonous population of cells. This area of atypia is less than 3 mm in extent and, therefore, fails to fulfill the extent criteria required to make a diagnosis of low grade DCIS. (B) Immunohistochemical staining with the myoepithelial marker smooth muscle myosin heavy chain (SMM-HC) highlights the area of ADH. (C) Higher power view shows the neoplastic proliferation forming rigid, 'punched-out' lumina. The constituent cells are uniform and contain regular, round, hyperchromatic nuclei. (D) High power view of SMM-HC in area of ADH.

of the lesion and in the encysting fibrous tissue of the duct wall.

PROGNOSIS AND THERAPY

Attempts at associating papillomas with malignancy, either as a precursor lesion or as a lesion that indicates an increased risk for subsequent malignancy, have been somewhat controversial. Haagensen stressed the importance of distinguishing solitary from multiple papillomas because they found the latter lesions were more likely associated with concurrent or subsequent development of breast carcinomas. Carter has demonstrated an association of multiple intraductal papillomas with breast carcinoma, both *in situ* and invasive.

Studies from the Nashville benign breast series have shown that the presence of a papilloma doubles the subsequent breast cancer risk relative to the general population, a level similar to other forms of proliferative breast disease without atypia. The presence of ADH, either within the papilloma or in adjacent breast parenchyma has striking risk implications, however. The subsequent breast cancer risk for these women was 7.5 times greater than the risk for women with papillomas without ADH. It was common for the women with ADH involving the papilloma to also have ADH in surrounding breast parenchyma, and in this situation the relative risk was even higher. The carcinomas that developed involved the ipsilateral breast in all but one case. This finding suggests that atypical hyperplasia within a papilloma may in fact be a precursor lesion, or marker of regional risk.

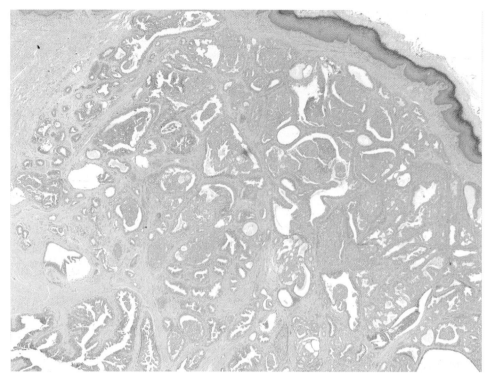

FIGURE 9-7
Nipple adenoma. The nipple epidermis overlies a mixture of an adenomatous and papillomatous proliferation with varying amounts of usual hyperplasia, enveloped in a fibrous stroma.

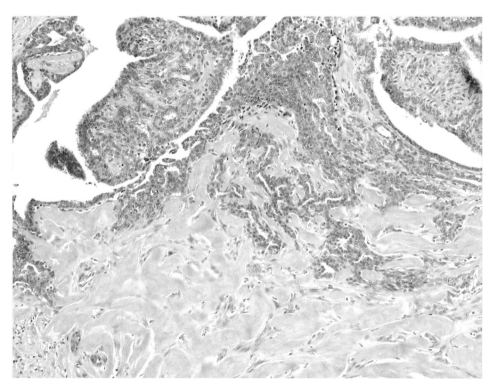

FIGURE 9-8
Sclerosis in a papilloma. Papilloma showing sclerosis of the fibrovascular cores. This should not be misinterpreted as invasive carcinoma.

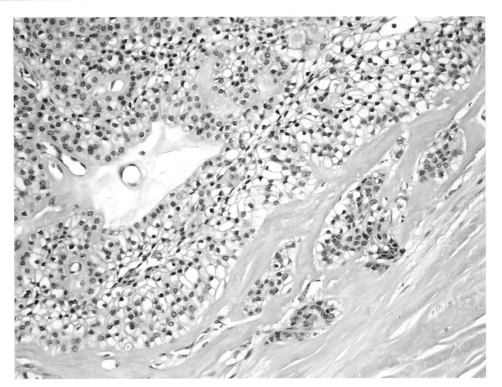

FIGURE 9-9
Pseudoinvasion in papillary DCIS. Medium power view showing entrapped epithelium within the sclerosed surrounding tissue, mimicking an invasive process. This often occurs following core biopsy of the lesion.

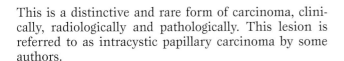

ENCYSTED NON-INVASIVE PAPILLARY CARCINOMA

This is a distinctive and rare form of carcinoma, clinically, radiologically and pathologically. This lesion is referred to as intracystic papillary carcinoma by some authors.

CLINICAL FEATURES

These uncommon lesions usually occur in the older population and may present with nipple discharge (up to 30% of patients), which is, on occasion, bloody. A palpable mass, sometimes reaching up to 10 cm in diameter is present centrally within the breast. Occasional cases are multiple and peripheral and are most often detected in screening programs.

RADIOLOGIC FEATURES

Mammographic evaluation shows a round circumscribed lesion, often initially thought benign. Examination by ultrasound shows a hypoechoic cystic lesion with posterior enhancement. Obvious papillary features

---

ENCYSTED NON-INVASIVE PAPILLARY CARCINOMA – FACT SHEET

Definition
▸ Distinctive mammary carcinoma with epithelial-lined fibrovascular cores

Incidence and Location
▸ Unusual, 1–2% of all breast cancers
▸ Usually central in the breast

Morbidity and Mortality
▸ Overall favorable prognosis

Gender, Race and Age Distribution
▸ Older and perimenopausal women
▸ Can be seen in males

Clinical Features
▸ Bloody nipple discharge
▸ Palpable mass

Radiologic Features
▸ Rounded, well defined mammographic lesion; may have microcalcification
▸ Hypoechoic, cystic lesion on ultrasound; may have microcalcification

Prognosis and Treatment
▸ Essentially cured by local excision with adequate margins if no DCIS is present in surrounding breast tissue

may be seen by ultrasound. Microcalcification may be seen with either radiographic modality.

PATHOLOGIC FINDINGS: GROSS AND MICROSCOPIC

On gross examination, a well-defined fibrous wall surrounds the papillary lesion. These lesions are quite distinct from the surrounding breast tissue. On average, they measure 1–3 cm but can reach vast diameters. A cystic space is usually demonstrable. Hemorrhagic areas are quite common.

Microscopic examination shows a monomorphic, evenly spaced population of cells completely occupying the papillary lesion. The epithelium either shows a single layer of well-oriented, monomorphic hyperchro-

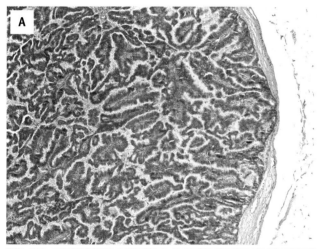

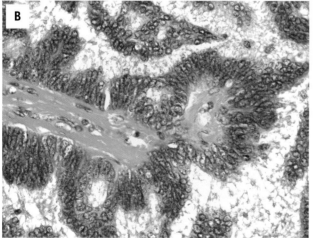

FIGURE 9-10

Encysted non-invasive papillary carcinoma. (A) Low power view showing the tall cell variant composed of fibrovascular cores lined by (B) a single layer of well-orientated hyperchromatic 'tall' columnar cells with loss of the normal myoepithelial cell layer.

ENCYSTED NON-INVASIVE PAPILLARY CARCINOMA – PATHOLOGIC FEATURES

Gross Findings
▶ Usually 1–3 cm, but can be vast
▶ Distinct from adjacent breast tissue
▶ Cystic spaces may be present
▶ Thick fibrous wall

Microscopic Findings
▶ Fibrovascular cores lined completely by DCIS or
▶ Fibrovascular cores lined by tall cell atypia
▶ At least focal, but often complete loss of the myoepithelial cell layer

Ultrastructural Features
▶ N/A

Fine Needle Aspiration Biopsy Findings
▶ Often bloody
▶ 3-D fibrovascular cores with increased cellularity
▶ Monotony of epithelial cells
▶ Unreliable in distinguishing from papilloma

Immunohistochemical Features
▶ Myoepithelial cell layer generally lost
▶ Estrogen receptor positive
▶ HER2/neu negative

Differential Diagnosis
▶ Papilloma partially involved by DCIS
▶ Invasive carcinoma versus pseudoinvasion

---

matic 'tall' columnar cells (tall cell atypia) (Figure 9-10) or complete replacement by recognizable patterns of DCIS, most often of cribriform (Figure 9-11) or solid pattern. There is loss of the normal myoepithelial layer within the tumor. Adequate and careful sampling is mandatory to rule out foci of invasion of the encysting wall. The adjacent breast tissue must also be sampled.

ANCILLARY STUDIES

Fine needle aspiration biopsy usually shows a very cellular specimen with distinctive fibrovascular cores lined by atypical epithelium. Grossly the specimens are often bloody or light brown. Fine needle aspiration is not very reliable in distinguishing papilloma from encysted non-invasive papillary carcinoma.

Encysted noninvasive papillary carcinoma is almost always estrogen receptor positive and there is usually absence of HER2/neu protein overexpression. Immunohistochemical stains for myoepithelial cells should show loss of this cell layer around the fibrovascular cores.

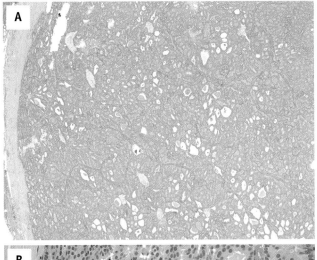

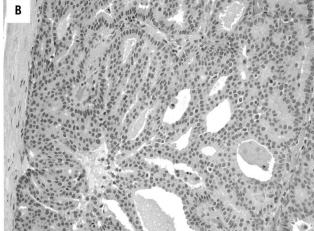

FIGURE 9-11

Encysted non-invasive papillary carcinoma. (A) Low power view showing a monomorphic, evenly spaced population of cells completely occupying the papillary lesion, giving rise to a cribriform pattern. (B) Higher power view showing a uniform neoplastic population of cells with rigid 'punched-out' lumina.

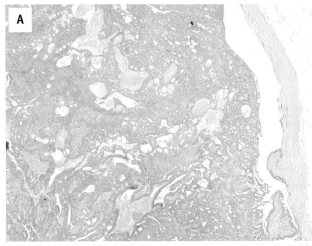

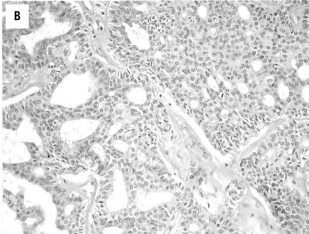

FIGURE 9-12

Ductal carcinoma in situ involving a papilloma. When the morphologic features of DCIS do not completely occupy the papilloma but are greater than 3 mm in extent, a diagnosis of DCIS involving a papilloma is made. (A) Low power view of a papillary lesion extensively, but not completely occupied by DCIS. (B) Higher power view shows the features typical of low grade DCIS with a uniform population of cells forming rigid lumina.

DIFFERENTIAL DIAGNOSIS

Included in the differential diagnosis is DCIS focally involving a papilloma. We diagnosis DCIS involving a papilloma based on the extent of the uniform population of cells. When the monomorphic, evenly placed cells, often with cribriform formations, cover an area greater than 3 mm but do not occupy the entire papilloma, DCIS is diagnosed (Figure 9-12). The DCIS is usually of low grade, but it can be intermediate grade.

As with benign papillomas, epithelial entrapment in the encysting fibrous tissue, a common occurrence, must not be diagnosed as invasive carcinoma. A useful rule of thumb is to withhold a diagnosis of invasive carci-noma unless invasion is seen outside the encysting fibrous tissue (Figure 9-13).

PROGNOSIS AND THERAPY

Encysted non-invasive papillary carcinoma has an overall favorable prognosis. Carter *et al* showed that encysted, non-invasive papillary carcinoma can be cured by local excision with adequate margins. Local excision was often unsuccessful however, if there was DCIS in the surrounding, non-papillary breast tissue, once again emphasizing the importance of careful and generous sampling of the tissue.

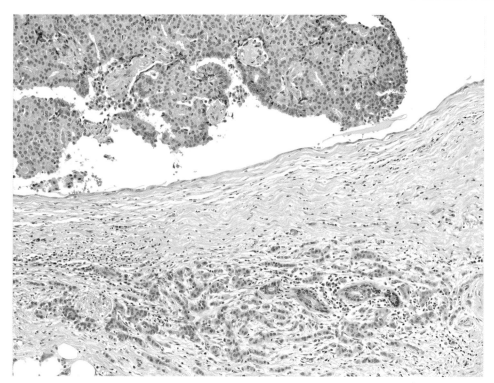

FIGURE 9-13

Encysted papillary carcinoma with invasion. Irregularly infiltrating cords and single cells with a surrounding desmoplastic response are seen to infiltrate beyond the encysting fibrous tissue.

SELECTED READING

Azzopardi JG, Salm R. Ductal adenoma of the breast: a lesion which can mimic carcinoma. J Pathol 1984;144:11–23.

Carter D. Intraductal papillary tumors of the breast: a study of 78 cases. Cancer 1977;39:1689–1692.

Ohuchi N, Abe R, Takahashi T, Tezuka F. Origin and extension of intraductal papillomas of the breast: a three-dimensional reconstruction study. Breast Cancer Res Treat 1984;4:117–128.

Ohuchi N, Rikiya A, Kasai M. Possible cancerous change of intraductal papillomas of the breast: a 3D reconstruction study of 25 cases. Cancer 1984;54:605–611.

Page DL, Salhany KE, Jensen RA, Dupont WD. Subsequent breast carcinoma risk after biopsy with atypia in a breast papilloma. Cancer 1996;78:258–266.

Rosen PP, Caicco AA. Florid papillomatosis of the nipple. A study of 51 patients, including nine with mammary carcinoma. Am J Surg Pathol 1986;10:87–101

Tavassoli FA, Norris HJ. A comparison of the results of long-term follow-up for atypical intraductal hyperplasia and intraductal hyperplasia of the breast. Cancer 1990;65:518–529.

10 Fibroepithelial Lesions, Including Fibroadenoma and Phyllodes Tumor

Sarah E Pinder · Anna Marie Mulligan · Frances P O'Malley

INTRODUCTION

Under the category of fibroepithelial lesions there are a number of unrelated entities which are composed of both stromal and epithelial components. Some of these lesions are recognized to be hyperplastic, such as fibroadenomas and fibroadenomatoid hyperplasia; others are neoplastic, such as phyllodes tumors. The inclusion of these disparate entities as one group of lesions is justified by their similarity in appearance as well as clinical presentation.

FIBROADENOMA

FIBROADENOMA – FACT SHEET

Definition
▸ A hyperplastic, benign fibroepithelial lesion of the breast composed of both stromal and epithelial components

Incidence
▸ Common

Gender, Race and Age Distribution
▸ Women in their 20s and 30s
▸ More common in Afro-Caribbean women

Clinical Features
▸ Mobile, painless, well-defined breast lump
▸ Asymptomatic, clinically impalpable
▸ Rarely undergoes infarction

Radiologic Features
▸ Well-defined mass with or without microcalcification
▸ Homogeneous hypoechoic mass on ultrasound

Prognosis and Treatment
▸ Surgical excision, without surrounding breast tissue
▸ Some recur; may develop further lesions in ipsilateral or contralateral breast

CLINICAL AND RADIOLOGIC FEATURES

This is a common lesion presenting as a mobile, painless well-defined breast lump, particularly in women in their thirties. Smaller clinically impalpable lesions may, however, be even more common and have even been suggested to be present in all breasts. Thus, a well-defined mass, with or without microcalcification, may be detected in women undergoing mammographic breast screening which may not have ever presented symptomatically. Ultrasonography shows a well-defined homogeneous hypoechoic mass.

Fibroadenomas are usually solitary, but in some patients bilateral or multiple lesions can be seen. It has been reported that this is more common in Afro-Caribbean women.

Rarely, fibroadenomas may undergo infarction; this is said to be more common in pregnant or lactating women. The consequent inflammatory reaction may mimic a more worrisome process and care should be taken not to misdiagnose malignancy, particularly in cytologic or frozen material from such lesions.

PATHOLOGIC FEATURES

GROSS FINDINGS

Macroscopically fibroadenomas are typically seen as well-defined masses which have been 'shelled-out' and thus are removed without surrounding breast tissue; they do not have a true capsule (Figure 10-1). They are round or ovoid, often gray in color. The cut surface is rubbery, often somewhat lobulated and duct structures within the lesion may be seen as slit-like spaces. Rarely the cut surface may appear myxoid. In older patients the lesion may be more fibrous and sclerosed. There is reasonable evidence that fibroadenomas are, at least to some extent, hormone dependent and some enlarge during pregnancy and then regress; it is certainly true that many appear to undergo atrophy after the menopause. The excised lesion is typically 1–3 cm in size but rare forms, typically in younger women/adolescents, may be up to 20 cm in size; the latter are often labelled as juvenile fibroadenomas, which is preferred to the term giant fibroadenoma.

FIBROADENOMA – PATHOLOGIC FEATURES

Gross Findings

▶ Well-defined masses, 1–3 cm in size; rarely up to 20 cm
▶ Round or ovoid, often gray in color
▶ No true capsule
▶ Rubbery cut surface, often lobulated with slit-like spaces
▶ Fibrous/sclerosed texture in older patients

Microscopic Findings

▶ Peri-canalicular and intra-canalicular types
▶ Stromal component loosely cellular, lacking cytologic atypia
▶ Epithelial component – compressed duct structures or tubules with epithelial and myoepithelial layers; may show epithelial hyperplasia; rarely atypical hyperplasia, lobular neoplasia or ductal carcinoma in situ
▶ Complex fibroadenomas show sclerosing adenosis, papillary apocrine change, epithelial calcifications or cysts >3 mm

Ultrastructural Features

▶ N/A

Fine Needle Aspiration Biopsy Findings

▶ Cellular specimen
▶ Abundant sheets and clumps of epithelial cells in a background of scanty stromal fragments and bare/stripped nuclei
▶ Epithelial cells may show mild atypia and discohesion

Immunohistochemical Features

▶ N/A

Differential Diagnosis

▶ Phyllodes tumor – increased stromal cellularity and atypia and true cleft-like spaces, mitoses more frequent
▶ Tubular adenoma
▶ Hamartoma

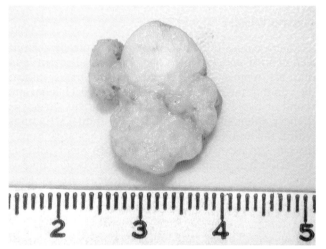

FIGURE 10-1

Fibroadenoma. Gross image of a fibroadenoma which has been shelled out without surrounding breast tissue. The lesion is well-defined with a homogeneous, lobulated cut surface.

MICROSCOPIC FINDINGS

The morphologic appearances vary and historically these lesions have been subdivided into pericanalicular and intra-canalicular types. There is no clinical or prognostic value to this sub-classification and some lesions may show a variety of the two patterns. Histologically in all fibroadenomas, the two components of stroma and epithelium (hence 'fibroepithelial lesion') are seen. However, the stromal growth in the intra-canalicular form compresses duct structures into slit-like spaces and surrounds them with a somewhat whorled appearance (Figure 10-2A,B). In the peri-canalicular type the stromal proliferation surrounds the breast epithelial component which forms ducts that are more tubular in appearance; these may appear somewhat disorganized as they do not form organoid, lobular structures (Figure 10-2C,D).

The epithelial portion of the lesion is formed from the normal constituents with an epithelial and underlying myoepithelial layer (Figure 10-3); the latter can be confirmed with the use of myoepithelial markers, such as smooth muscle myosin heavy chain. There may be epithelial hyperplasia within the fibroadenoma, particularly in young women, which may concern the inexperienced pathologist. However, it is not associated with any increased risk of subsequent carcinoma development. Squamous metaplasia of the epithelial component may be seen. Rarely atypical ductal hyperplasia, lobular neoplasia (Figure 10-4) or, very rarely, ductal carcinoma *in situ* may be seen in the epithelium of a fibroadenoma but care should be taken in making these diagnoses. Other benign changes in the epithelium such as papillary apocrine change, cysts and epithelial calcifications are not uncommon and sclerosing adenosis may be seen (Figure 10-5). Lesions with these benign changes have been called complex fibroadenomas. One study reported a slight, long-term, increased risk of subsequent breast carcinoma if these benign changes are present. However, this finding has not been confirmed, as yet, in other large cohorts. The presence of atypical hyperplasia within a fibroadenoma (Figure 10-6) does not appear to predict for its presence in the adjacent breast tissue and does not increase the subsequent risk for invasive breast cancer.

The stromal portion of the fibroadenoma is not markedly cellular and does not show cytologic atypia; if either of these features is seen, the diagnosis of phyllodes tumour should be considered (see below for differential diagnosis). The stroma is thus usually loosely cellular, formed from regular spindled cells, but may be myxoid, particularly in the younger woman (Figure 10-7A). Areas of hypercellularity may be seen within a fibroadenoma, however, typically the leaf-like architecture of a phyllodes tumor is absent or only poorly formed and these lesions are referred to as cellular fibroadenomas (Figure 10-7B). Areas of pseudo-angiomatous stromal hyperplasia, myoid metaplasia (Figure 10-8) and bizarre stromal giant cells (Figure 10-9) may be present within the stroma; the latter should not be mistaken for malignancy. In the older patient the stroma may be hyalinized and more fibrotic

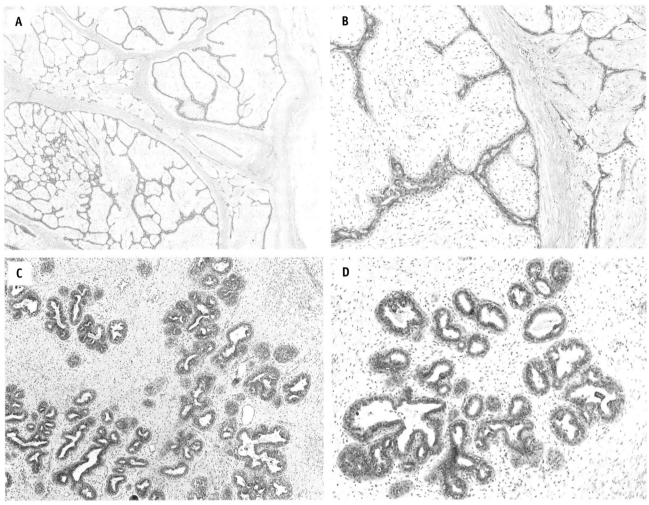

FIGURE 10-2

Fibroadenoma. (A,B) Intracanalicular growth pattern showing compressed duct structures as slit-like spaces, surrounded by stroma with a somewhat whorled appearance. (C,D) Pericanalicular growth pattern showing stromal proliferation surrounding disorganized epithelial tubular structures.

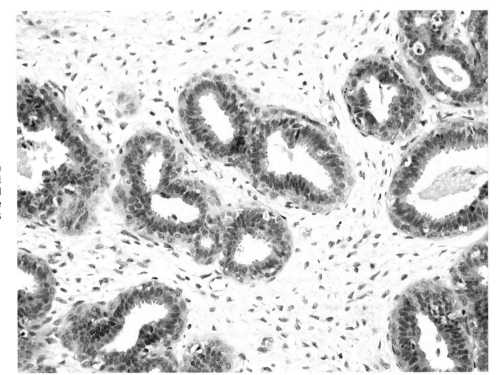

FIGURE 10-3

Fibroadenoma. The epithelial portion of the lesion is formed from normal constituents with an epithelial and underlying myoepithelial layer. The stroma is not hypercellular and lacks cytologic atypia.

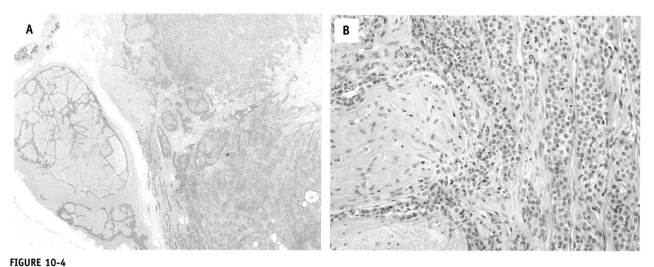

FIGURE 10-4

Lobular carcinoma in situ in a fibroadenoma. (A) Low power shows a fibroadenoma extensively involved by lobular carcinoma *in situ*. (B) At high power the slit-like ductal spaces are noted to be expanded by a neoplastic population of uniform cells.

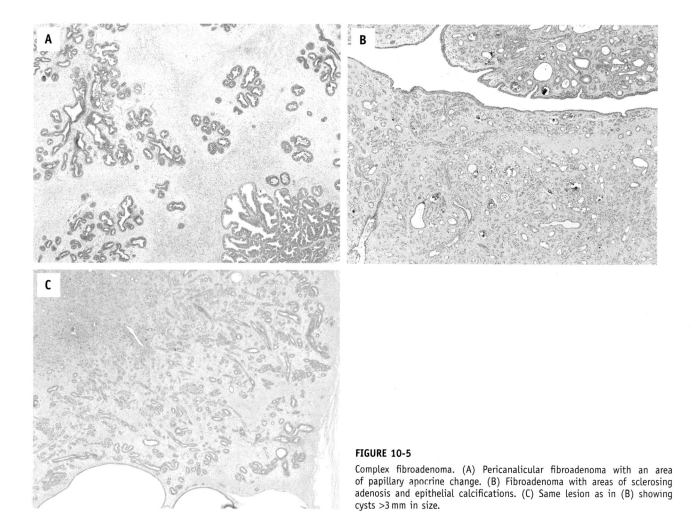

FIGURE 10-5

Complex fibroadenoma. (A) Pericanalicular fibroadenoma with an area of papillary apocrine change. (B) Fibroadenoma with areas of sclerosing adenosis and epithelial calcifications. (C) Same lesion as in (B) showing cysts >3 mm in size.

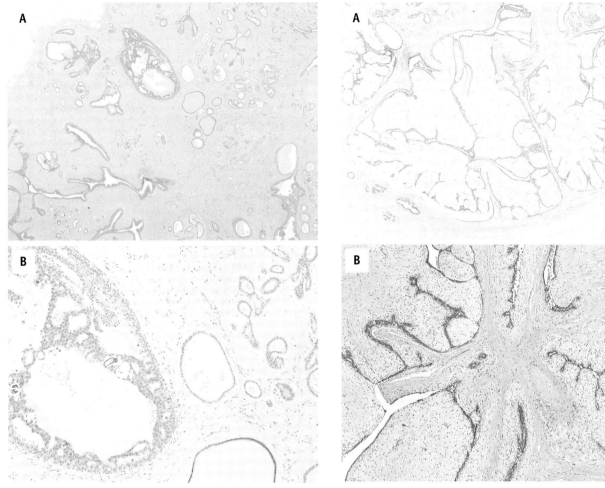

FIGURE 10-6

Fibroadenoma with atypical ductal hyperplasia. (A) Low power view with one duct showing atypical ductal hyperplasia. (B) Medium power of the atypical ductal hyperplasia.

FIGURE 10-7

Fibroadenoma. (A) The stroma is typically loosely cellular and lacks cytologic atypia, however, (B) a cellular fibroadenoma can show moderate stromal cellularity and may be difficult to distinguish from a benign phyllodes tumor.

(Figure 10-10). In patients in the older age group, microcalcification of the stroma is common.

ANCILLARY STUDIES

Additional studies such as ultrastructural or immunohistochemical examination is rarely undertaken on a fibroadenoma as they provide little assistance in differential diagnosis.

FINE NEEDLE ASPIRATION BIOPSY

Fine needle aspiration cytology commonly provides a cellular specimen with abundant sheets and clumps of regular epithelial cells in a background of scanty stromal fragments and prominent bare/stripped nuclei (Figure 10-11). The epithelial cells may show some mild increase in size and discohesion which, to the unwary, may be mistaken for carcinoma, particularly in a cellular sample (see Chapter 3).

DIFFERENTIAL DIAGNOSIS

The most important differential diagnosis is phyllodes tumor. Although fibroadenomas are more frequently seen in younger patients and are often of smaller size, these factors are not discriminatory and phyllodes tumors can be seen in women in their 30s. The key feature is the increase in stromal cellularity seen in the phyllodes tumor, with true cleft-like spaces. The stromal

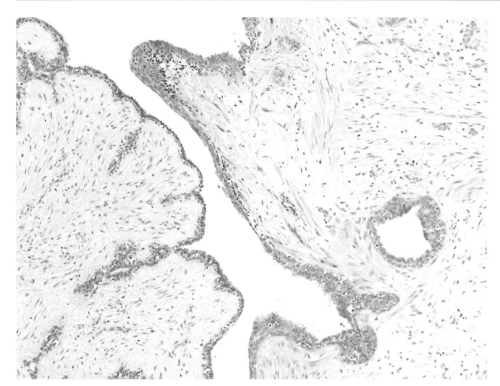

FIGURE 10-8
Fibroadenomatoid change with myoid metaplasia. The stroma shows elongated pink fibers, consistent with smooth muscle differentiation.

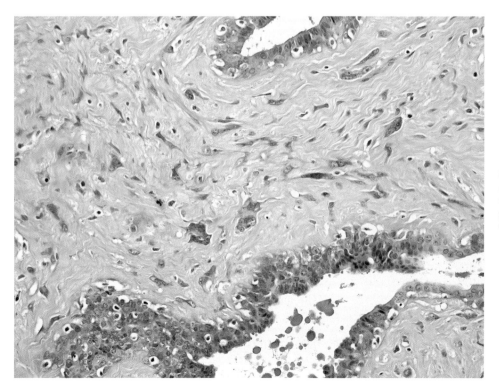

FIGURE 10-9
Fibroadenoma with bizarre giant cells in the stroma. The cells contain irregular, hyperchromatic nuclei; some cells are multi-nucleated.

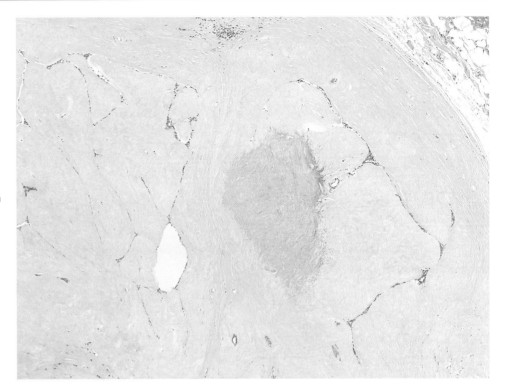

FIGURE 10-10

Hyalinized   fibroadenoma   with calcifications.

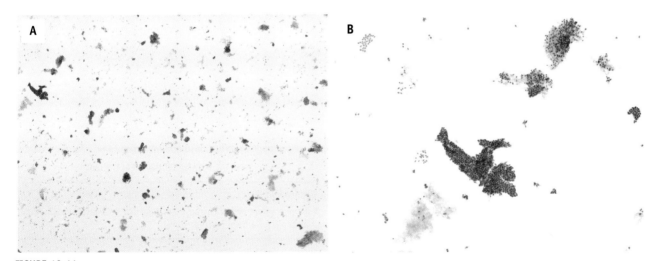

FIGURE 10-11

Fibroadenoma, fine needle aspiration. (A) Low power showing a highly cellular specimen composed of large clusters of epithelial cells in a background of stromal fragments and bipolar cells. (B) Higher power showing the complex, 'staghorn' configuration of an epithelial group. Stromal elements and individual bipolar cells are discernible in the background.

cells are more closely packed and may appear plump, rather than spindled in morphology, when compared to the fibroadenoma. Mitoses may be seen in the stroma or epithelium of the fibroadenoma, but are more frequent, and may indeed be prominent, in the stroma of a phyllodes tumor.

Other lesions which fall into the differential diagnosis include a tubular adenoma and a hamartoma (see below).

PROGNOSIS AND THERAPY

Fibroadenomas may be excised because of concern about the nature of the lesion or at the patient's request. As noted above, the lesion is most often 'shelled-out' without surrounding breast tissue. Some fibroadenomas will recur and some patients will develop further lesions elsewhere in the ipsilateral or contralateral breast.

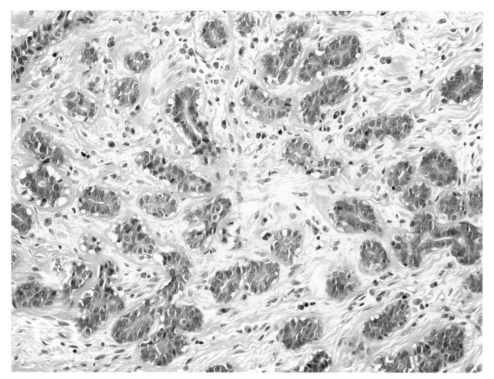

FIGURE 10-12
Tubular adenoma. Rounded ducts/ small tubular structures in a loosely cellular, vascularized stroma.

Women with non-complex fibroadenoma, without adjacent proliferative disease and without a family history of breast cancer are not at an elevated risk of breast cancer.

VARIANTS OF FIBROADENOMA

Many authorities consider a tubular adenoma to be a variant of a fibroadenoma. Indeed these are well-defined lesions composed of ductal/small tubular structures within a fibrovascular network of spindled cells of the same morphology as seen in the more 'typical' forms (Figure 10-12). Clinically the lesions are indistinguishable from other fibroadenomas.

Juvenile fibroadenomas most commonly occur in adolescents who present with a rapidly growing well-defined mass which may reach up to 20 cm in size. For this reason alone they may be considered clinically suspicious for malignancy. The macroscopic appearances are as for the more typical fibroadenoma. Histologically too, they are essentially similar, although the stroma may be more cellular. Epithelial proliferation is often more prominent and gynecomastoid-type hyperplasia may mimic ductal carcinoma *in situ* to the unwary (Figure 10-13). Cleft-like spaces are rarely seen, rather the ductal structures are more like the pericanalicular type of fibroadenoma and this feature may be helpful in distinguishing these lesions from phyllodes tumors. Fortunately, despite their large size, excision is curative with, typically, a good cosmetic result as the adjacent compressed normal breast tissue fills the excision site.

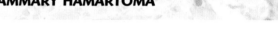

MAMMARY HAMARTOMA

CLINICAL AND RADIOLOGIC FEATURES

Hamartomas are seen in any age group but are commonest in the pre and peri-menopausal woman. The

---

MAMMARY HAMARTOMA – FACT SHEET

Definition
▶ Benign breast lesion composed of a variety of breast constituents arranged in a disorganized manner

Incidence and Location
▶ Uncommon

Gender, Race and Age Distribution
▶ Seen in any age group, but commonest in pre and peri-menopausal women

Clinical Features
▶ As for fibroadenoma

Radiologic Features
▶ Well-defined mass which may be centrally lucent on mammography

Prognosis and Treatment
▶ These are benign lesions
▶ Surgical excision is curative

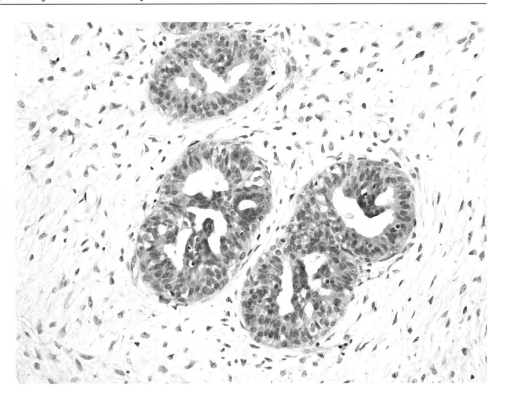

FIGURE 10-13
Juvenile fibroadenoma with gyneco-mastoid hyperplasia. Slender, tapering micropapillae project into the duct lumina. This is in contrast to the bulbous projections seen in atypical ductal hyperplasia.

clinical features are similar to those of a fibroadenoma. They present with a well-defined mobile mass or with a mammographically detected mass lesion which may be centrally lucent.

PATHOLOGIC FEATURES

GROSS FINDINGS

Hamartomas may vary in size but are typically a few centimeters in diameter. They are well-defined round masses with a rubbery fleshy cut surface and a gray or yellow color.

MICROSCOPIC FINDINGS

Breast hamartomas are composed of a variety of normal breast constituents with stroma surrounding duct and lobular structures (Figure 10-14A). These latter structures are disorganized with the lobules varying in size and merging with each other. The epithelial components are also microscopically normal with a single layer of epithelium overlying the myoepithelial component; epithelial hyperplasia is rare. The stromal portion of the lesion is often hyalinized and ill-defined, spreading around and through the lobular structures. Adipose tissue may be present; this may be prominent or, conversely, entirely absent. Smooth muscle may also be seen and such lesions in which this is marked have been classified as myoid hamartomas (Figure 10-14B).

MAMMARY HAMARTOMA – PATHOLOGIC FEATURES

Gross Findings
▶ Vary in size, typically a few centimeters in diameter
▶ Well-defined, round masses
▶ Rubbery, fleshy cut surface, gray or yellow in color

Microscopic Findings
▶ Disorganized ductal and lobular structures which vary in size and merge with each other
▶ Epithelial and myoepithelial layers; epithelial hyperplasia rare
▶ Surrounding stroma, often hyalinized with or without adipose tissue
▶ Smooth muscle may be seen

Ultrastructural Features
▶ N/A

Immunohistochemical Features
▶ N/A

Differential Diagnosis
▶ Fibroadenoma – more architectural organization seen and less cellular stroma
▶ Phyllodes tumor – cleft-like epithelial-lined spaces and more cellular stroma

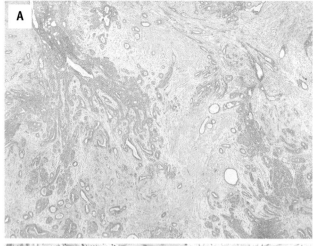

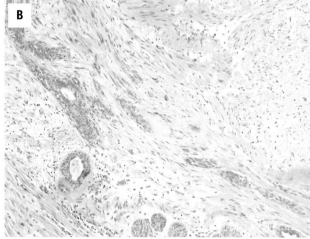

FIGURE 10-14
Myoid hamartoma. A variety of normal breast constituents are present with stroma surrounding disorganized duct and lobular structures. The epithelial components are microscopically normal. (B) Higher power view showing smooth muscle differentiation.

ANCILLARY STUDIES

Ancillary studies are rarely performed on these lesions. Immunohistochemistry can be undertaken to determine the extent of smooth muscle present but this is of no clinical importance.

DIFFERENTIAL DIAGNOSIS

The differential diagnosis of a hamartoma includes fibroadenoma and phyllodes tumor. Pragmatically, distinguishing a hamartoma from the former is not of great import; however, the hamartoma shows less architectural organization compared to the overall structure seen in the fibroadenoma, which also tends to have a less cellular stroma. Similarly, the stroma in the hamartoma is less cellular then in a phyllodes tumor and cleft-like epithelial-lined spaces are not seen.

PROGNOSIS AND THERAPY

Hamartomas are benign and excision is curative. Even if large, a good cosmetic result is invariably obtained. Exceptionally rarely, associated carcinoma in situ has been reported in these, as in other fibroepithelial lesions.

PHYLLODES TUMOR

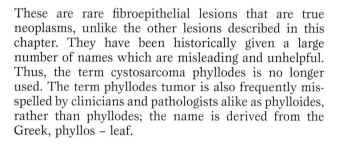

These are rare fibroepithelial lesions that are true neoplasms, unlike the other lesions described in this chapter. They have been historically given a large number of names which are misleading and unhelpful. Thus, the term cystosarcoma phyllodes is no longer used. The term phyllodes tumor is also frequently misspelled by clinicians and pathologists alike as phylloides, rather than phyllodes; the name is derived from the Greek, phyllos – leaf.

PHYLLODES TUMOR – FACT SHEET

Definition
▶ True fibroepithelial neoplasm composed of epithelial and stromal components

Incidence
▶ Rare, <1% of breast tumors

Gender, Race and Age Distribution
▶ Any age, but commonest in women in their 50s
▶ Rarely occur in young women

Clinical Features
▶ Rapidly growing but well-defined mass

Radiologic Features
▶ Well-defined mass on mammography
▶ Internal hyperechoic striations within a hypoechoic lesion on ultrasonography

Prognosis and Treatment
▶ Difficult to predict prognosis
▶ Vast majority benign
▶ 15–20% recur, depending upon completeness of excision
▶ Surgical excision with 10 mm margin of surrounding non-lesional tissue recommended in some centers
▶ Overt malignancy uncommon – high rates of recurrence reported in some series
▶ Metastases rare

CLINICAL AND RADIOLOGIC FEATURES

These are uncommon lesions which comprise less than 1% of breast tumors. They may occur at any age but are commonest in women in their 50s. While rare, they are described in young women, particularly in the Far East. Phyllodes tumors present typically with a rapidly growing but well-defined mass. Mammographically the lesion is also seen as a well-defined mass which on ultrasonography shows typical internal hyperechoic striations within a hypoechoic lesion.

PATHOLOGIC FEATURES

GROSS FINDINGS

Macroscopically phyllodes tumors vary in size from a few centimeters to 20 cm in diameter. They are well-defined, often lobulated lesions with a bosselated margin, although tongues of tumor may protrude into adjacent breast tissue. The most typical gross feature is the clefts seen on slicing within a tan or gray-brown whorled stroma. In malignant lesions the margin may be less well-defined and the clefts may be less obvious, particularly in forms with stromal overgrowth.

MICROSCOPIC FINDINGS

These are the quintessential fibroepithelial lesion; they are biphasic with clefts lined by a bilayer of epithelium and myoepithelium giving the leaf-like structures that contain a cellular stroma (Figure 10-15). The

---

PHYLLODES TUMOR – PATHOLOGIC FEATURES

Gross Findings
- Variable size from a few centimeters to 20 cm
- Well-defined, often lobulated; ill-defined in malignant lesions
- Cross-sectioning shows elongated clefts within a tan/gray-brown whorled stroma

Microscopic Findings
- Cellular stroma lined by an epithelial and myoepithelial bilayer, giving a leaf-like structure
- Benign lesions composed of cellular stroma, mild cytologic atypia and few mitoses (<5/10 HPF); margins well-defined; no stromal overgrowth
- Malignant lesions composed of markedly atypical stromal cells with abundant mitoses (>10/10 HPF); specific heterologous sarcomatous elements may be seen
- Borderline lesions composed of stroma with minimal to moderate cellular atypia with frequent mitoses (5–10/10 HPF); lack stromal overgrowth and infiltrative margins. Focal areas reminiscent of low grade fibrosarcoma may be seen

Ultrastructural Features
- N/A

Immunohistochemical Features
- Proliferation markers (e.g., MIB1) and other markers correlate with conventional classification but do not predict for recurrences and are not routinely used

Differential Diagnosis
- Benign phyllodes tumor: fibroadenoma and other benign fibroepithelial lesions
- Malignant phyllodes tumor: spindle cell metaplastic carcinoma – cytokeratins will stain constituent cells positive; pure sarcoma (make diagnosis with caution and only after extensive sampling)

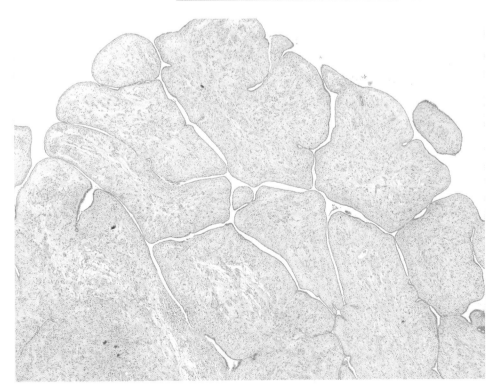

FIGURE 10-15

Phyllodes tumor. Low power view showing leaf-like structures.

stromal component is the important (neoplastic) portion of the lesion. A spectrum of appearances may be seen, varying from only slightly more cellular than that of a fibroadenoma, to frankly sarcomatous (Figure 10-16).

The majority of phyllodes tumors are benign and are composed of cellular stroma formed from spindled cells which are somewhat plump with mild cytologic atypia and few mitoses (less than 5 per 10 high power fields) (Figure 10-17). Occasional bizarre pleomorphic stromal

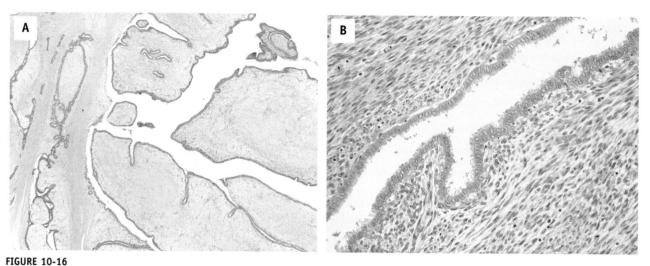

FIGURE 10-16

Phyllodes tumor. The stroma of a phyllodes tumor can vary from (A) slightly more cellular than a fibroadenoma with plumper stromal cells to (B) frankly sarcomatous.

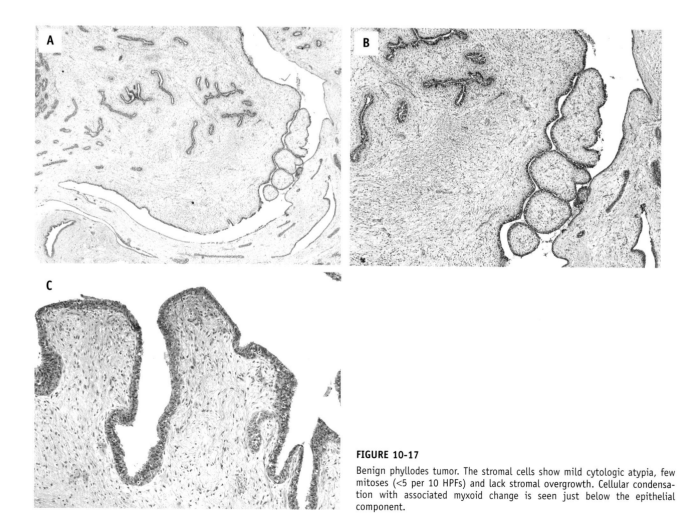

FIGURE 10-17

Benign phyllodes tumor. The stromal cells show mild cytologic atypia, few mitoses (<5 per 10 HPFs) and lack stromal overgrowth. Cellular condensation with associated myxoid change is seen just below the epithelial component.

cells may be seen but should not lead one to make the diagnosis of malignant phyllodes tumor in the absence of other features. The margin of the lesion is usually relatively well-defined and there is no stromal overgrowth.

At the other end of the phyllodes tumor spectrum are lesions composed of markedly atypical stromal cells with abundant mitoses (more than 10 per 10 high power fields) in which the stroma has out-grown the epithelial component and infiltrates into the adjacent parenchyma (Figure 10-18). Occasionally specific heterologous sarcomatous elements such as liposarcoma (Figure 10-19), chondrosarcoma or, indeed, osteosarcoma may be seen.

There is, however, a group of phyllodes tumors that cannot be readily consigned to the benign or the malignant categories. These lesions may show minimal to moderate stromal cell atypia without stromal overgrowth or infiltrative margins but in which mitoses are frequent (usually at least 5 per 10 high power fields) (Figure 10-20). Focal areas reminiscent of a low grade

fibrosarcoma may be seen, however, the majority of the stroma appears benign. These lesions are best classified as borderline phyllodes tumors.

In situ (ductal and lobular) and invasive carcinoma can occur in phyllodes tumor, although these changes are extremely rare (Figure 10-21).

ANCILLARY STUDIES

A number of studies have assessed a variety of immunohistochemical markers to attempt to describe methods of distinguishing cellular fibroadenomas from benign phyllodes tumors and to attempt to predict behaviour and more accurately classify phyllodes tumors. Proliferation indices using MIB1 monoclonal antibody to cell proliferation-associated Ki67 antigen have been used in

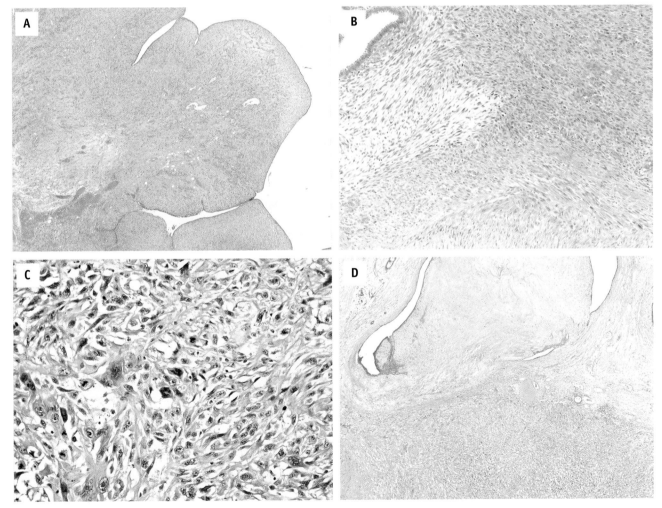

FIGURE 10-18

Malignant phyllodes tumor. (A) A well-defined leaf-like architecture with stromal overgrowth. The stroma predominates over the epithelial elements and is markedly hypercellular. (B) Malignant stroma showing a fibrosarcomatous appearance. (C) Marked cytologic atypia and abundant mitoses (>10 per 10 HPFs). (D) Heterogeneity is frequently seen within phyllodes tumors. Hyalinized stroma contrasts with the hypercellularity of the malignant stroma.

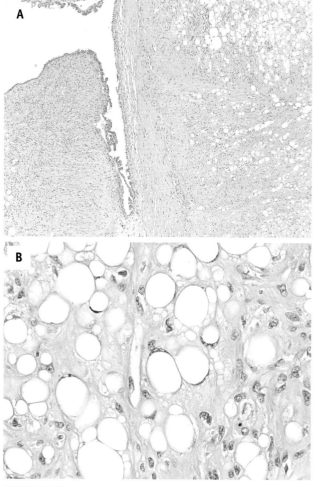

FIGURE 10-19

Malignant phyllodes tumor. (A) Liposarcomatous differentiation in a malignant phyllodes tumor. (B) High power view showing numerous lipoblasts.

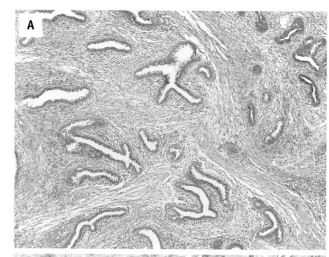

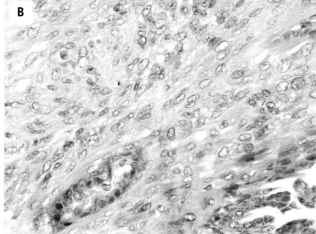

FIGURE 10-20

Borderline phyllodes tumor. (A) Medium power view showing stromal hypercellularity with (B) cytologic atypia. Mitoses are usually >5 per 10 HPFs. Stromal overgrowth and irregular margins are lacking.

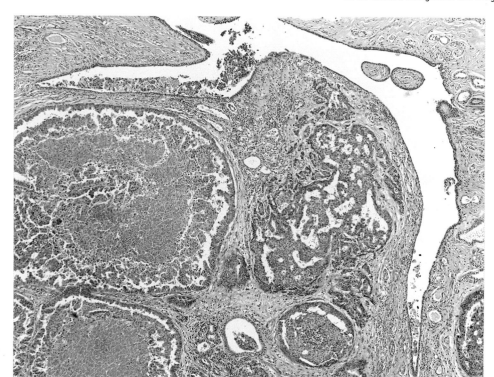

FIGURE 10-21

Ductal carcinoma in situ and invasive ductal carcinoma, no special type arising in a phyllodes tumor. The architecture of the underlying phyllodes tumor is recognizable but is extensively involved by invasive and in situ carcinoma.

study settings and show correlation with conventional classification. Many other markers, including p53, VEGF and CD10 have also been shown to correlate with categorization into benign, borderline and malignant categories. These have, however, not proven to be of practical help for diagnostic use. Similarly, although series have examined phyllodes tumors by flow cytometry and evaluated DNA ploidy and S-phase fraction, these do not add significantly to predicting outcome of these lesions.

DIFFERENTIAL DIAGNOSIS

As described above, the differential diagnosis of phyllodes tumor is, at one end of the spectrum, fibroadenoma and other benign fibroepithelial lesions. At the other end of the spectrum, malignant phyllodes tumors must be distinguished from metaplastic carcinoma and rarely, primary sarcomas of the breast. The differentiating features are described in Tables 10.1 and 10.2. In

TABLE 10-1

Features of fibroadenoma versus benign phyllodes tumor

Features	Fibroadenoma	Benign phyllodes tumor
Age distribution	Peak age 30 years	Peak age 50 years
Average size	1–3 cm, rarely up to 20 cm	Few cm up to 20 cm Rapidly growing
Gross appearance	Round/ovoid; gray Rubbery, lobulated cut surface Slit-like spaces	Well-defined, often lobulated Tan/gray whorled cut surface Elongated clefts
Margins	Circumscribed	Well-defined
Leaf-like architecture	Usually absent, may be focal	Well-formed
Cellularity (stroma)	Hypocellular* ± hyalinized	Cellular
Cellular atypia (stroma)	Absent	Mild
Mitoses	Rare	Few (<5/10 HPFs)
Recurrence rates	Some recur	15–20%

*Cellular fibroadenomas show a hypercellular stroma

TABLE 10-2

Features of benign, borderline and malignant phyllodes tumor (PT)

Features	Benign PT	Borderline PT	Malignant PT
Margins	Well-defined	Well-defined	Infiltrative
Cellularity	Cellular	Cellular	Cellular
Cellular atypia	Mild	Mild–moderate	Marked
Mitoses	Few (<5/10 HPFs)	Frequent (5–10/10 HPFs)	Abundant (>10/10 HPFs)
Stromal overgrowth	Absent	Absent	Often present
Heterologous elements	Absent	Absent	May be present

metaplastic carcinomas the malignant epithelial component tends to merge with the spindle cell element; whereas in phyllodes tumor, the epithelial component is benign and remains discrete from the spindle cell component. Cytokeratin immunohistochemistry can be particularly useful in highlighting the malignant epithelial spindle cells in metaplastic carcinoma.

Pure primary sarcomas of the breast are rare and include malignant fibrous histiocytoma, liposarcoma, leiomyosarcoma and, the exceptionally rare, osteosarcoma. The diagnosis of a pure sarcoma should only be made after thorough sampling of the lesion, as stromal overgrowth in a phyllodes tumor may result in the epithelial elements being very focal. Many lesions that have been reported as primary breast sarcoma represent malignant phyllodes tumor in which the epithelial elements have been missed. In addition, when phyllodes tumor recurs, it can do so as pure sarcoma, without epithelial elements; therefore, a history of a previous phyllodes tumor should be sought.

PROGNOSIS AND THERAPY

It is difficult to draw conclusions on the prognosis of phyllodes tumors from the literature as a variety of systems for classification have been used and in some series there appears to be an unlikely excess of malignant lesions. It should be re-iterated, that the vast majority of phyllodes tumors are benign and that the risk to the patient is of local recurrence rather than metastatic disease. In the vast majority of series, no metastatic disease and no deaths from benign phyllodes tumor are reported. The most powerful predictor of local recurrence is completeness of excision. Complete local excision is thus recommended for all phyllodes tumors with a rim of surrounding uninvolved breast tissue. In some centers a 10 mm margin of surrounding benign tissue is taken from around all phyllodes tumors, whether benign, borderline or malignant. However, this is not routine in all centers, particularly for lesions at the benign end of the spectrum. The data on rates of local recurrence are somewhat biased but approximately

15–20 % of lesions appear to recur; this figure is dependent on the adequacy of initial excision. Most local recurrences can be treated surgically, with malignant transformation being exceptionally rare. Similarly, most patients with local recurrences do not develop distant metastases.

The management of overtly malignant phyllodes tumors is difficult. High rates of local recurrence are reported in some series; although this ranges from a few percent to 60 % of patients with malignant lesions developing local recurrence of disease. Some groups would thus recommend mastectomy if a diagnosis of a malignant phyllodes tumor is made.

Review of the literature indicates that the likelihood of metastatic disease is, to some extent, related to overgrowth and cellularity of the stroma, as well as stromal cytologic atypia and mitotic frequency and, in some series, by the presence of necrosis. The reported rate of metastasis and death due to malignant phyllodes tumors varies enormously; from 0 % to 40 % for both metastasis and death.

SUGGESTED READINGS

Carter BA, Page DL, Schuyler P, *et al.* No elevation in long-term breast carcinoma risk for women with fibroadenomas that contain atypical hyperplasia. Cancer 2001;92:30–36.

Carter CL, Corle DK, Micozzi MS, *et al.* A prospective study of the development of breast cancer in 16,692 women with benign breast disease. Am J Epidemiol 1988;128:467–477

Diaz NM, Palmer JO, McDivitt RW. Carcinoma arising within fibroadenomas of the breast. A clinicopathologic study of 105 patients. Am J Clin Pathol 1991;95:614–622.

Dupont WD, Page DL, Parl FF, *et al.* Long-term risk of breast cancer in women with fibroadenoma. N Engl J Med 1994;331:10–15.

Elston CW, Ellis IO. Fibroadenoma and related conditions. In Elston CW, Ellis IO eds. The Breast Systemic Pathology Volume 13. Edinburgh: Churchill-Livingstone, 1998:147–186.

Fechner RE. Fibroadenoma and related lesions. In Page DL, Anderson TJ, eds. In Diagnostic Histopathology of the Breast. Edinburgh: Churchill Livingstone; 1987:72–85.

Rosen PP. Fibroepithelial Neoplasms. In Rosen's Breast Pathology, 2nd ed. Philadelphia: Lippincott-Williams and Wilkins; 2001:163–200.

Moffat CJ, Pinder SE, Dixon AR, *et al.* Phyllodes tumours of the breast: a clinicopathological review of thirty-two cases. Histopathology 1995;27:205–218.

11 Benign Stromal Lesions of the Breast

Frances P. O'Malley · Anita Bane · AM Mulligan · Sarah E. Pinder

INTRODUCTION

This chapter describes benign non-neoplastic and neoplastic entities that arise in the stroma of the breast. We focus on the most common lesions, but also describe some unusual lesions that present with characteristic findings. Pseudoangiomatous stromal hyperplasia (PASH) is a non-neoplastic lesion that can cause diagnostic problems. Amyloid, which occurs extremely rarely in the breast, enters into the differential diagnosis of stromal elastosis. Neoplastic lesions that are discussed are fibromatosis, a tumor that can behave in a locally aggressive fashion, and myofibroblastoma, an uncommon neoplasm that was initially thought to occur only in males, but has now been described in females. We briefly describe vascular lesions including hemangioma, angiomatosis and hemangiopericytoma. Granular cell tumors are addressed, highlighting the wide range of lesions that enter into the differential diagnosis of this rare benign tumor.

NON-NEOPLASTIC LESIONS

PSEUDOANGIOMATOUS STROMAL HYPERPLASIA

CLINICAL FEATURES

Pseudoangiomatous stromal hyperplasia is a distinct stromal lesion that was first described approximately 20 years ago. It generally occurs in pre-menopausal women, but has been reported in post-menopausal women who are on hormone replacement therapy. Several cases in males have also been described in association with gynecomastia. Most commonly PASH occurs as an incidental finding adjacent to other benign or malignant breast lesions but can present as a discrete, painless, mobile mass, clinically indistinguishable from a fibroadenoma. Occasionally, it can cause diffuse

enlargement of the breast. Rarely, peau d'orange and skin necrosis can develop when the lesion grows rapidly during pregnancy.

RADIOLOGIC FEATURES

Radiologically, PASH appears as a mass, not associated with calcification. The borders of the mass are usually well-circumscribed. Ultrasound examination reveals a well-defined hypoechoic lesion.

PATHOLOGIC FEATURES

GROSS FINDINGS

The lesion, ranging in size from 1 to approximately 7 cm, is firm and rubbery with a smooth external surface. The cut surface consists of homogeneous, fibrous, tan tissue.

MICROSCOPIC FINDINGS

PASH consists of anastomizing, angulated and slit-like spaces lined by slender spindle cells within a background of dense collagenous tissue (Figure 11-1). These characteristic findings are readily apparent under low power. The spindle cells lining the spaces are bland, showing no mitotic activity and the spaces are empty or contain an occasional red blood cell (Figure 11-2). The

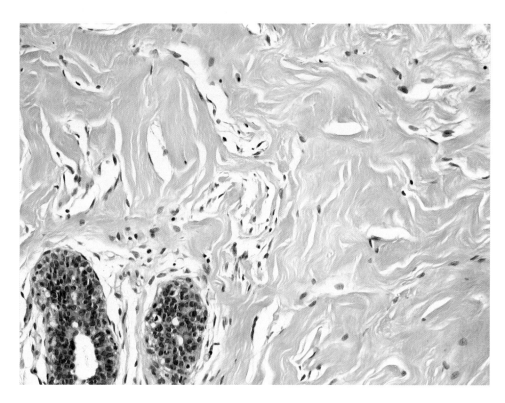

FIGURE 11-1
Pseudoangiomatous stromal hyperplasia (PASH). Medium power view showing anastomizing, angulated and slit-like spaces in a background of dense collagenous tissue.

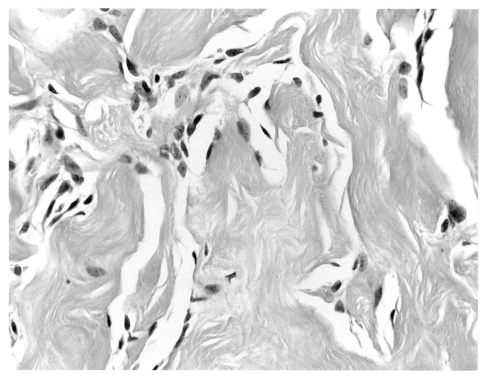

FIGURE 11-2
Pseudoangiomatous stromal hyperplasia (PASH). High power view showing bland, slender spindle cells lining the spaces. Mitotic activity is absent. The spaces are empty, or can contain an occasional red blood cell.

collagen and slit-like spaces extend into intralobular spaces. True vascular channels can be seen within the stroma.

ANCILLARY STUDIES

ULTRASTRUCTURAL FEATURES

The spindle cells have the ultrastructural characteristic of myofibroblasts, containing elongated cytoplasmic processes, a well-developed endoplasmic reticulum and a prominent Golgi apparatus. The intervening stroma consists of collagen fibrils.

IMMUNOHISTOCHEMISTRY

The myofibroblastic spindle cells lining the slit-like spaces are positive for vimentin, CD34 and actin and are uniformly negative for endothelial cell markers such as CD31 or factor VIII. They may show immunoreactivity for progesterone receptor (PR), but are negative for epithelial markers.

FINE NEEDLE ASPIRATION CYTOLOGY

Generally, a fine needle aspirate will yield a non-diagnostic or paucicellular specimen. The latter may contain bipolar spindle cells and scattered benign epithelial cells.

DIFFERENTIAL DIAGNOSIS

The most important differential diagnosis is low grade angiosarcoma. This is discussed in detail in Chapter 26. The relatively well-circumscribed appearance of PASH, lack of nuclear atypia, mitotic activity or destruction of breast ducts and lobules, as well as the lack of true vascular spaces, distinguish PASH from low grade angiosarcoma.

PROGNOSIS AND TREATMENT

Wide local excision is the treatment of choice. Recurrences may develop particularly if excision is incomplete.

OTHER NON-NEOPLASTIC LESIONS

Amyloid, which can be primary or secondary, has rarely been reported in the breast. It typically presents as a clinically or mammographically suspicious mass in an elderly woman. Microscopically, it is seen as an extracellular, homogeneous, eosinophilic substance in the fat, stroma and walls of ducts and vessels, which reveals apple green birefringence under polarized light on a Congo red stain. Excisional biopsy of primary amyloid is curative. The prognosis of secondary amyloid depends on the underlying systemic disease.

The main differential diagnosis of amyloid is stromal elastosis, which is the occurrence of abundant elastic fibers in the breast stroma. Elastosis can occur in an otherwise normal breast and appears to be associated with increasing age, although in this scenario, the elastic fibers are usually present in a periductal rather than stromal location. There are several benign lesions that may exhibit prominent stromal elastosis, such as radial scars/complex sclerosing lesions, and stromal elastosis may often accompany breast carcinoma. In the vast majority of these cases differentiating stromal elastosis from amyloid deposition is relatively easy. In difficult cases, the presence of stromal elastosis can be confirmed by highlighting the elastic fibers with an elastic stain such as the Verhoeff stain.

BENIGN NEOPLASTIC STROMAL LESIONS

FIBROMATOSIS

CLINICAL FEATURES

Fibromatosis is an infiltrating fibroblastic and myo-fibroblastic proliferation that can behave in a locally aggressive fashion if incompletely excised. However, it is not known to metastasize. It presents predominantly as a unilateral, painless, palpable, firm to hard mass which may be accompanied by skin dimpling and nipple retraction. Fibromatosis can occur at any age, most commonly in the forties, but cases have been reported in patients ranging from 13–80 years. It occasionally occurs as part of Gardner syndrome. There is a rare association with pregnancy, although hormonal factors are not thought to be important in the pathogenesis of the disease. There is a history of trauma in some cases.

FIBROMATOSIS – FACT SHEET

Definition
▶ An infiltrating spindle-cell proliferation composed of fibroblastic and myofibroblastic cells

Incidence and Location
▶ Rare
▶ Can occur in any quadrant. Rarely occurs in the sub-areolar region or the axillary tail

Age Distribution
▶ Age ranges varies from 13–80 years
▶ Most common in early to mid 40s

Clinical Features
▶ Usually presents as a painless, firm or hard mass
▶ Dimpling or retraction of the overlying skin can occur
▶ Occasionally occurs as part of Gardner syndrome
▶ Rare association with pregnancy, although hormonal factors are not thought to be important in the pathogenesis of the disease
▶ There is a history of trauma in some cases

Radiologic Features
▶ Typically appears as a stellate mass, resembling carcinoma
▶ Rarely the lesion presents with dense mammographic calcifications

Prognosis and Treatment
▶ Local recurrence occurs in up to 27 % of cases
▶ There are no histologic features that can help predict recurrence
▶ Wide local excision is the treatment of choice
▶ Hormonal therapy is of undetermined value

RADIOLOGIC FEATURES

Mammography may not reveal any abnormality, although a stellate lesion that mimics carcinoma may be identified. Rarely the lesion presents with dense mammographic calcifications.

PATHOLOGIC FEATURES

GROSS FINDINGS

The margins of the lesion are infiltrative and difficult to discern on gross examination. The cut surface reveals a firm consistency that is gray-yellow to gray-white in

---

FIBROMATOSIS – PATHOLOGIC FEATURES

Gross Findings
▶ Irregular, firm area of white/tan fibrous tissue
▶ Occasionally may produce well-circumscribed nodules
▶ There is a wide variation in size, ranging from <1 cm to 10 cm

Microscopic Findings
▶ Cells are spindle-shaped with oval or spindled, regular nuclei. There is minimal nuclear pleomorphism
▶ The cells are arranged in broad sheets or, occasionally, in a storiform or herringbone pattern
▶ Myxoid change or calcifications may be present
▶ There may be moderate to abundant deposition of collagen
▶ Mitoses are uncommon (<3/10 HPF)
▶ Lymphocytic infiltration is present at the periphery of the lesion in approximately 50 % of cases

Ultrastructural Features
▶ The spindle cells are composed of an admixture of fibroblasts with prominent rough endoplasmic reticulum, and myofibroblasts with intracytoplasmic myofibrils and dense bodies

Fine Needle Aspiration Biopsy Findings
▶ Usually of limited cellularity
▶ Uniform spindle cells are present in small clusters or dispersed singly
▶ Benign epithelial cells and lymphocytes may be present in the background

Immunohistochemical Features
▶ The cells stain positively with vimentin and may be positive with actin but are negative for cytokeratins, S100 protein, desmin, estrogen and progesterone receptors

Differential Diagnosis
▶ Scars from areas of healed fat necrosis or previous surgery
▶ Nodular fasciitis
▶ Myofibroblastoma
▶ Metaplastic carcinoma
▶ Fibrosarcoma
▶ Malignant fibrous histiocytoma

color. The lesion may range in size from less than 1 cm to greater than 10 cm.

MICROSCOPIC FINDINGS

Fibromatosis is characterized by bland spindle-shaped or oval cells (Figure 11-3B) arranged in broad sheets or fascicles and interlacing bundles, producing a storiform or herringbone pattern (Figure 11-3A). Myxoid change or calcifications may be present and there may be moderate to abundant deposition of collagen. The lesion irregularly infiltrates the adjacent breast parenchyma (Figure 11-4) and a lymphocytic infiltrate is present at the periphery of the lesion in approximately 50% of cases. Cellular atypia is classically absent and mitoses are uncommon with <3 mitoses per 10 HPF identified. Mitoses, if present, are more likely to be observed at the leading edge of the proliferation.

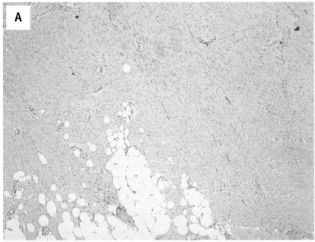
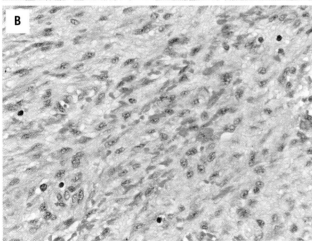

FIGURE 11-3

Fibromatosis. (A) Low power view showing sheets and fascicles of spindle cells in a mixed collagenous and myxoid stroma. (B) High power view showing bland spindle to oval cells, lacking atypia. Mitoses are uncommon (<3/10 HPF).

ANCILLARY STUDIES

ULTRASTRUCTURAL FEATURES

Fibromatosis consists of an admixture of fibroblasts, containing prominent rough endoplasmic reticulum, and myofibroblasts with intracytoplasmic myofibrils and dense bodies.

IMMUNOHISTOCHEMISTRY

The cells stain with vimentin (Figure 11-5) and may be positive with actin. They are uniformly negative for cytokeratins, S-100 protein, desmin and are usually negative for estrogen and progesterone receptors.

FINE NEEDLE ASPIRATION CYTOLOGY

The aspirates are usually of limited cellularity. Uniform spindle cells are dispersed singly or in clusters. Benign epithelial cells and lymphocytes may be present in the background.

DIFFERENTIAL DIAGNOSIS

It is important to distinguish fibromatosis from, at one end of the spectrum, benign lesions that have no potential to recur, and, at the other end of the spectrum, malignant lesions that may metastasize. A benign process that can mimic fibromatosis is a scar from an area of healed fat necrosis or surgery. Obtaining a history of previous surgery can be very helpful, although histologic clues, such as suture granulomata, may aid in the differential diagnosis. It may be particularly difficult to determine the presence of recurrence of fibromatosis after surgery. In this case one may need to rely on the extent of the lesion as indicating recurrence rather than reactive changes related to the surgery.

Nodular fasciitis may be difficult to differentiate from fibromatosis, although the more diffuse distribution of the inflammatory infiltrate in nodular fasciitis in contrast to the peripheral location of the inflammatory infiltrate in fibromatosis is a helpful distinguishing feature. In addition, nodular fasciitis is more mitotically active and more closely resembles granulation tissue. Also, the margins of nodular fasciitis are more circumscribed than one sees in fibromatosis.

Myofibroblastoma usually exhibits a circumscribed, non-infiltrative margin and contains thick bands of collagen in contrast to the interlacing fascicles of spindle cells that characterize fibromatosis.

Spindle-cell metaplastic carcinoma is an important malignant tumor that can mimic fibromatosis, particularly if the nuclei show only mild to moderate nuclear atypia. The recently described low grade metaplastic carcinoma with fibromatosis-like stroma can be exceedingly challenging to diagnose. Thus a low threshold for immunohistochemistry, including cytokeratin panels (34βE12, AE1/AE3), as well as p63, is required.

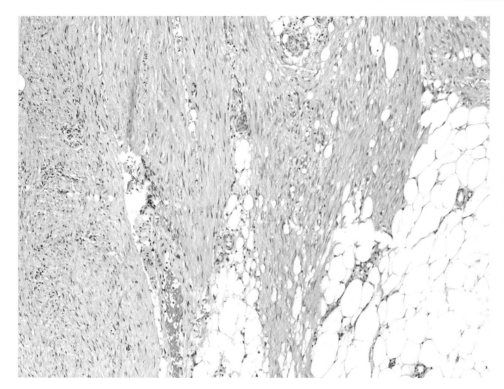

FIGURE 11-4

Fibromatosis. The margins are irregular with infiltration of the adjacent breast parenchyma and fat.

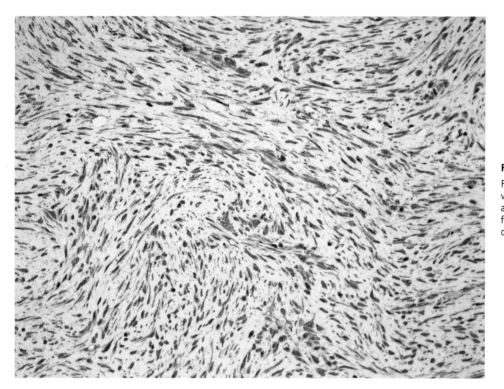

FIGURE 11-5

Fibromatosis. The cells stain with vimentin and may be positive with actin. They are uniformly negative for cytokeratins, S100 protein and desmin.

Fibrosarcoma can be distinguished from fibromatosis on the basis of greater cellularity, a significant degree of nuclear pleomorphism and abundant mitotic activity. Necrosis may also be evident in these lesions. Malignant fibrous histiocytoma, particularly if the lesion demonstrates storiform areas, is another rare entity that should be considered in the differential diagnosis. Like fibrosarcoma, these tumors demonstrate a greater degree of nuclear pleomorphism, cellularity and mitotic activity than fibromatosis.

TREATMENT AND PROGNOSIS

Wide local excision is the treatment of choice, although up to 27 % of lesions recur. Recurrences generally occur in the first 5 years. There are no histologic features that can help predict recurrence. Hormonal therapy is of undetermined value.

MYOFIBROBLASTOMA

Mammary myofibroblastoma is a rare benign tumor that is thought to arise from fibroblasts of the mammary stroma that are capable of multi-dimensional mesenchymal differentiation.

CLINICAL FEATURES

It presents as a solitary slowly growing painless mass in the breasts of men and women, aged between 40 and 87 years. The earlier reports showed an apparent predilection for older male patients. However, likely because of mammographic screening, lesions appear to occur at least as frequently in female patients. Multicentric and bilateral tumors have been reported.

RADIOLOGIC FEATURES

Radiologically these are well-circumscribed, often lobulated tumors devoid of microcalcifications.

MYOFIBROBLASTOMA – FACT SHEET

Definition
▶ These are benign mesenchymal lesions most likely derived from mammary stromal fibroblasts

Incidence and Location
▶ Rare lesions showing no reported predilection for any specific breast quadrant

Gender, Race and Age Distribution
▶ Occurs in males and females

Clinical Features
▶ Slowly growing painless mass

Radiologic Features
▶ Well-circumscribed mass lesion, devoid of calcifications

Prognosis and Treatment
▶ Local excision with clear margins is curative

PATHOLOGIC FEATURES

GROSS FINDINGS

Myofibroblastoma is characteristically a well-circumscribed tumor ranging in size from <1 cm to 10 cm. The mass is firm and rubbery with a bulging gray to white, whorled cut surface.

MICROSCOPIC FINDINGS

The tumor is generally well-circumscribed and composed of an admixture of oval to spindle-shaped cells arranged in fascicles and thick bands of eosinophilic collagen (Figure 11-6). The spindle cell tends to have elongated bland nuclei with eosinophilic cytoplasm and ill-defined cell borders. Necrosis is absent and mitoses are rare (<2 per 10 HPF). The tumor generally has a fatty component of variable extent. Scattered mast cells may be seen.

MYOFIBROBLASTOMA – PATHOLOGIC FEATURES

Gross Findings
▶ Circumscribed tumor mass of variable size
▶ Firm and rubbery with a white 'whorled' cut surface

Microscopic Findings
▶ Circumscribed edge
▶ Bland spindle cells arranged in fascicles
▶ Admixed thick, hyalinized collagen bands
▶ Variable admixture of adipose tissue and mast cells
▶ Necrosis is not present
▶ <2 mitoses per 10 HPF

Ultrastructural Features
▶ Myofibroblasts contain actin-like myofilaments and focal dense bodies

Fine Needle Aspiration Biopsy Findings
▶ Cellular specimens with bipolar spindle cells
▶ Cytologically bland nuclei with grooves

Immunohistochemical Features
▶ Positive immunoreactivity in the spindle cells for actin, desmin, CD34 and vimentin
▶ Estrogen, progesterone and androgen receptor positivity have been reported

Differential Diagnosis
▶ Fibromatosis
▶ Nodular fasciitis
▶ Spindle cell lipoma
▶ Metaplastic carcinoma
▶ Low-grade sarcoma

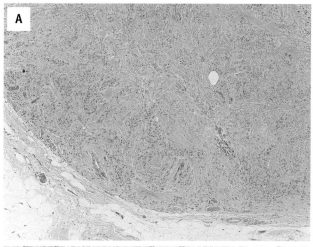

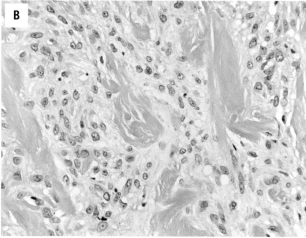

FIGURE 11-6

Myofibroblastoma. (A) Low power view showing a well-circumscribed tumor, composed of fascicles of spindle to oval cells with intervening thick bands of collagen. (B) Higher power shows the cells to have elongated bland nuclei with eosinophilc cytoplasm and ill-defined cell borders. Mitoses are rare (<2/10 HPF).

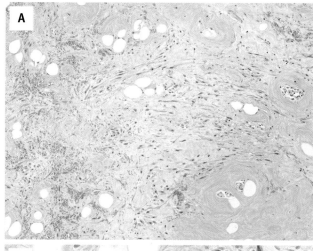

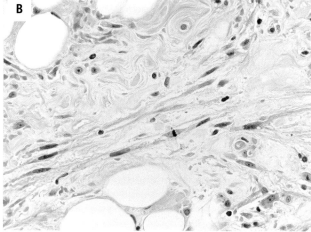

FIGURE 11-7

Nodular fasciitis. (A) Medium power showing a variably cellular infiltrate with prominent red blood cell extravasation. (B) Higher power shows spindle to round cells with frequent mitoses, embedded in a tissue culture-like stroma.

ANCILLARY STUDIES

ULTRASTRUCTURAL FEATURES

The myofibroblasts contain actin-like microfilaments measuring 5–7 nm in diameter, with focal dense bodies.

IMMUNOHISTOCHEMISTRY

Myofibroblasts show immunoreactivity for vimentin, smooth muscle actin, desmin and CD34. Estrogen receptor, progesterone receptor and androgen receptor positivity have also been reported.

FINE NEEDLE ASPIRATION CYTOLOGY

Myofibroblastomas often yield cellular aspirates composed of fascicles of bipolar spindle cells with smooth nuclear outlines, finely granular evenly dispersed chromatin and nuclear grooves.

DIFFERENTIAL DIAGNOSIS

Benign lesions that should be distinguished from myofibroblastomas include fibromatosis, nodular fasciitis and spindle cell lipoma. At the malignant end of the spectrum the major differential includes metaplastic carcinoma and low-grade sarcoma.

Fibromatosis can be distinguished from myofibroblastoma by its infiltrative margins and long, slender fascicles embedded in a variable amount of fibrous stroma as previously described. Fibromatosis may be actin positive but is negative for desmin and CD34.

Nodular fasciitis is characterized by spindle to round plump cells with frequent mitoses, embedded within a myxoid, tissue culture-like stroma, containing an inflammatory lymphocytic component, extravasated red blood cells and foci of microcystic change (Figure 11-7). Lesional cells tend to be diffusely positive for actin, may show focal CD34 positivity, but are generally negative for desmin.

Spindle cell lipoma is composed of a population of bland spindle cells with intervening ropey bundles of collagen and variable amounts of admixed adipose tissue. This lesion tends to have more admixed fat than myofibroblastoma and the spindle cells are positive for CD34 but generally negative for actin and desmin. A recent finding that myofibroblastoma shares the same cytogenetic abnormalities previously considered characteristic of spindle cell lipoma (13q deletion and 16q deletion) raises the possibility that the two lesions are related.

Difficulty may also arise in distinguishing myofibroblastoma from spindle cell metaplastic carcinoma although the margins of metaplastic carcinoma are infiltrative. As discussed previously a cytokeratin panel can be particularly useful in differentiating these lesions.

Low-grade fibrosarcoma/malignant fibrous histiocytomas are composed of spindled cell with variable cytologic atypia, with a herringbone and/or storiform growth pattern with possible admixed histiocytes and multinucleated giant cells. Immunohistochemistry reveals diffuse vimentin staining with only focal smooth muscle actin and CD34 positivity.

TREATMENT AND PROGNOSIS

Local excision with clear margins is curative. Recurrences or metastases have not been reported.

BENIGN VASCULAR LESIONS OF THE BREAST

HEMANGIOMA

CLINICAL FEATURES

Hemangiomas may occur in males or females with a wide age range (18 months to 82 years). They may present as palpable mass lesions, imaging-detected abnormalities or as incidental findings (perilobular hemangiomas) in benign breast biopsies.

RADIOLOGIC FEATURES

Capillary hemangiomas display a well-defined, lobulated heterogeneous appearance on mammography.

Ultrasound of such lesions reveals a hypoechoic solid lesion.

PATHOLOGIC FEATURES

GROSS FINDINGS

The majority of clinically apparent lesions are well circumscribed with a reddish brown spongy appearance. They vary in size from 0.4–2 cm.

MICROSCOPIC FINDINGS

Symptomatic hemangiomas may be of the cavernous, capillary or venous subtype.

Cavernous hemangiomas consist of a mesh of dilated thin-walled vessels lined by flattened endothelial cells. Blood or thromboses distend the vessels (Figure 11-8).

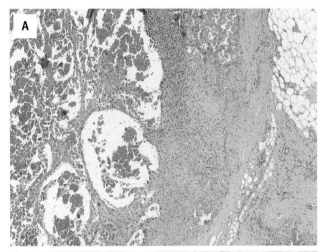

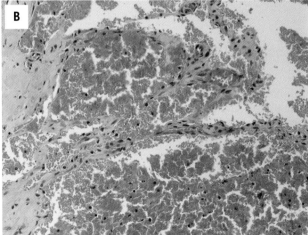

FIGURE 11-8

Hemangioma. (A) Low power view of a cavernous hemangioma showing a mesh of dilated thin-walled vessels containing blood. (B) Higher power showing vascular channels lined by endothelial cells, some of which have hyperchromatic nuclei. Papillary endothelial hyperplasia is not a feature. Mitoses are absent.

Capillary hemangiomas consist of a collection of small vessels in a lobular configuration arranged around a central feeding vessel. The endothelial cells lining the vessels may have hyperchromatic nuclei. Venous hemangiomas consist of vessels with muscular walls of varying thickness. Incidental, perilobular hemangiomas contain thin-walled vessels lined by flattened endothelial cells arranged in a haphazard manner in the interlobular stroma. Extension into the adjacent adipose tissue may be seen.

ANCILLARY STUDIES

IMMUNOHISTOCHEMISTRY

The endothelial cells stain for CD31 and factor VIII.

DIFFERENTIAL DIAGNOSIS

As the majority of vascular lesions arising in the breast (rather than in the overlying skin), are malignant, angiosarcoma is the most important lesion in the differential diagnosis. Angiosarcomas are composed of vessels of varying caliber exhibiting an anastomosing growth pattern with infiltrative borders. There is usually papillary endothelial hyperplasia with variable degrees of nuclear atypia and increased mitotic activity.

Atypical hemangiomas are usually small, are relatively well-circumscribed and are composed of broadly anastomosing vascular channels. In contrast to hemangiomas, they may demonstrate mild nuclear atypia, but lack overt histologic characteristics of angiosarcoma as described above.

PROGNOSIS AND TREATMENT

Complete excision is warranted with careful examination to rule out low grade angiosarcoma. Recurrences are not reported.

ANGIOMATOSIS

CLINICAL FEATURES

Angiomatosis is a rare lesion presenting as a breast mass. Most cases have been described in women between 19 and 61 years. However, it can occur at birth.

PATHOLOGIC FEATURES

GROSS FINDINGS

This usually presents as a poorly circumscribed mass, but it may not have an obvious vascular appearance. Size is variable, with the largest documented case measuring 22 cm.

MICROSCOPIC FINDINGS

It is composed of thin-walled, small to large caliber blood or lymphatic vessels, which diffusely extend into the breast parenchyma. Intralobular growth is not evident.

DIFFERENTIAL DIAGNOSIS

Angiomatosis may be very difficult to differentiate from low grade angiosarcoma. However, there is no evidence of endothelial atypia in angiomatosis and lobules are not disrupted.

TREATMENT AND PROGNOSIS

As these lesions can locally recur, complete excision with long-term follow-up is recommended.

HEMANGIOPERICYTOMA

CLINICAL FEATURES

Presentation is usually as a mass lesion. Patients are usually women aged between 22 and 67 years, but it has been described in a young boy.

PATHOLOGIC FEATURES

GROSS FINDINGS

Hemangiopericytomas are well-circumscribed, firm lesions ranging in size from 1–19 cm. The cut surface is pale gray to pink, predominantly solid with focal cystic or myxoid areas.

MICROSCOPIC FINDINGS

The tumor is composed of closely packed, spindle shaped cells with indistinct cell margins arranged around thin-walled irregular branching vessels. The latter may have a 'staghorn' configuration (Figure 11-9).

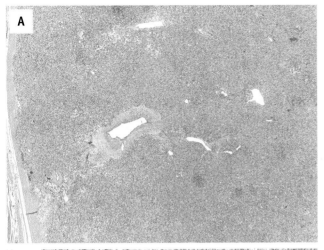

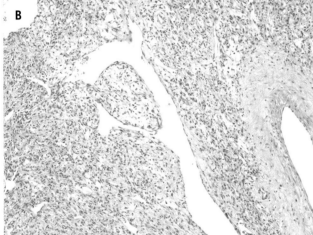

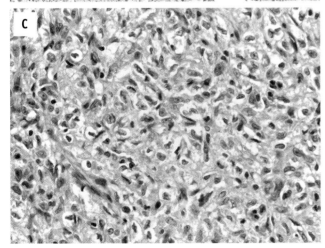

FIGURE 11-9

Hemangiopericytoma. (A) Low power view showing a well-circumscribed, cellular lesion with prominent thin-walled vessels, many of which (B) show a 'staghorn' (irregular branching) configuration. (C) High power view showing spindle shaped cells with indistinct cell margins.

ANCILLARY STUDIES

ULTRASTRUCTURAL FEATURES

Electron microscopy shows an admixture of pericytes and endothelial cells. The former are characterized by an incomplete basal lamina and the presence of complex cytoplasmic processes with pinocytotic vesicles.

IMMUNOHISTOCHEMISTRY

The spindle cells are vimentin and actin positive and the endothelial cells stain with CD31, CD34 and factor VIII. A reticulin stain outlines the spindle cells and vascular spaces.

FINE NEEDLE ASPIRATION CYTOLOGY

Aspiration cytology shows clumps of spindle cells with abundant capillaries. However, these findings are not specific.

PROGNOSIS AND TREATMENT

Complete excision is recommended. A 'high grade' variant, characterized by mitotic activity (>5 mitoses per 10 HPF) and necrosis is recognized and potentially may recur or metastasize.

BENIGN GRANULAR CELL TUMOR

BENIGN GRANULAR CELL TUMOR – FACT SHEET

Definition
▶ A neoplastic proliferation of cells derived from Schwann cells of peripheral nerves

Gender, Race and Age Distribution
▶ Occurs predominantly in women between 30 and 50 years
▶ Approximately 10 % of cases occur in males

Clinical Features
▶ Generally presents as a firm, painless mass
▶ Can occur anywhere in the breast parenchyma, axillary tail or in the subcutaneous tissue
▶ Occasionally nipple inversion or skin retraction can be associated with superficial lesions

Radiologic Features
▶ Typically produces a stellate mass that is difficult to distinguish from a carcinoma
▶ Calcifications are generally absent

Prognosis and Treatment
▶ Treatment involves wide local excision
▶ Local recurrence may occur if the lesion has been incompletely excised
▶ <1 % of all granular cell tumors are malignant. Wide local excision is also the treatment of choice for malignant lesions. There does not appear to be a role for chemotherapy or radiotherapy

CLINICAL FEATURES

This uncommon tumor of putative Schwann cell origin, frequently simulates carcinoma, both clinically and radiologically. It occurs in both males and females over a wide age range, 17–73 years, but is most common in middle-aged women. The tumor presents as a slowly growing painless mass and, while the lesions are usually solitary, multifocal and bilateral cases have been reported. The tumor can arise anywhere within the breast.

RADIOLOGIC FEATURES

Mammography reveals a mass lesion, which can be stellate or well-circumscribed, but is usually devoid of calcifications. Ultrasonography confirms a hypoechoic mass with acoustic shadowing.

PATHOLOGIC FEATURES

BENIGN GRANULAR CELL TUMOR – PATHOLOGIC FEATURES

Gross Findings
▸ These lesions present as a firm or hard mass
▸ The borders of the mass may be ill-defined or well-circumscribed
▸ The cut surface is white/gray or yellow/tan
▸ The mass is usually <2 cm in maximum dimension

Microscopic Findings
▸ The tumor is composed of solid nests or sheets of cells with abundant eosinophilic cytoplasmic granules which are diastase resistant and PAS positive
▸ The cells are large and round or polygonal in shape
▸ Mitotic activity is generally absent
▸ The cells have prominent nucleoli and moderate nuclear atypia may be present
▸ The cells often encompass small nerves
▸ The margins of the lesion are infiltrative

Ultrastructural Features
▸ The cells contain myelin figures and numerous lysosomes
▸ Some cells may contain triangular membrane-bound structures composed of microtubules and microfibrils

Fine Needle Aspiration Biopsy Findings
▸ The aspirate is usually cellular and contains single cells and may readily be confused with a malignancy

Immunohistochemical Features
▸ The tumor cells are strongly positive for S100 protein and vimentin and are negative for cytokeratin, estrogen and progesterone receptor proteins

Differential Diagnosis
▸ Granulomatous inflammatory reaction
▸ Invasive carcinoma with apocrine features
▸ Metastatic renal cell carcinoma
▸ Metastatic malignant melanoma
▸ Alveolar soft part sarcoma

GROSS FINDINGS

Granular cell tumors form a yellowish, white solid mass with irregular or well-defined borders.

MICROSCOPIC FINDINGS

The tumor is composed of sheets, nests or cords of large oval or polygonal cells with abundant granular eosinophilic cytoplasm, with small round nuclei (Figure 11-10). The cellular aggregates are separated by prominent fibrous septae and may appear to infiltrate irregularly into the adjacent breast parenchyma. Mitoses are rare and pleomorphism unusual.

ANCILLARY STUDIES

SPECIAL STAINS

The cytoplasmic granules are positive for PAS and are diastase resistant.

IMMUNOHISTOCHEMISTRY

The large cells stain positively for S100 protein, NSE and vimentin; CD68 and CEA positivity is variable. Estrogen receptor and progesterone receptors and cytokeratins are negative.

ULTRASTRUCTURAL FEATURES

Granular cells contain abundant secondary lysosomes in the cytoplasm and replicated basal lamina around the granular cells. Some cells may contain triangular membrane-bound structures composed of microtubules and microfibrils.

FINE NEEDLE ASPIRATION CYTOLOGY

Fine needle aspirates of granular cell tumors are cellular with cohesive groups of cells with a syncytial appearance and dispersed single cells. The cells contain abundant, finely eosinophilic granular cytoplasm and small round to slightly oval nuclei. Bare bipolar cells of stromal or myoepithelial type are absent. This, combined with the increased cellularity, may be confused with malignancy.

DIFFERENTIAL DIAGNOSIS

The differential diagnosis is diverse, including inflammatory, benign and malignant lesions, most notably inflammatory fat necrosis, apocrine carcinoma, secretory carcinoma, the alveolar variant of lobular carcinoma, alveolar soft part sarcoma, malignant melanoma and metastatic renal cell carcinoma.

Inflammatory fat necrosis may form a mass lesion, leading to radiologic, cytologic and surgical evaluation. The mass is composed of an admixture of foamy

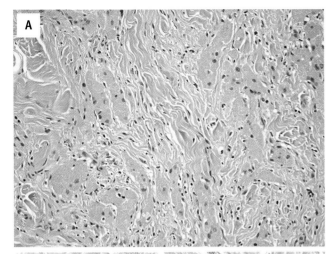

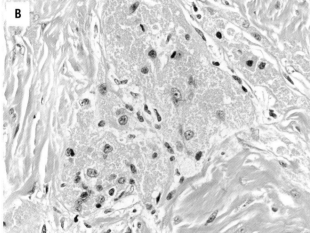

FIGURE 11-10

Granular cell tumor. (A) Medium power view showing nests and cords of large oval/polygonal cells, separated by prominent fibrous septae, giving the appearance of irregular infiltration of the breast parenchyma. (B) High power of the component cells containing abundant granular eosinophilic cytoplasm, with small round nuclei.

histiocytes, multinucleated giant cells engulfing fat and a scattering of lymphocytes. As the lesion ages, fibrosis becomes apparent. The cells are CD68 positive, but negative for S100 protein.

Apocrine carcinoma can be confused with granular cell tumor as both have an infiltrative growth pattern and cells with abundant granular, eosinophilic cytoplasm. However, the overtly malignant nuclear features in apocrine carcinoma should help in the differential diagnosis and the malignant cells will show cytokeratin and EMA positivity.

Secretory carcinoma of the breast is an extremely rare low grade carcinoma predominantly affecting children and younger adults, but can occur at any age. The solid variant, in particular, may be confused with granular cell tumor. It is composed of a solid proliferation of neoplastic cells characterized by large amounts of pale staining cytoplasm; mucin filled intracytoplasmic lumina abound. The nuclei are ovoid and have small nucleoli. Immunopositivity for cytokeratins is a useful adjunct.

Alveolar soft part sarcoma is an uncommon sarcoma of contentious histogenesis. It is composed of an organoid arrangement of tumor cells, rounded or polygonal in shape with cytoplasm of varying density. Thin-walled sinusoidal vascular spaces permeate between tumor nests. Early suggestions that it was related to paraganglioma or Schwann cells have been discounted and more recently a possible skeletal muscle origin has been favored, based on the immunohistochemical demonstration of various muscle associated-proteins, especially desmin.

Malignant melanoma can be distinguished from granular cell tumor by the presence of cytoplasmic melanin granules and immunoreactivity for HMB45 and Melan A, in addition to S100 protein positivity.

Metastatic renal cell carcinoma, of conventional type, is known for its ability to metastasize to unusual sites. A prior history of renal cell carcinoma or a renal mass are helpful clinical indicators. Morphologically the tumor cell nuclei are typically more pleomorphic than those usually observed in granular cell tumor and their cytoplasm is generally clear and voluminous. Immunopositivity for cytokeratin is another distinguishing feature.

PROGNOSIS AND TREATMENT

Wide local excision with tumor-free margins is the treatment of choice. Malignant granular cell tumors have been reported and the treatment is similar, as these tumors appear to be insensitive to current chemotherapeutic agents as well as to radiotherapy.

SUGGESTED READINGS

Adeniran A, Al-Ahmadie H, Mahoney MC, Robinson-Smith TM. Granular cell tumor of the breast: a series of 17 cases and review of the literature. Breast J 2004;10:528–531.

Brogi E. Benign and malignant spindle cell lesions of the breast. Semin Diagn Pathol 2004;21:57–64.

Damiani S, Dina R, Eusebi V. Eosinophilic and granular cell tumors of the breast. Semin Diagn Pathol 1999;16:17–25.

Dunne B, Lee AH, Pinder SE, et al. An immunohistochemical study of metaplastic spindle cell carcinoma, phyllodes tumor and fibromatosis of the breast. Hum Pathol 2003;34:1009–1015.

Elston CW, Ellis IO, eds. The Breast, 3e. Volume 13 Systemic Pathology Series. Edinburgh: Churchill Livingstone, 1998.

Gobbi H, Simpson JF, Borowsky A, et al. Metaplastic breast tumors with a dominant fubromatosis-like phenotype have a high risk of local recurrence. Cancer 1999;85:2170–2182.

Luo JH, Rotterdam H. Primary amyloid tumor of the breast: a case report and review of the literature. Mod Pathol 1997;10:735–738.

McMenamin ME, DeSchryver K, Fletcher CD. Fibrous lesions of the breast: a review. Int J Surg Pathol 2000;8:99–108.

Page DL, Anderson TJ, eds. Diagnostic Histopathology of the Breast. Edinburgh: Churchill Livingstone 1987.

Powell CM, Cranor ML, Rosen PP. Pseudoangiomatous stromal hyperplasia (PASH). A mammary stromal tumor with myofibroblastic differentiation. Am J Surg Pathol 1995;19:270–277.

Rocken C, Kronsbein H, Sletten K, et al. Amyloidosis of the breast. Virchows Arch 2002; 440:527–535.

12

Diseases of the Nipple

Anita Bane · Anna Marie Mulligan · Frances P O'Malley

INTRODUCTION

The nipple–areola complex is centrally placed in the breast and contains abundant sensory nerve endings, sebaceous glands and apocrine glands. The collecting ducts, which represent the terminal component of the lobar branching duct system of the breast, open onto the nipple. Immediately beneath the nipple these collecting ducts dilate to form the lactiferous sinuses, which are surrounded by interweaving fascicles of smooth muscle continuous with the musculature of the nipple.

Reflecting the anatomy of the nipple, the most common clinical disorders of the nipple arise from the stratified squamous epithelium of the external nipple or the ductal epithelium lining the collecting ducts and lactiferous sinuses. Rarer developmental anomalies will be mentioned for completeness.

DEVELOPMENTAL ANOMALIES

The most common developmental anomaly of the nipple is the presence of an accessory nipple, a condition known as polythelia. The nipple–areola complex and the underlying breast parenchyma are derived embryologically from the mammary line (primitive milk streak), which extends on each side of the body from axilla to groin. Normally the distal two-thirds of this line disappear by the seventh or eighth week in utero, leaving the proximal one third in place from which the nipple and breast develop. Rarely accessory nipples develop, and can be found anywhere along the line of the primitive milk streak.

DISEASES OF THE SQUAMOUS EPITHELIUM OF THE NIPPLE

DERMATITIS

The keratinizing stratified squamous epithelium of the nipple is susceptible to all forms of dermatitis that affect the skin in general. The clinical relevance of chronic dermatitis of the nipple, more specifically eczema, lies in distinguishing it from Paget's disease.

DISEASES OF THE DUCTAL EPITHELIUM

PAGET'S DISEASE OF THE NIPPLE

Paget's disease of the nipple, so named after the seminal observations of Sir James Paget, describes the presence of malignant glandular epithelial cells within the squamous epithelium of the nipple. It is invariably associated with an underlying ductal carcinoma, either DCIS or invasive. It is estimated that Paget's disease occurs in 1–4.3 % of all breast cancers.

CLINICAL FEATURES

The clinical manifestations of Paget's disease are dependent on the extent of involvement of the epidermis by the malignant glandular epithelial cells. The nipple may appear normal or show changes ranging from mild erythema to the classic description of eczematous weeping and crusting. Retraction of the nipple may also be present. This change may extend to involve the areola and adjacent epidermis of the breast proper. Age at presentation is highly variable and ranges from 26–88; 50–60 % of breasts with Paget's disease will have a palpable tumor in the underlying breast parenchyma.

RADIOLOGIC FEATURES

In the nipple–areolar region the significant findings include thickening of the nipple. Underlying calcifications with or without a mass lesion may be observed.

PAGET'S DISEASE - FACT SHEET

Definition
▶ The presence of malignant glandular epithelial cells within the squamous epithelium of the nipple

Incidence
▶ 1–4.3% of all breast cancers (invasive and *in situ*)

Age Distribution
▶ Age 26–88 years

Clinical Features
▶ Normal, mild erythema or eczematous weeping and crusting

Radiologic Features
▶ Thickening of the nipple
▶ Underlying calcifications/mass lesion

Prognosis and Treatment
▶ Determined by the extent and grade of the associated carcinoma
▶ Treatment dictated by associated carcinoma

PAGET'S DISEASE - PATHOLOGIC FEATURES

Gross Findings
▶ The nipple may vary from being macroscopically normal to being erythematous and ulcerated
▶ Dilated ducts may be seen deep to the nipple
▶ A mass lesion may be present in the breast parenchyma

Microscopic Findings
▶ Malignant glandular cells are seen within the squamous epithelium
▶ These cells may be seen singly in all layers of the epidermis or they may cluster in the basal layers
▶ Cytologically they are large with pleomorphic nuclei and abundant eosinophilic cytoplasm

Ultrastructural Features
▶ Paget's cells contain intracytoplasmic lumens with microvilli and tight junctions or desmosomes, features that characterize glandular epithelial cells

Immunohistochemical Features
▶ The cells stain with EMA, low molecular weight cytokeratin (e.g., CAM5.2), CEA and they contain PAS positive diastase resistant mucin globules in their cytoplasm
▶ They may express ER and PR protein and frequently (>90%) show HER2/neu protein overexpression
▶ The cells are negative with HMB45, Melan-A and other melanocytic markers

Differential Diagnosis
▶ Malignant melanoma
▶ Bowen's disease/carcinoma *in situ*
▶ Basal cell carcinoma
▶ Clear cell change
▶ Toker cells

PATHOLOGIC FEATURES

MACROSCOPIC FINDINGS

The gross changes present in the resected specimen reflect those observed clinically, and range from a normal nipple to eczematous ulceration. The underlying breast parenchyma may show an infiltrative mass lesion or dilated ducts.

MICROSCOPIC FINDINGS

The defining histologic feature of Paget's disease is the presence of malignant glandular epithelial cells within the squamous epithelium of the nipple. These cells are frequently clustered in the basal epidermis but may occur singly in the more superficial layers. Cytologically they are large cells with abundant eosinophilic cytoplasm that may contain phagocytosed melanin granules. The nuclei tend to be pleomorphic, often exhibiting prominent nucleoli with a variable mitotic rate (Figure 12-1). The underlying lactiferous ducts contain ductal carcinoma *in situ* (DCIS), cytologically similar to the Paget's cells. The *in situ* carcinoma may extend to a variable degree into the underlying ductal system and frequently has comedo type necrosis. An accompanying invasive carcinoma may be found. The reminder of the nipple epithelium shows varying degrees of hyperplasia, hyperkeratosis, inflammation and ulceration.

ANCILLARY STUDIES

IMMUNOHISTOCHEMISTRY

Paget's cells stain positively for EMA, low molecular weight cytokeratins and CEA and their cytoplasm contains diastase resistant PAS positive globules consistent with mucin (Figure 12-2). They may be estrogen (ER) and progesterone receptor (PR) positive, resembling the immunoprofile of the underlying DCIS, which is invariably of high nuclear grade. They frequently overexpress HER2/neu protein. Paget's cells do not stain for HMB45 or Melan-A and the vast majority of cases will also be negative for S100 protein.

ULTRASTRUCTURAL STUDIES

Electron microscopic studies of Paget's cells have confirmed the glandular nature of these neoplastic cells. They show intracytoplasmic lumens with micovilli, together with the tight junctions or desmosomes that

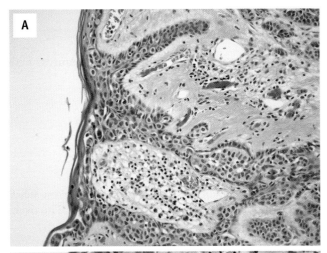

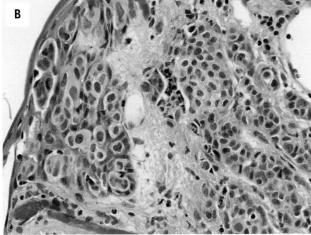

FIGURE 12-1

Paget's disease of the nipple. Malignant glandular epithelial cells within the squamous epithelium of the nipple. The cells are clustered in the basal epidermis and also occur singly, more superficially. The cells are large with pleomorphic nuclei, prominent nucleoli and abundant eosinophilic cytoplasm.

characterize all epithelial cells. This test is not required in routine diagnostics.

DIFFERENTIAL DIAGNOSIS

The differential diagnosis of suspected Paget's disease in a skin biopsy includes malignant melanoma, Bowen's disease/squamous carcinoma in situ and clear cell change.

MALIGNANT MELANOMA

Malignant melanoma cells show cytoplasmic pigmentation, frequently exhibit nesting at the dermo-epidermal junction and 'buck shot' spread through the overlying epidermis. Immunohistochemical staining for S100 protein, HMB45 and Melan-A are positive and negative staining for epithelial markers confirm the neural crest origin of these cells.

BOWEN'S DISEASE/SQUAMOUS CARCINOMA IN SITU

Extensive replacement of the nipple epidermis by Paget's cells can simulate Bowen's disease. However, Bowen's disease is not associated with an underlying malignancy. In addition, Bowen's disease is usually positive for high molecular weight cytokeratins and negative for HER2/neu protein overexpression.

CLEAR CELL CHANGE

Clear cells constitute a non-neoplastic alteration of benign keratinocytes. They can be distributed throughout the epidermis although are more frequent in the

FIGURE 12-2

Paget's disease of the nipple, DPAS. The cytoplasm of Paget's cells contain diastase resistant PAS positive globules, consistent with mucin.

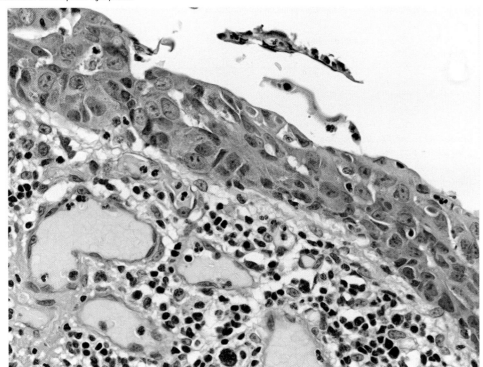

basal and mid epidermal layers. Cytologically, they have bland nuclei with cytoplasmic clearing.

PROGNOSIS AND THERAPY

The prognosis of Paget's disease is determined by the extent and grade of the associated carcinoma. Similarly, the features of the associated carcinoma dictate the appropriate therapy.

NIPPLE ADENOMA

The nipple adenoma has several synonyms including nipple duct adenoma, florid papillomatosis, papillomatosis of the nipple, subareolar duct papillomatosis or erosive adenomatosis. The number of alternative names parallels the variety of morphologic features that may be seen in this benign entity.

CLINICAL FEATURES

Nipple adenoma may occur in all age categories and in both sexes but it is most common in women in their fifth decade. Presenting symptoms include erosion of the nipple, serosanguinous nipple discharge or a mass lesion underlying the nipple.

RADIOLOGIC FEATURES

The mammographic and sonographic features may suggest carcinoma.

PATHOLOGIC FEATURES

MACROSCOPIC FINDINGS

The typical macroscopic finding is of a firm mass with irregular edges, simulating a carcinoma. The overlying epidermis may be ulcerated or scaly.

MICROSCOPIC FINDINGS

Nipple adenomas have been subdivided by some authors into 3–4 variant forms, depending on the dominant microscopic findings. These categories are somewhat arbitrary and are of no prognostic significance. Indeed, most adenomas show composite features to include an adenomatous proliferation of glandular structures set within a desmoplastic stroma with a pseudoinfiltrative edge and florid epithelial hyperplasia

---

NIPPLE ADENOMA – FACT SHEET

Definition
▶ A benign papillomatous and/or adenomatous proliferation of epithelial glands

Incidence and Location
▶ Uncommon
▶ Usually unilateral

Gender, Race and Age Distribution
▶ Women in their fifth decade

Clinical Features
▶ Erosion of the nipple
▶ Serosanguinous nipple discharge
▶ Mass lesion under nipple

Radiologic Features
▶ May be suggestive of carcinoma

Prognosis and Treatment
▶ Complete surgical excision
▶ Recurrences have been reported after incomplete excision

NIPPLE ADENOMA – PATHOLOGIC FEATURES

Gross Findings
▶ Irregular, firm area simulating a carcinoma
▶ Overlying epithelium may be scaly or ulcerated

Microscopic Findings
▶ Adenomatous proliferation of glandular structures set within the nipple stroma
▶ The glandular structures may be expanded by papillary epithelial proliferations
▶ Epithelial hyperplasia of usual type, squamous metaplasia and apocrine metaplasia may be present
▶ Focal necrosis, overlying epithelial ulceration and an inflammatory cell infiltrate are variable features

Fine Needle Aspiration/Cytologic Findings
▶ Cellular specimen showing an admixture of benign epithelial and myoepithelial cells
▶ Epithelial atypia may be present, particularly in cases showing surface ulceration

Immunohistochemical Features
▶ The glandular structures are all lined by a layer of myoepithelial cells which can be stained with actin, smooth muscle myosin, S100 protein, calponin or p63

Differential Diagnosis
▶ Central papilloma
▶ Subareolar abscess
▶ Adenocarcinoma

without atypia (Figure 12-3). Variants of epithelial hyperplasia, such as gynecomastoid and compact hyperplasia frequently occur in nipple adenomas (Figures 12-4 and 12-5). These patterns can be confused with atypical ductal hyperplasia, but lack the architectural rigidity. Superimposed squamous metaplasia and/or apocrine metaplasia (Figure 12-6) with or without cyst formation may be evident. Other histologic features include myoepithelial hyperplasia, necrosis (Figure 12-7), which should not be misinterpreted as indicative of DCIS, and a variable mitotic activity. The overlying squamous epithelium of the nipple may be hyperplastic or ulcerated. Concurrent ulceration of the overlying epithelium may add an inflammatory cell infiltrate.

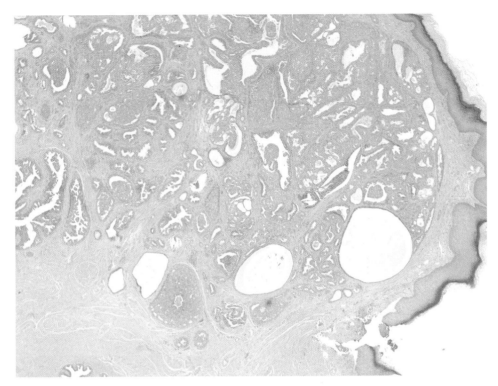

FIGURE 12-3

Nipple adenoma. Low power view showing an adenomatous proliferation of glandular structures, beneath the epidermis with a pseudoinfiltrative edge.

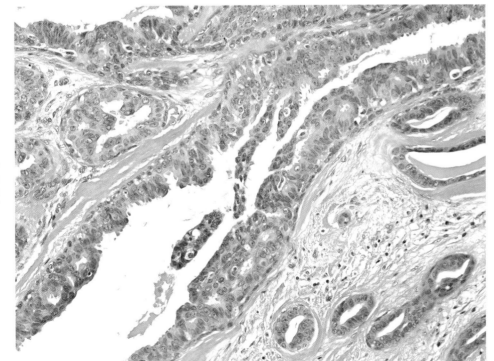

FIGURE 12-4

Nipple adenoma. Medium power showing gynecomastoid hyperplasia within a duct. The hyperplastic cells form long, tapered, finger-like projections within the duct.

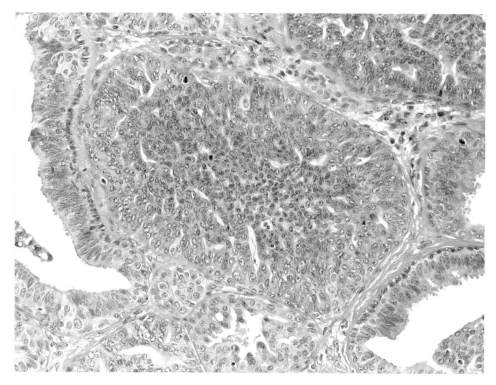

FIGURE 12-5

Nipple adenoma. High power showing compact hyperplasia with a duct.

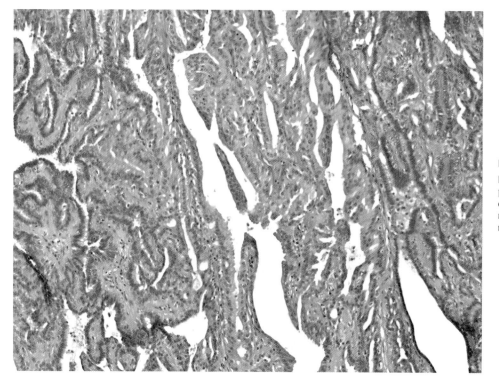

FIGURE 12-6

Nipple adenoma with apocrine metaplasia. Cells with abundant pink cytoplasm and centrally placed round nuclei, indicative of apocrine metaplasia.

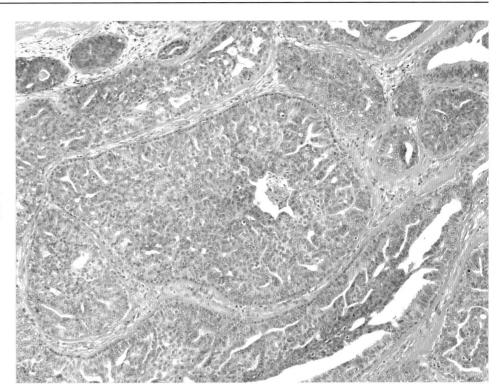

FIGURE 12-7
Nipple adenoma with necrosis. Necrosis can occur within benign ducts and should not be misinterpreted as ductal carcinoma *in situ*.

ANCILLARY STUDIES

IMMUNOHISTOCHEMISTRY

Immunohistochemical staining for myoepithelial cells will reveal the presence of these cells surrounding the proliferative glands.

CYTOLOGY

A nipple adenoma can be examined cytologically by scrapings from an ulcerated nipple surface or alternatively from an FNA of the subareolar mass lesion. Both methods usually reveal a cellular specimen containing a variable admixture of glandular and myoepithelial cells. The cellularity, necrosis and variable inflammatory infiltrate may be misinterpreted as atypia or even carcinoma and caution is advised.

DIFFERENTIAL DIAGNOSIS

The differential diagnosis includes central papilloma, subareolar abscess and adenocarcinoma.

CENTRAL PAPILLOMA

The central solitary papilloma grows within the dilated milk duct and is usually confined by it, so it has

---

SYRINGOMATOUS ADENOMA – FACT SHEET

Definition
▶ A locally invasive tumor of the nipple/areola, morphologically similar to syringoma of the skin
▶ Postulated to differentiate towards intra-epidermal eccrine sweat ducts

Incidence and Location
▶ Rare
▶ Unilateral

Gender, Race and Age Distribution
▶ 11–74 years (average 40 years)

Clinical Features
▶ Firm, discrete mass in the nipple and subareolar region
▶ Pain and nipple discharge variable

Radiologic Features
▶ Stellate, subareolar mass-like lesion on mammography

Prognosis and Treatment
▶ Complete surgical excision with adequate margins
▶ Recurrence has been reported

a much more circumscribed and better delineated border with the surrounding parenchyma. The lesion has true, well-developed fibrovascular cores as opposed to the adenotic growth pattern of a nipple adenoma.

SUBAREOLAR ABSCESS

A subareolar abscess is easily distinguishable from a nipple adenoma as it is composed of an admixture of inflammatory cells in a reparative fibrovascular stroma with parenchymal disruption.

ADENOCARCINOMA

Adenocarcinoma under the nipple, like adenocarcinomas of the remainder of the breast, is composed of glands or islands of malignant epithelium devoid of a myoepithelial cell layer, infiltrating adjacent parenchyma in an irregular manner.

PROGNOSIS AND THERAPY

Complete surgical excision, which usually requires removal of the nipple, is the treatment of choice. Recurrences following incomplete excision have been reported. Association with carcinoma is rare, but has been reported, particularly in males.

SYRINGOMATOUS ADENOMA

Syringomatous adenoma is a locally invasive tumor of the nipple/areolar region, which is morphologically similar to syringoma of the skin. Syringoma of the skin has been postulated as a tumor showing differentiation towards intra-epidermal eccrine sweat ducts. Similar histogenesis has been proposed for syringomatous adenoma of the nipple.

CLINICAL FEATURES

The presenting symptom is usually a firm discrete mass in the nipple and subareolar region. Pain and nipple discharge are variable features. Age range of presentation is from 11–74 years, with an average age of 40 years.

RADIOLOGIC FEATURES

Mammography reveals a stellate subareolar mass-like lesion

PATHOLOGIC FEATURES

MACROSCOPIC FINDINGS

The lesion appears as a firm ill-defined mass in the nipple/areolar region, ranging in size from 1–3 cm. Small cysts may be visible on the cut surface.

MICROSCOPIC FINDINGS

The tumor is composed of glands, nests and cords of cells permeating between the muscle bundles of the nipple stroma (Figure 12-8). The stroma may vary from normal to fibrotic to edematous. The glands are often angulated, reminiscent of those in tubular carcinoma; however, the neoplastic cells lining the glandular structures are arranged in two layers: a luminal layer and a basal cell layer (Figure 12-9). The latter may contain smooth muscle actin filaments but a consistent myoepithelial layer is not a feature. The luminal cells may show squamous differentiation with keratin pearl and keratin cyst formation. Cytologically, the neoplastic cells are bland with scant amounts of eosinophilic cytoplasm and round regular nuclei with scant mitotic activity. Connection with the overlying epidermis may occasionally be observed, as may perineural invasion.

DIFFERENTIAL DIAGNOSIS

The differential diagnosis includes tubular carcinoma, nipple adenoma and low grade adenosquamous carcinoma.

SYRINGOMATOUS ADENOMA – PATHOLOGIC FEATURES

Gross Findings
▶ Irregular, ill-defined gray white mass of variable size
▶ Small cysts may be visible on the cut surface

Microscopic Findings
▶ Glands, cords and nests of cells haphazardly permeate the nipple stroma
▶ The neoplastic cells are arranged in two layers, luminal and basal
▶ The cells exhibit minimal nuclear pleomorphism, contain scant quantities of eosinophilic cytoplasm and mitotic figures are rare
▶ Squamous differentiation of the luminal cells with keratin cyst formation is frequently observed
▶ Perineural growth and permeation of fat may be seen and is not indicative of malignancy

Immunohistochemical Features
▶ The luminal cells stain with CEA and the basal cells display actin positivity

Differential Diagnosis
▶ Tubular carcinoma
▶ Nipple adenoma
▶ Low grade adenosquamous carcinoma

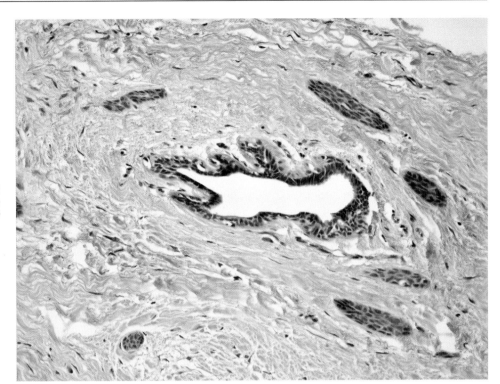

FIGURE 12-8

Syringomatous adenoma. Nests and cords of cells typically permeate between the muscle bundles of the nipple stroma.

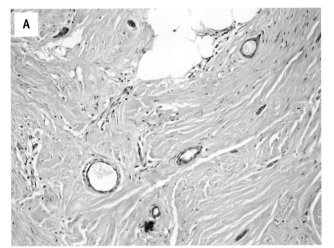

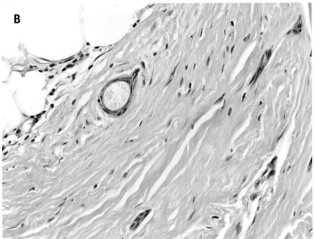

FIGURE 12-9

Syringomatous adenoma. (A) Angulated glands, reminiscent of those in tubular carcinoma are seen; however, (B) the neoplastic cells lining the glandular structures are arranged in two layers.

TUBULAR CARCINOMA

Tubular carcinoma, a special type of breast cancer, rarely involves the nipple region. It consists of tear drop-shaped glands lined by a single layer of low grade neoplastic cells devoid of squamous differentiation, set in a fibrotic stroma (see Chapter 18).

NIPPLE ADENOMA

The nipple adenoma, as previously described, forms a mass lesion that displaces the nipple stroma. The nipple adenoma is abundantly cellular with florid epithelial hyperplasia without atypia, together with foci of apocrine and squamous metaplasia. Keratin pearls are unusual.

LOW GRADE ADENOSQUAMOUS CARCINOMA

Low grade adenosquamous carcinoma is a rare tumor, which principally involves the breast parenchyma rather than the overlying nipple. It is composed of a variable admixture of malignant glands and nests of squamous cells with squamous pearls and keratin cyst formation, set in a 'fibromatosis like' stroma. Like other invasive mammary carcinomas, a myoepithelial layer is absent.

PROGNOSIS AND THERAPY

Complete surgical excision with adequate margins is the treatment of choice. Recurrence has been reported.

SUGGESTED READINGS

Ellis IO, CW Elston, SE Pinder. Papillary lesions. In: CW Elston, IO Ellis. The Breast. Churchill Edinburgh: Livingstone 1998; p133–146

Rosen, PP. Papilloma and related benign tumors. In: Rosen PP ed. Rosen's Breast Pathology. New York: Lippincott Williams & Wilkins 2001; p77–119.

Tavassoli FA. Diseases of the nipple. In: Tavassoli FA ed. Pathology of the Breast. New York: McGraw-Hill 1999; p731–762.

Tavassoli FA, Devilee P. Pathology and Genetics of Tumors of the Breast and Female Genital Organs. World Health Organisation of Classification of Tumors. Lyon. IARC Press 2003.

13

Fibrocystic Change and Columnar Cell Lesions

Bruce J Youngson

FIBROCYSTIC CHANGE

CLINICAL FEATURES

The term 'fibrocystic change' (FCC) refers to a constellation of benign breast changes that are currently considered to represent normal, but exaggerated, hormonally mediated breast tissue responses. FCC replaces a wide variety of synonymous terms used previously that implied an underlying pathology to this process (i.e., fibrocystic disease, fibrous mastopathy, mammary dysplasia, Schimmelbusch's disease, chronic cystic mastitis, and so on).

FCC is extremely common, with more than one-third of females 20–45 years of age showing some evidence of this condition on physical examination. In autopsy series, microscopic evidence of FCC has been found in approximately 60 % of grossly normal breasts. FCC generally affects pre-menopausal women and is the commonest cause of a breast lump in females under 50 years of age. The risk of developing FCC appears to be increased in women who have conditions that result in a preponderance of estrogenic hormones. Hyperestrogenism has been implicated in both the development and proliferation of the terminal ductulo-lobular unit epithelium, as well as the accompanying stromal fibrosis that is thought to cause relative obstruction of the breast ductules in this condition. In the presence of persistent, hormonally mediated, cyclic epithelial secretion, the obstructed ductules gradually dilate and form cysts, while the proximal lobules involute. Some workers have suggested that apocrine metaplasia is an initial event in FCC, with microcysts developing as a result of the secretory activity of these cells. In the absence of hormonal replacement therapy, FCC symptomatology (i.e., premenstrual swelling with pain and tenderness), generally ceases one to two years following the menopause as the cystic changes of FCC gradually involute.

RADIOLOGIC FEATURES

Mammographically, the breast tissue may show increased density secondary to stromal fibrosis. Microcalcifications may be present. Ultrasound examination demonstrates multiple cysts and fibrosis.

PATHOLOGIC FEATURES

GROSS FINDINGS

Breast tissue that demonstrates FCC will generally show fibrosis with blue-dome or clear cysts that may range in size from less than a mm in diameter to greater than 2 cm in diameter. These changes are variable in extent, but are usually multifocal and bilateral (Figure 13-1).

FIBROCYSTIC CHANGE – FACT SHEET

Definition
▸ A constellation of benign, hormonally mediated breast changes that include cyst formation, stromal fibrosis, and mild epithelial hyperplasia without atypia

Incidence and Location
▸ More than one-third of females 20–45 years of age
▸ 60 % of grossly normal breasts (autopsy series) show microscopic evidence of FCC
▸ Usually bilateral and multifocal

Morbidity and Mortality
▸ Cyclic (premenstrual) breast pain and tenderness
▸ Breast lumpiness (FCC is the commonest cause of a breast mass in females <50 years old)
▸ No increased risk for subsequent carcinoma development

Clinical Features
▸ Lumpy, premenstrually painful breasts

Prognosis and Treatment
▸ FCC symptomatology generally ceases 1–2 years following menopause
▸ Hormonal manipulation (BCP)

FIBROCYSTIC CHANGE – PATHOLOGIC FEATURES

Gross Findings

▶ Blue dome or clear cysts with stromal fibrosis
▶ May form a mass lesion

Microscopic Findings

▶ Cysts, apocrine metaplasia, stromal fibrosis, mild epithelial hyperplasia without atypia

Ultrastructural Findings

▶ Not helpful or applicable

Fine Needle Aspiration Biopsy Findings

▶ Cohesive fragments of bland ductal epithelium, cyst debris with macrophages, apocrine metaplastic cells

Immunhistochemical Features

▶ Not helpful or applicable

Differential Diagnosis

▶ Any breast mass with fibrosis (malignancy, sclerosing adenosis, apocrine lesions, inflammatory/reactive processes, and so on)

MICROSCOPIC FINDINGS

The characteristic histologic changes of non-proliferative FCC include stromal fibrosis, dilated/ectatic ducts with cyst formation, apocrine metaplasia and mild epithelial hyperplasia without atypia (Figure 13-2). Florid epithelial hyperplasia of usual type (a proliferative disease) is discussed in Chapter 14.

The cyst-lining epithelium may be attenuated, but the normal outer myoepithelial cell layer associated with it always remains. Typically, many of the cysts demonstrate apocrine metaplasia, a metaplastic change where the lining epithelial cells have abundant, granular eosinophilic cytoplasm, apical cytoplasmic snouts that protrude into the lumen, and round, basally to centrally located nuclei that often have a prominent nucleolus. The apocrine cell layer may be flat or form papillae. This latter has been described as papillary apocrine change. The papillary clusters of the apocrine cells most often taper and do not interconnnect, but complex patterns of prolonged arcades as well as anastomosing arrays of these cells may be seen.

PROGNOSIS AND THERAPY

There is no increased risk for the subsequent development of breast carcinoma in women with non-proliferative FCC, including mild usually ductal hyperplasia (i.e., hyperplasia where the epithelial proliferation is more than two, but not more than four cells in thickness). The non-surgical treatment of FCC consists mainly of hormonal manipulation, with the goal being to provide symptomatic relief from the breast pain and tenderness, and prevent progression. Oral contraceptives (BCP) have been used to treat FCC with success rates of 70–90 %. The use of oral or percutaneous progesterone during the luteal phase of the menstrual cycle has also been reported to result in symptomatic improvement of FCC in 80–85 % of cases. Surgery rarely (if ever) has any role in the management of FCC, other than to provide a definitive histologic diagnosis in the investigation and treatment of a breast mass or radiologic lesion.

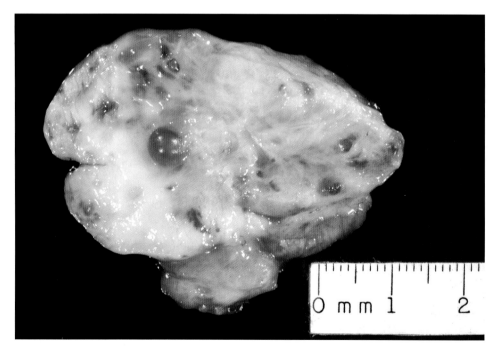

FIGURE 13-1

Fibrocystic changes (gross). Breast tissue with gross fibrosis and cyst formation characteristic of fibrocystic changes.

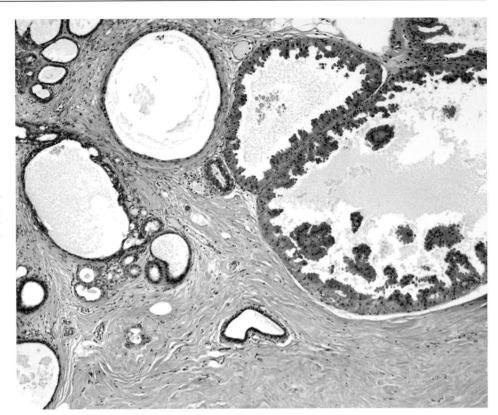

FIGURE 13-2

Fibrocystic changes. Low power view of nonproliferative fibrocystic changes showing cysts, apocrine metaplasia, papillary apocrine metaplasia and stromal fibrosis.

COLUMNAR CELL LESIONS

CLINICAL FEATURES

Columnar cell change (CCC) or columnar cell hyperplasia (CCH) are histologic findings characterized by the presence of columnar epithelial cells lining the terminal ductulo-lobular unit (TDLU). Columnar cell alterations have been recognized for many years by histopathologists, and have been described under a variety of different names, including blunt duct adenosis, columnar alteration of lobules, columnar metaplasia, hyperplastic terminal groupings, atypical lobules type A, columnar cell hyperplasia, columnar alteration with prominent apical snouts and secretions (CAPSS), pretubular hyperplasia, and atypical cystic lobules.

Columnar cell lesions (CCLs) are often multifocal, and typically occur in premenopausal women 35–50 years of age. Of particular importance is the fact that columnar cell change is a finding being encountered with increasing frequency in surgical pathology practice due to its tendency to be associated with mammographic microcalcifications. Unfortunately, the confusion created by a lack of standardized terminology and the dearth of reliable data regarding its clinical significance have created difficulties in both the pathologic diagnosis and clinical management of this entity. Recently, the

World Health Organization (WHO) Working Group on the Pathology and Genetics of Tumours of the Breast (2003) introduced the term 'flat epithelial atypia' (FEA) for columnar lesions exhibiting low grade cytologic atypia, but lacking the architectural complexity to qualify as atypical ductal hyperplasia (ADH) or low grade ductal carcinoma in situ (DCIS); it has yet to be determined how widely used this term will become.

PATHOLOGIC FEATURES

GROSS FINDINGS

Columnar cell lesions are not identifiable macroscopically, but are often associated with FCC.

MICROSCOPIC FINDINGS

Columnar cell alterations include a spectrum of changes that range from uncomplicated CCC/CCH, through CCC/CCH with atypia (flat epithelial atypia). Although some columnar cell lesions may appear to exhibit a progressive spectrum of morphologic alterations, this does not necessarily imply a biologic continuum, or that progression along the observed spectrum is inevitable. For practical purposes, non atypical CCL may be broadly placed into one of two groups, CCC or CCH.

COLUMNAR CELL LESIONS – FACT SHEET

Definition

▶ Columnar cell change (CCC): Presence of columnar epithelial cells lining the TDLU
▶ Columnar cell hyperplasia (CCH): Presence of columnar epithelial cells more than 2 cells thick lining the TDLU
▶ CCC/CCH with atypia (flat epithelial atypia): CCC/CCH with the presence of cytologic atypia insufficient for ADH/DCIS by classical criteria
▶ Columnar cell lesion (CCL): A lesion showing CCC/CCH

Incidence and Location

▶ Incidence not well established, commonly associated with FCC and microcalcifications
▶ Bilateral/multifocal

Morbidity and Mortality

▶ No known morbidity
▶ Atypia appears to confer an increased risk of malignancy that is not well defined

Gender, Race and Age Distribution

▶ Premenopausal women 35–50 years old

Clinical Features

▶ Often identified on mammography with microcalcification, no symptomatic lesion

Prognosis and Treatment

▶ Controversial and evolving
▶ Most authors suggest that CCL with atypia (flat epithelial atypia) on core biopsy be followed by excisional biopsy to allow an intensive search for a more significant lesion (i.e., ADH/DCIS/invasive carcinoma)
▶ If CCL with atypia (flat epithelial atypia) is found on excisional biopsy, the specimen should probably be submitted *in toto* for histologic examination with multiple levels cut from the blocks showing CCL with atypia

---

COLUMNAR CELL LESIONS – PATHOLOGIC FEATURES

Gross Findings

▶ No specific gross findings (often associated with FCC, but a histopathologic diagnosis)

Microscopic Findings

▶ Columnar cell change (CCC): Presence of columnar epithelial cells lining the TDLU
▶ Columnar cell hyperplasia (CCH): Presence of columnar epithelial cells more than 2 cells thick lining the TDLU
▶ CCC/CCH with atypia (flat epithelial atypia): CCC/CCH with the presence of cytologic atypia insufficient for ADH/DCIS by classical criteria

Ultrastructural Findings

▶ None of relevance

Fine Needle Aspiration Biopsy Findings

▶ Often those of FCC with prominent columnar cells, but none specific to this diagnosis

Immunohistochemical Features

▶ None of significant diagnostic value

Differential Diagnosis

▶ Benign apocrine lesions (apocrine metaplasia, apocrine hyperplasia)
▶ Cystic hypersecretory lesions (cystic hypersecretory hyperplasia, cystic hypersecretory carcinoma)
▶ Clinging carcinoma (DCIS)

Columnar cell changes: In CCC, the normal epithelial cell layer of the TDLU is replaced by one or two layers of taller columnar epithelial cells that have basal nuclei and apical cytoplasmic snouts. The nuclei are oriented in a regular fashion perpendicular to the basement membrane, are uniform, oval to elongated, and have evenly dispersed chromatin without conspicuous nucleoli. Mitotic figures are rare. No cytologic or architectural atypia is present and the normal myoepithelial cell and basement membrane layer are retained. There may be some mild stromal proliferation adjacent to the affected TDLU. Instead of the normal, rounded acinar configuration of the TDLU, the acini are variably dilated and take on a larger, irregularly branching appearance (Figure 13-3). Microcalcification of luminal secretions is common in columnar cell lesions and is most often the reason for its detection.

Columnar cell hyperplasia: The term columnar cell hyperplasia is used to describe an alteration of TDLUs with the same features described above for CCC, but where the columnar cells show cellular stratification with more than two cell layers (Figure 13-4). The nuclei retain a bland appearance and, for the most part, a perpendicular orientation to the basement membrane. Crowding/overlapping of nuclei in these hyperplastic foci may give the appearance of hyperchromasia. Architecturally, the hyperplastic columnar cells may form small mounds, tufts, or short micropapillations similar to that seen in gynecomastia. Apical luminal cytoplasmic snouts may be quite prominent and luminal microcalcifications are common, sometimes having a morphologic appearance similar to that of psammoma bodies (Figure 13-5). When architectural and cytologic atypia are not present, CCH is not currently recognized to carry with it any significant risk of subsequent development of breast cancer.

CCC/CCH with atypia (flat epithelial atypia): Cytologic atypia may be encountered in lesions with the architectural features of either CCC or CCH that ranges from subtle (i.e., relatively rounded or ovoid rather than elongated nuclei with a slight increase in the nuclear: cytoplasmic ratio, slight margination of chromatin, variably prominent nucleoli, and loss of polarity) to more overt (Figure 13-6). A resemblance of the columnar cells in cases to the cells forming the tubules of a tubular carcinoma has been noted by some authors. Depending on

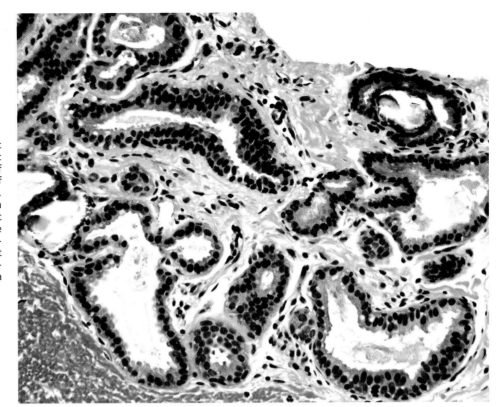

FIGURE 13-3

Columnar cell changes. Terminal duct lobular unit acini showing cystic dilatation with one or two layers of lining epithelium consisting of columnar cells with crowded, basal, oval to elongated nuclei with a uniform chromatin pattern, and that are oriented perpendicular to the basement membrane. Luminal cytoplasmic snouts with some flocculent intraluminal secretion and microcalcifications are also present. No atypia is seen.

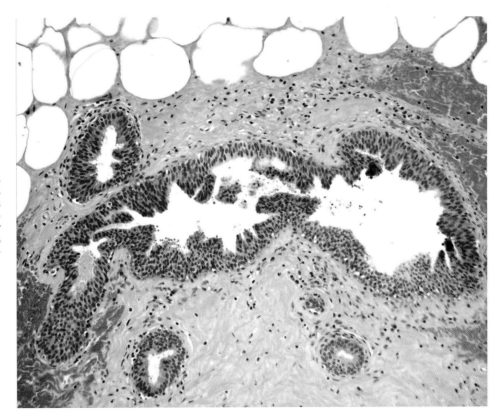

FIGURE 13-4

Columnar cell hyperplasia. Ductules lined by more than two cell layers of columnar cells with features as described in Figure 13-1. Architecturally, the hyperplastic columnar cells are forming small mounds, tufts and short micropapillations. No cytologic or architectural atypia is seen.

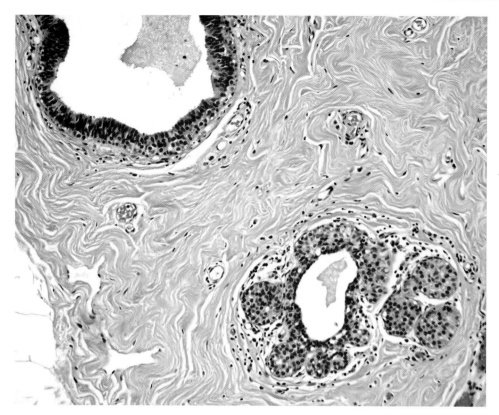

FIGURE 13-5

Columnar cell hyperplasia with adjacent atypical lobular hyperplasia. Ductule showing columnar cell hyperplasia without atypia but with adjacent ALH. An association between some CCL and lobular neoplasia has been noted by several authors.

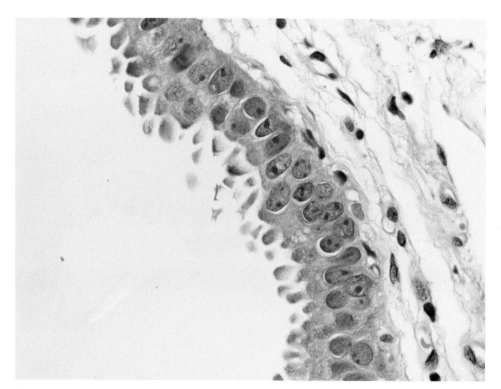

FIGURE 13-6

Flat epithelial atypia. High power showing atypical cells with rounded nuclei, nucleoli and prominent apical shouts. There is no evidence of architectural complexity.

the number of cell layers present, columnar cell lesions of this type are designated as columnar cell change with atypia or columnar cell hyperplasia with atypia (Figure 13-7). Using the terminology recently described by the WHO Working Group on the Pathology and Genetics of Tumours of the Breast both lesions would be classified as flat epithelial atypia. Some cases of CCC with atypia may not be evident on low power examination due to the lack of significant cellular proliferation and the subtle nature of the cytologic atypia; it may only be on high power examination that such subtle atypia is appreciated. High grade cytologic atypia (i.e., the extreme nuclear pleomorphism and other nuclear features present in high grade DCIS) is not a feature of CCC/ CCH with atypia or flat epithelial atypia. The presence of such high grade nuclear features requires a diagnosis of DCIS to be made, even if the cells comprise only a single cell layer; typically, high grade DCIS exhibiting other architectural patterns is also present. Given that an element of subjectivity exists in such cytologic/ histologic assessments, difficulties and controversies in assigning a diagnostic category to some borderline lesions may be a significant practical problem. As we gain more experience with these types of lesions, and as long term clinical follow-up data becomes available, hopefully a classification system based on more objective criteria will become available.

ADH/DCIS: Some columnar cell lesions exhibit cytologic and architectural atypia such as rigid bridging, bars, arcades, cribriform spaces with sieve-like fenestrations or well developed micropapillations. The most prudent approach to such lesions is to categorize them as either ADH or DCIS depending upon the severity and extent of the cytologic and architectural features present according to classical criteria.

IMMUNOHISTOCHEMISTRY

Although there are no immunohistochemical stains that are particularly helpful in further defining or classifying the above lesions, there are a number of recent studies that have looked at the immunohistochemical profile of the cells comprising columnar cell lesions. Most of the epithelial cells of columnar cell lesions (both with and without atypia) appear to express cytokeratin 19 (a low molecular mass keratin), while the high molecular mass keratins (e.g., cytokeratin 5 and 6, 34BE12) are not expressed. Estrogen and progesterone receptor proteins also appear to be highly expressed in the majority of columnar cell lesions. In at least one study, Ki-67 expression has also been noted to be low, suggesting that the cells of columnar cell lesions (even in those with atypia) have a low proliferative rate. The cells of CCL have also been noted to express GCDFP-15, a marker of apocrine differentiation, a finding that correlates with their cytologic features which also suggest apocrine differentiation. The immunoreactivity of these cells for bcl-2 and estrogen receptor protein contrasts that seen in usual benign apocrine cells.

FIGURE 13-7

Atypical ductal hyperplasia (ADH) arising in a background of columnar cell changes and columnar cell hyperplasia with atypia (flat epithelial atypia). A number of acini show a complex cellular proliferation with the formation of bridges and fenestrations sufficient for a diagnosis of ADH.

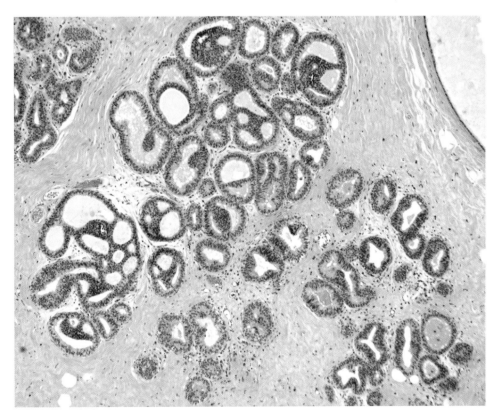

DIFFERENTIAL DIAGNOSIS

Benign apocrine lesions such as apocrine metaplasia and proliferative apocrine lesions must be distinguished from columnar cell lesions. Although the cytoplasm of the cells of both apocrine lesions and CCL is somewhat eosinophilic and granular, and feature luminal cytoplasmic snouts, the cells of apocrine lesions possess more abundant, granular, and eosinophilic cytoplasm. The nuclei of columnar cell lesions at the benign end of the spectrum also tend to be ovoid, while those of apocrine lesions tend to be round and often possess a single prominent nucleolus. Hobnail type cells, with prominent apical snouting and flocculent luminal secretions, while seen in some columnar cell lesions, are not typical of apocrine lesions.

Columnar cell lesions should also be distinguished from the spectrum of cystic hypersecretory proliferations that include hyperplasia and carcinoma. Although both CCL and cystic hypersecretory proliferations are prone to micropapillary growth patterns, cystic hypersecretory proliferations are characterized by sparse microcalcifications and intraluminal accumulation of eosinophilic secretions that resemble thyroid colloid. CCL tend not to accumulate conspicuous secretions and are often associated with microcalcifications. Carcinomas arising from cystic hypersecretory intraductal carcinoma are usually poorly differentiated, whereas CCLs with atypia may be seen associated with tubular carcinoma.

CLINICAL SIGNIFICANCE

An association between some columnar cell lesions and lobular neoplasia (i.e., atypical lobular hyperplasia and lobular carcinoma *in situ*), low grade DCIS and invasive tubular carcinoma has been noted by a number of authors. Whilst in many cases, the atypical columnar cell lesions have been identified in geographically separate surrounding tissue, in some cases, merging or coexistence of the two lesions have been noted. It is not uncommon for various combinations of the columnar cell lesions discussed above to coexist in the same area, and while CCC/CCH with atypia (flat epithelial atypia) may exist as an isolated lesion, it may coexist with areas of ADH or DCIS. The presence of CCC/CCH with atypia should alert the pathologist to the possibility of, and prompt an intensive search for, a more significant lesion.

Brogi *et al.* looked at the frequency and distribution of a CCL with atypia that they termed 'atypical cystic lobules' in 54 consecutive breast biopsies that contained ALH or LCIS and found CCL with atypia in 60 % of the biopsies with LCIS and 46 % of the biopsies with ALH. Although CCL with atypia was usually identified in areas geographically separate from the lobular neoplasia, coexistence of the lobular neoplasia and CCL with atypia was observed in a small number of cases. Fraser *et al.* looked at 100 consecutive breast biopsies performed for microcalcifications and identified columnar cell lesions they termed 'columnar cell alteration with prominent apical snouts and secretions' or 'CAPSS' in 42 % of those cases. Microcalcifications were associated with CAPSS in 72 % of cases. In some of the cases a spectrum of changes ranging from CAPSS without atypia to CAPSS with atypia to areas of low grade DCIS were noted. Among the 16 cases in which both CAPSS and DCIS co-existed, the two lesions were located in either the same or adjacent TDLU in 81 % of the cases, suggesting a relationship between these lesions. Other studies have noted a strong association of CCC, CCH and flat epithelial atypia with cribriform/micropapillary DCIS and invasive breast cancer. Furthermore, increasing numbers of foci of CCL were strongly associated with cribriform/micropapillary DCIS, invasive breast carcinoma, and LCIS.

Rosen has noted that patients with tubular carcinoma often have associated with them foci of columnar cell hyperplasia in the adjacent breast tissue that sometimes even merges with the invasive carcinoma, and has suggested that 'tubular carcinoma might sometimes arise when the hyperplastic lesion has transformed to intraductal carcinoma'. Goldstein and O'Malley examined 32 tubular carcinomas, 41 grade I invasive ductal carcinomas with DCIS, 40 grade III invasive ductal carcinomas, 20 low grade DCIS, and 80 cases with fibrocystic changes, to determine the significance of CCL with atypia. In 17 of these cases, atypical columnar cell lesions were identified: 14 tubular carcinomas and 3 grade 1 invasive ductal carcinomas. CCL with atypia was identified at the periphery of the invasive carcinomas and adjacent to the DCIS, providing further support for a relationship between CCL with atypia and malignancy.

Studies that have microdissected breast specimens that displayed the entire spectrum of CCC through DCIS including invasive carcinoma were able to demonstrate a gradient of progressive genetic changes manifesting allelic loss damage that also provides support for the hypothesis that CCL are morphologic precursors to invasive carcinoma.

The few available clinical follow-up studies suggest that the risk of developing subsequent breast carcinoma in patients with CCL with atypia is considerably lower than that seen with low grade DCIS.

Based on these, and a number of other observations, it would appear likely that at least some columnar cell lesions, particularly those that demonstrate architectural or cytologic atypia, may represent a precursor lesion of, or risk factor for, low grade DCIS or invasive carcinoma, particularly tubular carcinoma. Given the dearth of clinical follow-up studies addressing the relationship of the various columnar cell lesions and malignancy however, additional long term follow-up studies are essential before any definitive conclusions are reached.

PROGNOSIS AND THERAPY

The management recommendations for a patient whose breast biopsy shows CCL are somewhat controversial and will continue to evolve as more information on these lesions becomes available. Based on the currently available data, most recommend that a diagnosis of CCL without atypia on core biopsy does not warrant formal excisional biopsy.

However, there is recent data indicating that when CCL with atypia (flat epithelial atypia) is present in a core biopsy, that approximately one-third of subsequent formal excisional biopsies will demonstrate significant pathology (i.e., ADH, DCIS or invasive carcinoma) and thus most recommend follow-up excisional biopsy in cases of core biopsy diagnosis of CCL with atypia.

There are no currently available data to suggest that the presence of CCL without atypia in an excisional biopsy specimen requires additional pathologic examination of the tissue or special follow-up treatment. However, most experts recommend that the presence of CCL with atypia (flat epithelial atypia) in an excisional biopsy specimen requires a thorough pathologic search for more significant lesions (i.e. ADH, DCIS or invasive carcinoma) in the tissue. This would include obtaining additional levels from the block(s) showing the flat epithelial atypia, and submission of the remaining tissue for histologic examination.

SUGGESTED READINGS

Fibrocystic Changes

Ciatto S, Biggeri A, Del Turco MR, *et al*. Risk of breast cancer subsequent to gross cystic disease. Eur J Cancer 1990;26:555–557.

Haagensen DE Jr. Is cystic disease related to cancer? Am J Surg Pathol 1991;15:687–694.

London SJ, Connolly JL, Schnitt SJ, Colditz GA. A prospective study of benign breast disease and the risk of breast cancer. J Am Med Assoc 1992;267:941–944.

Love SM, Gelman RS, Silen W. Fibrocystic 'disease' of the breast – a non-disease. N Engl J Med 1982;307:1010–1014.

Pastides H, Kelsey JL, LiVolsi VA, *et al*. Oral contraceptive use and fibrocystic disease with special reference to its histopathology. J Natl Cancer Inst 1983;71:5–9.

Vilanova JR, Simon R, Alvarez J, Rivera-Pomar JM. Early apocrine change in hyperplastic cystic disease. Histopathology 1983;7:693–698.

Vorherr H. Fibrocystic breast disease: Pathophysiology, pathomorphology, clinical picture, and management. Am J Obstet Gynecol 1986;154:161–179.

Columnar Cell Lesions

Brogi E, Oyama T, Koerner FC. Atypical cystic lobules in patients with lobular neoplasia. Int J Surg Pathol 2001;9:201–206.

Fraser JL, Raza S, Chorny K, *et al*. Columnar alteration with prominent apical snouts and secretions: a spectrum of changes frequently present in breast biopsies performed for microcalcifications. Am J Surg Pathol 1998;22:1521–1527.

Goldstein NS, O'Malley BA. Cancerization of small ectatic ducts of the breast by ductal carcinoma in situ cells with apocrine snouts: a lesion associated with tubular carcinoma. Am J Clin Pathol 1997;107:561–566.

Otterbach F, Bankfalvi A, Bergner S, *et al*. Cytokeratin 5/6 immunohistochemistry assists the differential diagnosis of atypical proliferation of the breast. Histopathology 2000;37:232–240.

Oyama T, Iijima K, Takei H, *et al*. Atypical cystic lobule of the breast: an early stage of low-grade ductal carcinoma in situ. Breast Cancer 2000;7:326–331.

Page DL KM, Jensen RA. Hypersecretory hyperplasia with atypia in breast biopsies. What is the proper level of clinical concern? Pathol Case Rev 1996;1:36–40.

O'Malley FP, Moshin SK, Badve S, *et al*. Interobserver reproducibility in the diagnosis of flat epithelial atypia. Mod Pathol 2006;19:172–179.

Rosen PP. Columnar cell hyperplasia is associated with lobular carcinoma in situ and tubular carcinoma. Am J Surg Pathol 1999;23:1561.

Rosen PP. Rosen's Breast Pathology 2nd ed. Philadelphia: Lippincott, Williams and Wilkins, 2001.

Schnitt SJ and Vincent-Salomon A. Columnar cell lesions of the breast. Advan Anat Pathol 2003;10:113–124.

Shaaban AM, Sloan JP, West CR, *et al*. Histopathologic types of benign breast lesions and the risk of breast cancer: case–control study. Am J Surg Pathol 2002;26:421–430.

Tavassoli FA, Devilee P. Pathology and Genetics of Tumours of the Breast and Female Genital Organs. World Health Organisation of Classification of Tumours. Lyon. IARC Press 2003.

14

Usual Epithelial Hyperplasia and Atypical Ductal Hyperplasia

Beverley A Carter · David L Page · Frances P O'Malley

INTRODUCTION

Epithelial hyperplasias are patterns of epithelial cell increase and are commonly present in breast biopsies. These reproducibly recognizable histologic patterns are linked with validated epidemiological outcomes and therefore have consistent clinical relevancy. Without the uniform application of criteria, consistency in diagnosis is unlikely; when the criteria discussed below are used for their diagnoses, agreement between pathologists reaches over 90 %.

EPITHELIAL HYPERPLASIA OF USUAL TYPE

Consistent with its definition elsewhere in the body, epithelial hyperplasia of the breast may be understood to mean an increased number of cells relative to a basement membrane. Thus, the increased number of glands without a concomitant increase relative to the basement membrane would not constitute hyperplasia but rather adenosis. Hyperplasia represents an increased number of cells above the basement membrane, and because this number is normally two, the presence of three or more cells above the basement membrane constitutes hyperplasia.

The intent of the term usual is to denote that these are the common patterns of cytology and cell relationships seen in epithelial hyperplasias. The usual type or common patterns of hyperplasia have been termed ductal in the past largely to contrast them with lobular neoplasia. Because these lesions regularly occur within acini of lobular units, the designation *ductal* should not

---

EPITHELIAL HYPERPLASIA OF USUAL TYPE – FACT SHEET

Definition
▶ Increase in number of epithelial cells in breast ducts and lobules
▶ No specific patterns of atypical hyperplasia

Incidence and Location
▶ 20–30% of women undergoing breast biopsy
▶ Either breast, any quadrant

Gender, Race and Age Distribution
▶ Found largely in the latter stages of the pre-menopausal years

Clinical Features
▶ None specific, outside of age and gender

Radiologic Features
▶ Microcalcifications occasionally
▶ Usually found incidentally to other lesions

Prognosis and Treatment
▶ Less than twice the risk of future development of breast cancer in ensuing 20 years
▶ Risk for either breast
▶ Mammographic surveillance

EPITHELIAL HYPERPLASIA OF USUAL TYPE – PATHOLOGIC FEATURES

Gross Findings
▶ None specific

Microscopic Findings
▶ 3 or more cells above basement membrane
▶ Variable cell composition
▶ Variable architecture
▶ Variable nuclei
▶ Irregular slit-like lumina connected in 3-D

Ultrastructural Features
▶ N/A

Fine Needle Aspiration Biopsy Findings
▶ Variable cell population
▶ Cells may be arranged in complex architectural arrangements
▶ Nuclei are small and round to oval
▶ Myoepithelial cells are conspicuous within epithelial groups

Immunohistochemical Features
▶ Cells are generally positive with high molecular weight cytokeratin

Differential Diagnosis
▶ ADH
▶ DCIS

be interpreted as a cell of origin or a site of occurrence. Proliferative lesions in true ducts are unusual and are papillomas characteristically (Figure 14-1).

CLINICAL FEATURES

These changes are largely present in the latter premenopausal years. Moderate and florid examples of usual epithelial hyperplasia are seen in 20–30 % of breast biopsies. There is some relationship to increased density on mammograms.

RADIOLOGIC FEATURES

There are no specific associations of usual hyperplasia with calcifications or other mammographic patterns. Occasionally, microcalcifications can lead to mammographic detection of usual hyperplasia, but it is almost always a part of another radiologically identified lesion such as radial scar, complex sclerosing lesion, adenosis or microcysts.

PATHOLOGIC FEATURES: GROSS AND MICROSCOPIC

Hyperplasia of usual type is generally not identified grossly.

On histologic examination, mild epithelial hyperplasia is characterized by a proliferation of cells in a lobular unit or duct of no more than three to four cells above the basement membrane (Figure 14-2). Mild epithelial hyperplasia is not associated with any subsequent increased breast cancer risk.

Hyperplastic lesions that reach five or more cells above the basement membrane and tend to cross and distend the space or spaces in which they occur are called moderate epithelial hyperplasia. The term *florid* is used for more pronounced changes, but there are no reliable criteria separating the moderate and florid categories (Figure 14-3). Separation of these categories is not necessary, however, as in follow-up studies the breast cancer risk between these two groups was found to be similar.

Epithelial hyperplasias of usual type are lobulocentric and may distend the individual elements of an enlarged lobular unit in various ways. The pattern is similar throughout an individual lobular unit, but often differs quite obviously from the patterns seen in adjacent or nearby units.

The histologic features that characterize epithelial hyperplasia of usual type are a mild variation of size, shape and placement of cells. The nuclei are haphazardly arranged in the involved spaces. Nuclei immediately adjacent to each other may vary in terms of

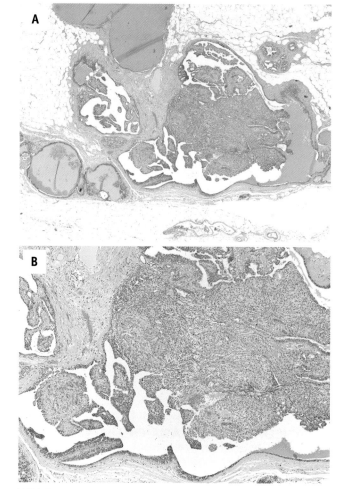

FIGURE 14-1
Florid epithelial hyperplasia of usual type in a papilloma. (A) Low power view showing ducts expanded by a papillary lesion, showing marked cellularity. (B) On higher power, the typical streaming pattern of florid epithelial hyperplasia of usual type is seen. Prominent cellular overlapping is present.

roundness, oval nature and nuclear density. Groups of, often, oval cells exhibit patterns of swirling or streaming, representing parallel arrangements, which maintain intercellular adhesion. Secondary lumina are often present within the spaces and are irregular or slit-like in shape. These intercellular spaces are usually spindled because in three dimensions they interconnect. Secondary lumina, particularly in larger, more cellular lesions, may be present peripherally, immediately above the cells that surmount the basement membrane of the containing space (Figure 14-4).

ANCILLARY STUDIES

Immunohistochemical stains consisting mostly of different keratins have been indicated as an adjunct to the differential diagnosis of atypical hyperplasia and usual

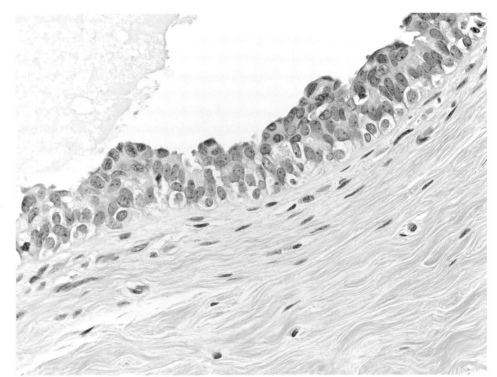

FIGURE 14-2

Mild epithelial hyperplasia. Medium power showing a proliferation of cells within a duct, of no more than four cells above the basement membrane.

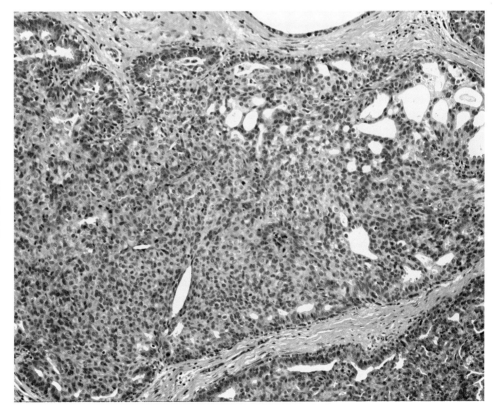

FIGURE 14-3

Florid epithelial hyperplasia of usual type. Pronounced epithelial hyperplasia within a duct, with extension of the proliferation across the duct. A streaming pattern of growth is readily identifiable.

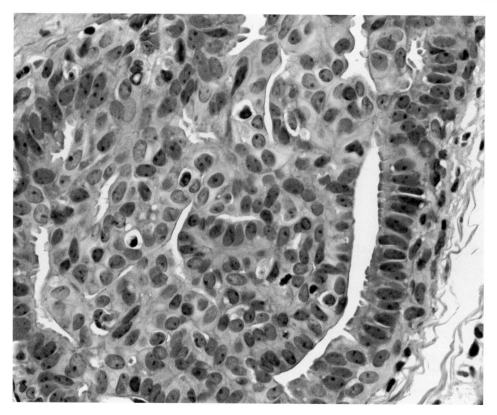

FIGURE 14-4

Florid epithelial hyperplasia of usual type. High power view showing a mild variation in the size and shape of cells. The nuclei haphazardly occupy the involved spaces. Secondary lumina assume an irregular or slit-like shape.

epithelial hyperplasia. This is further discussed in Chapter 25. We have not found such stains to be of defining aid in borderline cases and rely more upon extensiveness of change in order to make a diagnosis of a meaningful clinical type. Most importantly, although of biologic interest, these stains have not been clinically verified with regard to subsequent breast cancer risk. There has been some interest in recent years in different cytokeratins and their variant patterns. Their major utility has been to define the uniformity of cell populations, which is an element of atypical ductal hyperplasia, discussed in the next section.

DIFFERENTIAL DIAGNOSIS

The most important differential diagnoses for the usual patterns of epithelial hyperplasia are its confusion with atypical ductal hyperplasia or low grade ductal carcinoma *in situ*. Failing to diagnose minor examples of epithelial hyperplasia of usual type of mild, or even florid degrees, is of little concern because they are essentially benign with an indication of no or slight increased risk of developing breast cancer. The pattern of florid epithelial hyperplasia of usual type most often confused with low grade ductal carcinoma in situ is the compact pattern. In compact florid hyperplasia, the variegated shapes and varied patterns of the nuclei of florid hyperplasia are compactly arranged with little intervening

cytoplasm. Often, the nuclei are somewhat pyknotic (Figures 14-5 and 14-6). When one defaults to thinking about cellular pleomorphism as an ominous indicator, then overdiagnosis occurs. We have found that this over-diagnosis is most common in intra-operative frozen section samples and thick sections as they appear as a solid population of cells obscuring the intercellular slit-like spaces. Also, low grade DCIS will involve contiguous lobular units and ducts, unlike florid epithelial hyperplasia.

Hyperplasia of usual type in limited or small core biopsies, particularly in a background of sclerosis, as well as some cytologic samples, may present confusion because of the polymorphous cytologic features. A single enlarged lobular unit or a radial scar may be largely involved with florid epithelial hyperplasia and because it is present in many spaces, this may also be over-diagnosed as ductal carcinoma *in situ* (Figure 14-7). Such examples are regularly less than 3 or 4 mm in greatest dimension and lack the even placement of cells which is characteristic of atypical ductal hyperplasia and low grade ductal carcinoma in situ.

PROGNOSIS AND THERAPY

The clinical significance of moderate/florid epithelial hyperplasia rests in the demonstration of a slight increased relative risk (1.5 to 2 times) of subsequent

FIGURE 14-5

Compact hyperplasia. The nuclei of florid hyperplasia are compactly arranged with little intervening cytoplasm, giving the impression of a second population of cells.

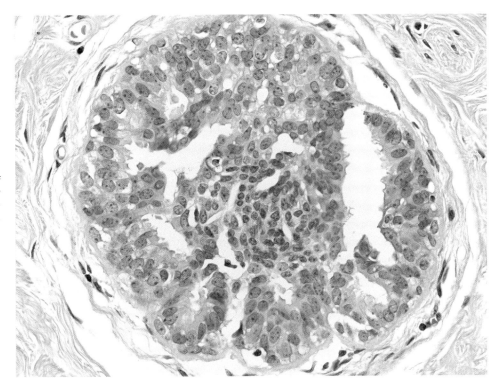

FIGURE 14-6

Compact hyperplasia. These compactly arranged cells can extensively fill a duct. The nuclei appear hyperchromatic and are somewhat pyknotic.

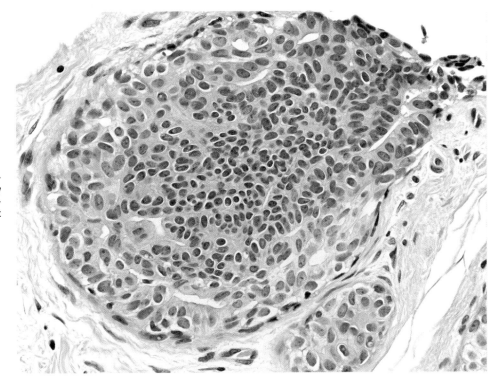

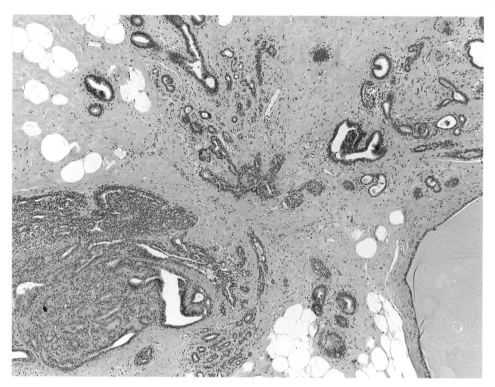

FIGURE 14-7

Florid epithelial hyperplasia of usual type in a radial scar. A large lobular unit in the bottom left of the picture is involved by florid epithelial hyperplasia of usual type, which can lead to over-diagnosis as ductal carcinoma *in situ*.

invasive breast carcinoma in the ensuing 5–15 years, compared to women matched for age who had no breast biopsy. This is particularly true in peri-menopausal women. Even in this age group the risk is not of clinical significance beyond that of indicating a need for continued mammographic surveillance. The risk of cancer is at any site, in either breast. The absolute risk is sometimes more clinically relevant, example: a 40-year-old woman has a 1/1000 risk of cancer in one year. A doubling of this risk is usually not perceived as meaningful.

The clustering of radial scars and co-occurrence of sclerosing adenosis with usual hyperplasia may further elevate risk of future development of breast cancer beyond that associated with these lesions alone. There is some promise that some markers might further stratify the risk in hyperplastic lesions of increased cellularity. Several markers have been tested, but none have been sufficiently validated for clinical use.

ATYPICAL DUCTAL HYPERPLASIA

The intent of the term atypical ductal hyperplasia (ADH) is to indicate a group of fairly specific histologic patterns that have been shown to implicate an increased risk of later breast cancer development. Despite histologic similarity with minute examples of DCIS, ADH has a very different clinical implication.

ATYPICAL DUCTAL HYPERPLASIA – FACT SHEET

Definition
▶ Fairly specific histologic patterns of epithelial hyperplasia that imply elevated risk of breast cancer

Incidence and Location
▶ Approximately 10 % of screen directed biopsies
▶ Either breast, any quadrant

Gender, Race and Age Distribution
▶ Late 40s
▶ Screening programs

Clinical Features
▶ None specific

Radiologic Features
▶ Non-specific, usually microcalcifications or as a part of a mammographically more distinct lesion

Prognosis and Treatment:
▶ 4–5 times relative risk of breast cancer in 10–15 years after biopsy
▶ Mammographic surveillance is appropriate treatment

The atypical hyperplastic lesions have some of the same features as those of carcinomas in situ but either lack a major defining feature of the carcinoma or have the features in lesser extent, primarily by limited extent within the primary spaces or partial involvement of lobular unit(s) (Figure 14-8).

ATYPICAL DUCTAL HYPERPLASIA – PATHOLOGIC FEATURES

Gross Findings
▸ N/A

Microscopic Findings
▸ Most often a solitary lesion
▸ Confined to a single lobular unit
▸ Seldom larger than 3 mm
▸ At least focally a uniform cell population and architectural features of low grade DCIS
▸ Evenly spaced cells with hyperchromatic nuclei

Ultrastructural Features
▸ N/A

Fine Needle Aspiration Biopsy Findings
▸ Variable cellularity
▸ Epithelial cells may have a monotonous appearance
▸ Nuclei have fine chromatin and inconspicuous nucleoli
▸ There is loss of cohesion

Immunohistochemical Features
▸ Cells are usually negative with high molecular weight cytokeratin

Differential Diagnosis
▸ Low grade DCIS
▸ Epithelial hyperplasia

CLINICAL FEATURES

The average age of the women with ADH is late 40s, similar to that of usual hyperplasia. There is no specific clinical presentation, and it may be diagnosed as part of a breast screening strategy. Approximately 10 % of biopsies taken as part of a mammographic screening program contain ADH and/or ALH.

RADIOLOGIC FEATURES

ADH has no specific mammographic features. It may present as microcalcifications of indeterminate significance, but rarely presents as a symptomatic breast lesion. It is usually associated with more mammographically distinct lesions such as radial scars or papillomas.

PATHOLOGIC FEATURES: GROSS AND MICROSCOPIC

ADH is generally not detected grossly.

The lower boundary of ADH is the florid pattern of usual hyperplasia with focal areas of cellular uniformity and even placement of cells. These cells are usually

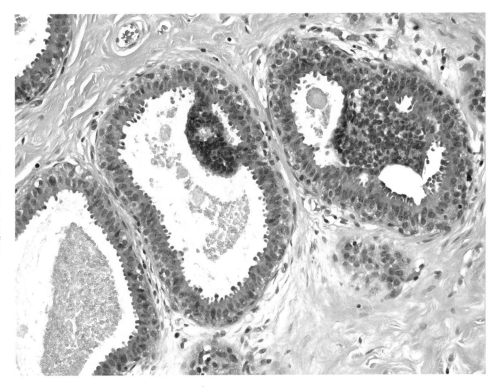

FIGURE 14-8
Atypical ductal hyperplasia. Partial involvement of two ducts by a neoplastic population of cells, with the formation of rigid bridges and bars. The neoplastic cells are identical to those seen in low grade ductal carcinoma *in situ*, however, they do not reach the minimum criteria required for this diagnosis, on the basis of partial involvement and limited extent.

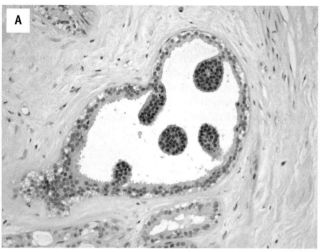 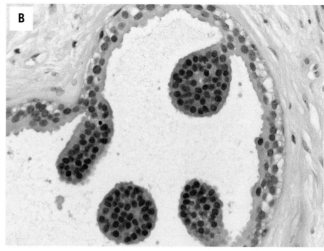

FIGURE 14-9

Atypical ductal hyperplasia, micropapillary type. (A) Medium power shows a duct partially involved by a neoplastic population of cells forming micropapillae. (B) High power shows the hyperchromatic, evenly placed nuclei of the neoplastic cell population within the micropapillary structures. A dual cell population is evident, with columnar cells along the periphery of the duct, making the changes insufficient for a diagnosis of low grade ductal carcinoma *in situ*.

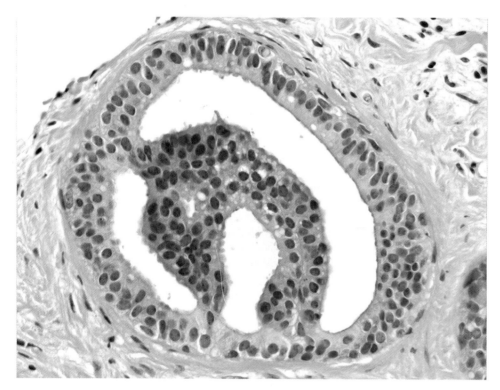

FIGURE 14-10

Atypical ductal hyperplasia. Partial involvement of a duct with a uniform population of cells forming a rigid cribriform archicture. A second cell population of columnar cells lines the remainder of the duct.

hyperchromatic (Figures 14-9 and 14-10). At the upper boundary, the same features present in low grade DCIS are evident, but in a less developed form. Because the criteria of ADH are derived from those of DCIS, histologic criteria for the latter must be understood. Two major criteria are required for the diagnosis of DCIS (low grade). First, a uniform population of neoplastic cells must populate the entire basement membrane-bound space. Furthermore, this alteration must involve at least two such spaces (Figure 14-11). An adjunct to assessing the extent of involvement has been put forth by Tavassoli and Norris. They consider lesions smaller than 2 mm as ADH, with a resulting moderate increase in later cancer development. Another helpful secondary criterion is hyperchromatic nuclei which highlight the nuclear uniformity criterion, but may not be present in all cases. The pattern of high grade DCIS (comedo pattern) is not even discussed here because its characteristic extreme nuclear atypia is far beyond the patterns seen in ADH.

ANCILLARY STUDIES

In fine needle aspiration biopsies ADH can be specifically diagnosed only when rigid intercellular patterns are seen, but is not reliably separated from low grade DCIS.

Differentiating cytokeratins may be helpful in identifying uniform populations of cells in hyperplasic lesions of the breast, but the data is preliminary and not accepted as standard of practice.

DIFFERENTIAL DIAGNOSIS

The main differential diagnoses of atypical ductal hyperplasia are usual epithelial hyperplasia and, more importantly, low grade DCIS. The differentiating characteristics are included in Table 14-1 and Figure 14-12.

Some cases of ADH share features with the so-called clinging carcinoma described by Azzopardi. A study from northern Italy suggests a considerable overlap of clinging carcinoma with ADH in histologic patterns and in risk of subsequent cancer development. Most students of breast pathology do not believe that the diagnosis of clinging carcinoma (monomorphic type) as a form of DCIS is appropriate because it obviously indicates a different behavior from that expected from classic forms of DCIS.

PROGNOSIS AND THERAPY

The link of specific histologic patterns to a moderate magnitude of breast cancer risk depends on the use of defined criteria. This link of ADH lesions to risk is the result of a group of studies that sought to restrict the term to a small number of histologic patterns that have

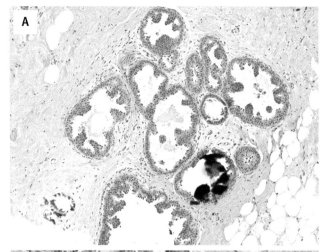
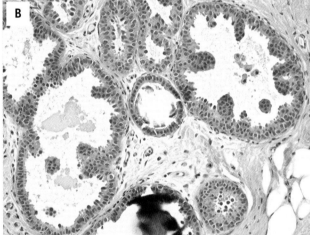

FIGURE 14-11
Low grade DCIS. (A) Low power view showing multiple ducts, completely involved by a population of neoplastic cells, showing a micropapillary growth pattern and (B) consisting of uniform cells with hyperchromatic nuclei. Microcalcifications are present within involved ducts.

FIGURE 14-12
Diagrammatic representation comparing low grade ductal carcinoma in situ, atypical hyperplasia and florid epithelial hyperplasia of usual type. The lumina in DCIS are rigid and punched out. In ADH, some of the lumina share this structure, however, some poorly defined and slit-like spaces are also seen. In fluid epithelial hyperplasia of usual type (FEHUT) rigid lumina are absent and the secondary lumina are poorly formed. The cells of DCIS and ADH lie perpendicular to the lumina, are uniform and have distinct cell borders. Compared with this, cells of FEHUT run parallel with the lumina, show indistinct cell borders and overlap.

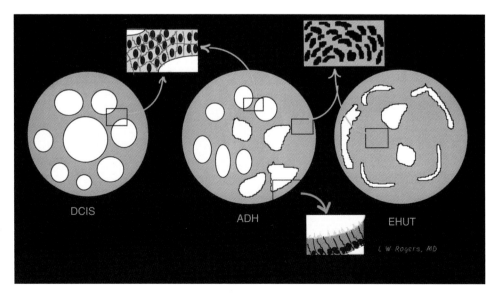

TABLE 14-1

Differentiating characteristics of epithelial hyperplasia of usual type, atypical ductal hyperplasia, and low grade ductal carcinoma *in situ*.

	Epithelial hyperplasia of usual type	Atypical ductal hyperplasia	Low grade ductal carcinoma *in situ*
Size	–Variable, rarely extensive –Usually lobulocentric	–Less than 2 membrane bound spaces or 2 mm –Usually confined to a single lobular unit	May be extensive
Cellular composition	Varied	Uniform cell population at least focally	Uniform
Architecture	–Irregular cell placement –Streaming/swirling patterns	At least focal patterns of DCIS	Micropapillary, cribriform or solid
Lumina	Irregular, slit-like, can be peripheral, connected in 3-D	Focal well-formed spaces	Well-defined punched out spaces throughout (if cribriform)
Nuclei	Unevenly spaced, varying shape and size	Usually hyperchromatic, uniform nuclei	Evenly spaced

some of the same features as the analogous carcinoma in situ lesions.

ADH is associated with a 4–5 times relative risk of developing breast cancer in the ensuing 10–15 years after breast biopsy. The absolute risk of developing cancer in women with ADH after age 40–45 is approximately 10 % in the first 15 years. The risk of cancer is at any site and in either breast.

Regular mammographic follow up of both breasts is the recommended treatment. Prophylactic mastectomies are only indicated in genetically extremely high-risk women for whom surveillance is unacceptable.

SUGGESTED READINGS

Bassett L, Winchester DP, Caplan RB, et al. Stereotactic core-needle biopsy of the breast: a report of the Joint Task Force of the American College of Radiology, American College of Surgeons, and College of American Pathologists. CA Cancer J Clin 1997;47:171–190.

Ely KA, Carter BA, Jensen RA, et al. Core biopsy of the breast with atypical ductal hyperplasia: a probabilistic approach to reporting. Am J Surg Pathol 2001;25:1017–1021.

Fitzgibbons PL, Henson DE, Hutter RV. Benign breast changes and the risk for subsequent breast cancer: an update of the 1985 consensus statement. Cancer Committee of the College of American Pathologists. Arch Pathol Lab Med 1998;122:1053–1055.

London SJ, Connolly JL, Schnitt SJ, Colditz GA. A prospective study of benign breast disease and the risk of breast cancer. J Am Med Assoc 1992;267(7):941–4.

Page DL, Rogers LW. Combined histologic and cytologic criteria for the diagnosis of mammary atypical ductal hyperplasia. Hum Pathol 1992;23(10):1095–7.

Page DL, Jensen RA, Simpson JF. Premalignant and malignant disease of the breast: the roles of the pathologist. Mod Pathol 1998;11:120–128.

Schnitt SJ, Connolly JL, Tavassoli FA, Fechner RE, Kempson RL, Gelman R, et al. Interobserver reproducibility in the diagnosis of ductal proliferative breast lesions using standardized criteria. Am J Surg Pathol 1992;16:1133–1143.

Schnitt SJ. Benign breast disease and breast cancer risk: morphology and beyond. Am J Surg Pathol 2003;27:836–841.

Tavassoli FA, Norris HJ. A comparison of the results of long-term follow-up for atypical intraductal hyperplasia and intraductal hyperplasia of the breast. Cancer 1990;65:518–529.

15

Atypical Lobular Hyperplasia (ALH) and Lobular Carcinoma *in situ* (LCIS) Including 'Pleomorphic Variant'

Timothy W Jacobs

Atypical lobular hyperplasia (ALH) and lobular carcinoma *in situ* (LCIS) are relatively uncommon lesions which have been shown to confer an increased risk of subsequent breast cancer. The features of classic LCIS were originally described over 60 years ago by Foote and Stewart (1941) who used the term 'carcinoma *in situ*' to suggest similarities to ductal carcinoma in situ (DCIS), in part because the constituent cells resembled those found in invasive lobular carcinoma. More recently in situ carcinomas with ambiguous histologic features have been recognized. One of these variants, pleomorphic LCIS (PLCIS), exhibits the growth pattern of classic LCIS but is composed of larger and more pleomorphic cells. Because ALH and LCIS have identical cytologic features and are defined histologically by differing degrees of distention of involved spaces, some authorities have advocated using the term lobular neoplasia to encompass both entities. The term lobular intraepithelial neoplasia (LIN) has also been proposed to include the morphologic spectrum of classic ALH and LCIS through PLCIS, however this classification scheme has not found widespread epidemiologic or clinical applicability.

CLINICAL FEATURES

There are no clinical features diagnostic of ALH or LCIS and therefore these lesions are usually incidental microscopic findings in breast tissue removed for other reasons. Consequently, their true incidence in the general population is unknown but estimated to be between 1 and 3.6 %. The incidence of PLCIS is unknown but is certainly far lower. LCIS is most commonly found in pre-menopausal women with a mean age of occurrence of 44–46 years. ALH and LCIS are often multicentric (approximately 50 % of cases) and frequently bilateral (up to 30 % of cases). These lesions are considered generalized risk factors for subsequent breast cancer, since cancers that develop are usually not at the same site in the ipsilateral breast and may also occur in the contralateral breast. The relative risk (compared to controls) of subsequent cancer is approximately 4 to 5 times for ALH and 8 to 10 times for LCIS. This translates (depending on the patient population) to an absolute risk of breast cancer in relation to LCIS of

---

ALH, LCIS, PLCIS – FACT SHEET

Definition

▸ Group of breast lesions characterized cytologically by dyshesive uniform cells with eccentric nuclei, frequently with intracytoplasmic mucin vacuoles
▸ ALH and LCIS distinguished by degree of extension of involved spaces
▸ PLCIS characterized by larger, more pleomorphic cells

Incidence and Location

▸ True incidence unknown, estimated 1–3.6 % for ALH and LCIS; PLCIS far lower
▸ Often multicentric, frequently bilateral

Morbidity and Mortality

▸ ALH and LCIS are generalized risk factors for subsequent breast cancer (relative risk of 4–5 times for ALH, 8–10 times for LCIS)
▸ PLCIS natural history is unknown; may behave like DCIS

Gender, Race and Age Distribution

▸ ALH and LCIS more common in premenopausal women (mean 44–46 years)
▸ PLCIS might be slightly older (limited data available)

Clinical Features

▸ No specific clinical features
▸ Usually incidental microscopic finding in tissue removed for other reasons

Radiologic Features

▸ ALH and LCIS: no specific radiologic features. Calcifications often nearby or in ductal-lobular unit or lesion secondarily involved.
▸ PLCIS may calcify especially if necrosis present
▸ Mass lesions only if secondarily involved by ALH, LCIS or PLCIS (e.g, fibroadenoma)

Prognosis and Treatment

▸ ALH and LCIS are considered risk lesions, with conservative treatment aimed at risk reduction, such as close observation, selective estrogen antagonists (e.g. Tamoxifen).
▸ Excision of positive surgical margins and eradication of individual lesions is not required
▸ Core needle biopsy with incidental ALH or LCIS need not be excised provided adequate imaging-pathology correlation. Lesions to excise include those with accompanying high risk lesions (such as ADH), poor imaging-pathology correlation, and where the histologic features of the ALH/LCIS are ambiguous

ALH, LCIS, PLCIS – PATHOLOGIC FEATURES

Gross Findings

▸ No specific features

Microscopic Findings

▸ Distention of involved lobules by a dyshesive, uniform proliferation of round cells with eccentric cytoplasm
▸ Cells frequently contain intracytoplasmic mucin vacuole, often 'targetoid'
▸ Classic, type 'A' cells 1–1.5 times the size of a lymphocyte; type 'B' cells are larger, twice the size of a lymphocyte, often with nucleoli, but still uniform and not pleomorphic.
▸ Individual cells of ALH and LCIS identical; distinguished by degree of distention of involved space: at least 50% of spaces in a TDLU filled and distended in LCIS
▸ PLCIS has dyshesive growth pattern of LCIS, but cells are larger (4 times size of a lymphocyte), more pleomorphic, mitoses may be found, necrosis can be present.

FNAB Features

▸ Smears may contain characteristic atypical-appearing cells, present predominantly singly and may erroneously be called suspicious for carcinoma. However, cellularity is often low.
▸ PLCIS may pose particular diagnostic problems because of the dyshesive pleomorphic cells present.

Immunohistochemical Features

▸ ALH, LCIS and PLCIS are uniformly negative for E-cadherin
▸ Most are positive for estrogen and progesterone receptor, negative for HER2/neu
▸ PLCIS has higher proliferation rate (Ki-67 index) and more likely p53 positive versus classic ALH/LCIS

Differential Diagnosis

▸ Invasive carcinoma (particularly when secondarily involving a sclerosing lesion such as radial scar or sclerosing adenosis)
▸ Myoepithelial cells
▸ Fixation artifact with 'pseudo-dyshesion'
▸ Ductal carcinoma in situ (DCIS)

approximately 1–2% per year with a lifetime risk of approximately 30–40%. The time to cancer from an initial biopsy with LCIS is relatively long (compared to DCIS) and ranges from 15–30 years, depending on the study.

Invasive carcinomas that develop may be infiltrating ductal or infiltrating lobular carcinoma. However, the incidence of infiltrating lobular carcinoma occurring with LCIS is significantly greater than without. This fact, together with more recent reports indicating that ipsilateral carcinomas are three times more common than contralateral carcinomas, suggest that ALH and LCIS may also be precursor lesions in addition to risk factors. Current and ongoing molecular studies support this notion. However, the distinguishing features between which particular ALH/LCIS lesions are direct precursors and which are generalized risk factors are not known at the present time.

RADIOLOGIC FEATURES

ALH and LCIS have no distinct radiologic features. When these lesions are found in biopsies targeting mammographically detected microcalcifications, the histologic calcifications are usually present in normal tissue adjacent to areas of LCIS or in terminal duct lobular units (TDLU) secondarily involved by LCIS. Nonetheless, ALH and LCIS may 'present' because of targeted calcifications closely associated in up to 40% of cases. In addition, rather than presenting as a mass lesion *per se*, LCIS may involve sclerosing adenosis causing architectural distortion on mammography, or a fibroadenoma causing a mass lesion on ultrasound examination. Therefore, when ALH or LCIS are detected on limiting sampling techniques such as core needle biopsy (CNB), careful radiologic-pathologic correlation is crucial to ensure adequate diagnostic tissue has been obtained. In contrast to classic ALH and LCIS, PLCIS may present with calcifications similar to that of DCIS, particularly if central (comedo-type) necrosis is found.

PATHOLOGIC FEATURES

GROSS FINDINGS

In keeping with the clinical and imaging features, classic ALH and LCIS are not associated with specific gross findings, apart from lesions secondarily involved (e.g. fibroadenoma involved by LCIS).

MICROSCOPIC FINDINGS

LCIS is characterized by distention of involved lobules by a uniform proliferation of dyshesive small cells, with small, uniform, round-to-oval nuclei (approximately 1 to 1.5 times the size of a lymphocyte) showing relatively homogeneous chromatin and absent or inconspicuous nucleoli. The nuclei are often eccentrically placed and the cytoplasm is usually pale to lightly eosinophilic. The cells often contain intracytoplasmic mucin vacuoles which are occasionally large enough to produce signet ring cell forms (Figure 15-1). The intracytoplasmic mucin may have a characteristic 'targetoid' appearance seen as a darker central 'dot' surrounded by a clearer halo. LCIS cases with these features constitute the classical type or 'type A'. LCIS cases may be characterized by cells with more abundant cytoplasm, slightly larger nuclear size (up to twice the size of a lymphocyte), slightly more variation in nuclear size and shape, and with nucleoli and are then classified as 'type B' LCIS (as originally described by Haagensen and by Azzopardi) (Figure 15-2). Occasionally, type A and type B LCIS cells may involve a single space.

The individual cells of LCIS and ALH are morphologically identical and the distinction between these lesions is based on the degree of involvement of the TDLU, with less extensive involvement in ALH compared to LCIS. However, the diagnostic criteria vary

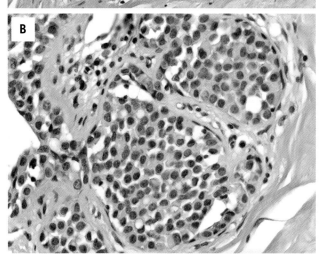

FIGURE 15-1

LCIS involving a terminal duct lobular unit: (A) low power showing distention of the acini and pagetoid involvement of the terminal duct by a uniform population of dyshesive small cells; (B) at higher power, note the eccentrically placed cytoplasm and small round-oval nuclei with homogeneous chromatin and inconspicuous nuclei. Note the presence of an intracytoplasmic mucin vacuole in several cells. These constitute 'classic' or 'type A' LCIS cells.

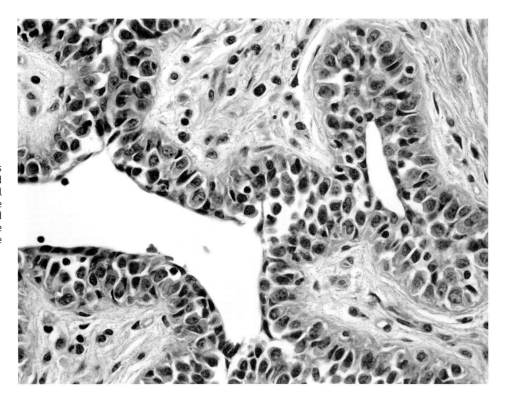

FIGURE 15-2

These LCIS cells insinuate themselves between the native epithelial and basement membrane/myoepithelial cell layer in a pagetoid fashion. The cells are slightly larger with mild variation in nuclear size and shape with nucleoli and are known as 'type B' cells.

amongst authors. The most widely used definition is that of Page and Anderson, requiring at least 50 % of spaces in a given TDLU to be filled and distended by the characteristic cells for a diagnosis of LCIS (Figure 15-3). The clinical relevance of this cut-off is supported by outcome studies demonstrating a two fold difference in risk of subsequent cancer for LCIS versus ALH. Therefore, making a distinction between ALH and LCIS rather than using a combined term of 'lobular neoplasia' might be more clinically and epidemiologically appropriate.

ALH or LCIS may involve extralobular ducts either solidly or, more commonly, in a 'pagetoid' fashion insinuating themselves between the native luminal epithelial cells of the duct and the myoepithelial cells and basement membrane layer (Figures 15-2 and 15-4). Of note, the diagnosis of ALH or LCIS is based on the characteristic cytologic features and dyshesive growth pattern of the constituent cells rather than their location (i.e.,

within a lobule or duct), and therefore LCIS involving a duct must not be erroneously interpreted as DCIS. As alluded to above, ALH and LCIS may secondarily involve otherwise benign lesions such as sclerosing adenosis, radial scar (see Chapter 8), fibroadenoma or collagenous spherulosis (Figure 15-5), raising the differential diagnosis of invasive carcinoma or DCIS in the latter (see below). Apart from signet ring cell features (Figure 15-6), other cytologic variants include LCIS with clear cell change, apocrine metaplasia, myoid change, as well as the pleomorphic variant known as pleomorphic LCIS (PLCIS).

PLCIS exhibits the characteristic dyshesive growth pattern of LCIS, but the individual cells have larger nuclei (3–4 times the size of a lymphocyte), with marked pleomorphism (at least two- to three fold variation in nuclear size with irregularity) and frequently have prominent nucleoli. Although the nuclei are usually eccentrically placed, the nuclear-cytoplasmic ratio is

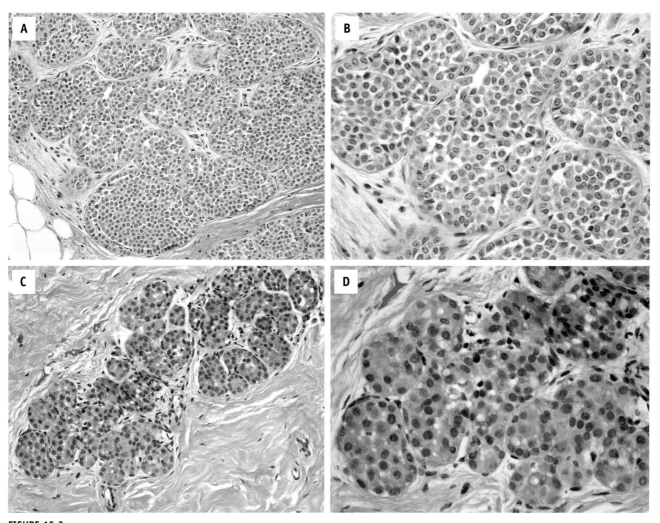

FIGURE 15-3
LCIS versus ALH: (A, B) LCIS by definition consists of characteristic dyshesive, uniform cells filling and distending more than 50 % of the spaces in this terminal duct lobular unit. (C, D) In ALH, although the cells are morphologically similar to those in LCIS, there is no distention of the acinar spaces (by definition <50 %).

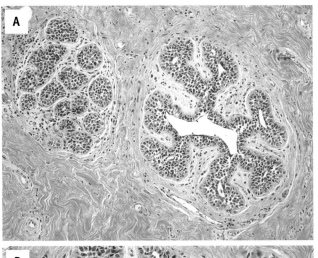

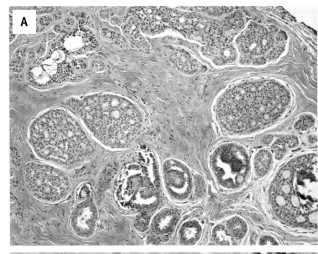

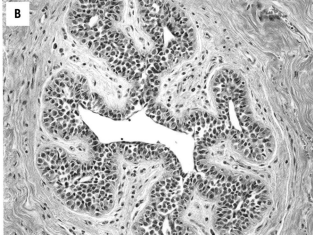

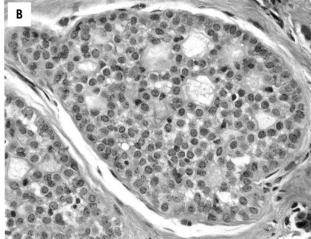

FIGURE 15-4

ALH involving a terminal duct lobular unit: (A) low power showing the lobular acini at left and terminal duct at right involved by ALH; (B) high power showing a cross-section of the terminal duct with ALH cells present in a pagetoid fashion.

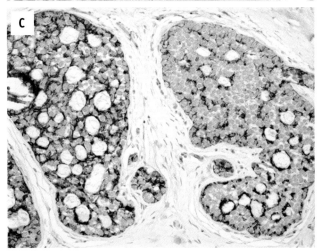

FIGURE 15-5

LCIS involving collagenous spherulosis: (A) low power appearance of fenestrated duct spaces, mimicking cribriform DCIS due to the uniform cell population; (B) high power view showing the characteristic dyshesive, small and uniform cells of LCIS undermining the spherules of collagenous spherulosis. These spherules are surrounded by an irregular cuticle, unlike cribriform DCIS, where the true lumens of the fenestrations are smooth and comprise the apical surfaces of component neoplastic cells; (C) E-cadherin immunostain with LCIS cells negative and residual scaffolding of collagenous spherulosis positive.

increased, and unlike classic LCIS, mitoses may be present (Figures 15-7 and 15-8). The cytologic features are similar to those found in the individual cells of high grade DCIS. Necrosis may be present and is often central within the involved space, similar in appearance to that found in comedo-pattern DCIS (Figure 15-9). Unlike classic LCIS, PLCIS may contain calcifications, particularly if there is apoptosis and/or necrosis present. Although spaces may be involved by these pleomorphic cells to varying degree, the term PLCIS is used for all lesions and the term 'pleomorphic ALH' is not generally favored. PLCIS may be seen as an isolated lesion or in association with invasive carcinoma. The cytomorphologic features of PLCIS are similar irrespective of the presence of an associated invasive component. When infiltrating lobular carcinoma is present, this may be classic or pleomorphic type.

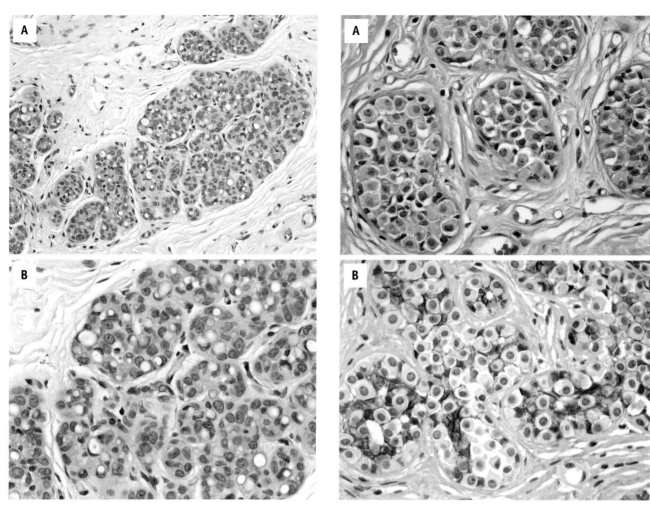

FIGURE 15-6

ALH with signet ring features: (A) low power of the involved terminal duct lobular unit and (B) high power showing intracytoplasmic vacuoles distended with mucin, which compresses the nuclei resulting in a signet ring cells.

FIGURE 15-7

Pleomorphic LCIS (PLCIS): (A) the characteristic dyshesive growth pattern of LCIS is present, but the cells have larger nuclei which are pleomorphic with prominent nucleoli. Note that the nuclei are eccentric and occasional intracytoplasmic vacuoles are seen; (B) Immunohistochemistry for E-cadherin: the PLCIS cells are negative, while the residual acinar epithelial cells are positive.

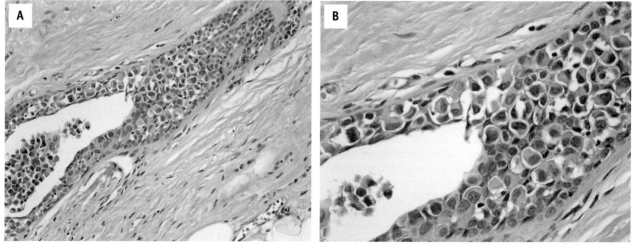

FIGURE 15-8

Pleomorphic LCIS (PLCIS) involving a duct in a pagetoid fashion: Although the dyshesive pagetoid growth pattern is characteristic of LCIS (A), the individual cells are markedly pleomorphic and may mimic those of high grade DCIS (B).

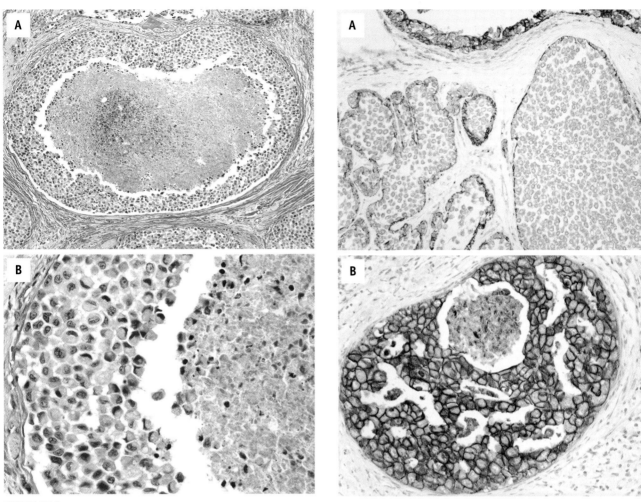

FIGURE 15-9
Pleomorphic LCIS (PLCIS) with central (comedo-type) necrosis

FIGURE 15-10
E-cadherin immunostaining: (A) LCIS is E-cadherin negative (note the residual positive staining ductal epithelium serving as an internal control); (B) DCIS (high nuclear grade with necrosis) is E-cadherin positive with strong circumferential membrane staining.

ANCILLARY STUDIES

Expression of the cell membrane adhesion molecule E-cadherin is lost in the vast majority of cases of LCIS and infiltrating lobular carcinoma but not in most DCIS or infiltrating ductal/no special type carcinoma (Figure 15-10). Therefore, analysis of E-cadherin protein expression by immunohistochemistry has shown promise in the categorization of *in situ* lesions, particularly those which are histologically ambiguous (see Differential Diagnosis section). Of note, mutations in the E-cadherin gene have been found in approximately 50 % of lobular carcinomas, most of which result in non-functional proteins predominantly involving the extracellular domain. Loss of heterozygocity (LOH) at 16q22 occurs in 63–87 % of lobular carcinomas involving the region of the E-cadherin locus (16q22-1). In addition, transcriptional silencing of the E-cadherin promoter by methylation has been reported. A recent study has suggested that immunohistochemistry using antibody

34betaE12 (toward high molecular weight cytokeratins) stains LCIS positive and DCIS negative, however the findings remain to be validated by other investigators. Classic LCIS and PLCIS show some similarities and some differences with regard to immunophenotype. Similar to classic LCIS, PLCIS has been shown to be E-cadherin negative by immunohistochemistry (Figure 15-7).

Both classic LCIS and PLCIS are positive for estrogen and progesterone receptor expression in the majority of cases (up to 90–100 %). The majority of PLCIS cases are negative for HER2/neu overexpression (up to 4 % positive in one study) while classic LCIS has been shown to be uniformly negative. In contrast to classic LCIS, PLCIS has a higher proliferation rate (measured by Ki-67 immunostaining) and more likelihood of positivity for p53 protein (25 % PLCIS versus 0 % LCIS cases). Recent findings suggest that cases of PLCIS have similar cytomorphologic features and biomarker expression profiles irrespective of the presence or absence of accompanying invasive carcinoma.

FINE NEEDLE ASPIRATION BIOPSY

Because the cells of ALH and LCIS are dyshesive, these may be aspirated by fine needle. Smears usually show the characteristic lobular cells present singly or in small clusters. The presence of moderately atypical, dyshesive cells may lead to a suspicious diagnosis being rendered and based on the cytomorphology the smears may be impossible to distinguish from carcinoma. However, the cellularity is usually not as high as overt invasive carcinoma. FNA of PLCIS may be even more problematic due to the dyshesive pleomorphic cells present.

DIFFERENTIAL DIAGNOSIS

The major differential diagnostic considerations for classic ALH and LCIS are discussed below:

INVASIVE CARCINOMA

ALH and LCIS may involve benign lesions such as sclerosing adenosis or radial scar, mimicking invasive carcinoma. Recognizing the morphologic features of the underlying benign sclerosing lesion as well as the presence of myoepithelial cells surrounding the nests of atypical glands are keys to the correct diagnosis. Immunohistochemistry for myoepithelial markers such as p63 and smooth muscle myosin heavy chain is useful in difficult cases where the morphology of the involved benign lesion is not clear-cut. Sclerosing lesions involved by PLCIS may be particularly diagnostically challenging due to the pleomorphism of the neoplastic cells (Figure 15-11) (see Chapter 8 for a detailed discussion of sclerosing lesions). In addition, a TDLU involved by ALH/LCIS may be sclerotic and/or tangentially sectioned, leading to confusion with invasive lobular carcinoma (Figure 15-12). A benign TDLU involved by ALH maintains the normal duct and lobular/acinar architecture and is well circumscribed. In contrast, the cells of invasive lobular carcinoma percolate haphazardly without regard to the normal ductolobular architecture. As with any non-invasive process, recognition of the presence of myoepithelial cells is key to the correct diagnosis.

MYOEPITHELIAL CELLS

Myoepithelial cells may be confused with the cells of ALH/LCIS particularly when the latter involve TDLUs or extralobular ducts in a pagetoid fashion (Figure 15-13). The clear appearing myoepithelial cell cytoplasm that often surrounds the nucleus may give an illusion of a dyshesive cell. However, the characteristic small, round-to-ovoid, pyknotic-appearing nucleus of the myoepithelial cells differs from that of the ALH/LCIS cell which tends to be slightly larger, less intensely basophilic, with courser chromatin and not as smoothly contoured round/ovoid. Furthermore, in contrast to the clear indiscernible cytoplasm of the myoepithelial

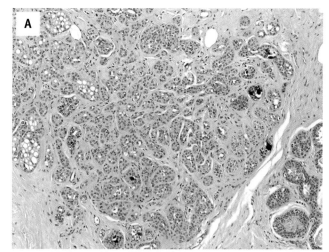

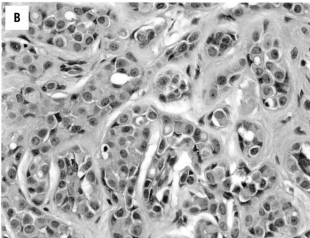

FIGURE 15-11

PLCIS involving sclerosing adenosis: (A) low power, showing the characteristic lobulocentric pattern of the involved sclerosing adenosis. Note calcifications; (B) high power demonstrating the dyshesive pleomorphic cells with eccentric nuclei and intracytoplasmic mucin vacuoles, present in nests within a sclerotic stroma. Note the surrounding myoepithelial cells.

cell, the eosinophilic cytoplasm of the ALH/LCIS cell is usually easily identified and is eccentric and in close contiguity to the nucleus. The cells of ALH/LCIS are truly dyshesive with a clear space surrounding both the nucleus and cytoplasm. In histologically challenging cases, immunohistochemistry for the myoepithelial markers is useful, particularly for p63 which is a nuclear antigen.

FIXATION ARTIFACT WITH 'PSEUDODYSHESION'

Occasionally the epithelial cells within a TDLU, duct or benign lesion (such as fibroadenoma) may appear dyshesive due to tissue fixation artifact, mimicking ALH. Recognition that this 'pseudodyshesion' involves all epithelial cells to varying degree in a particular area of a tissue section is a useful discriminating feature, in contrast to ALH where only the individual cells are dyshesive. In addition, with fixation artifact, residual

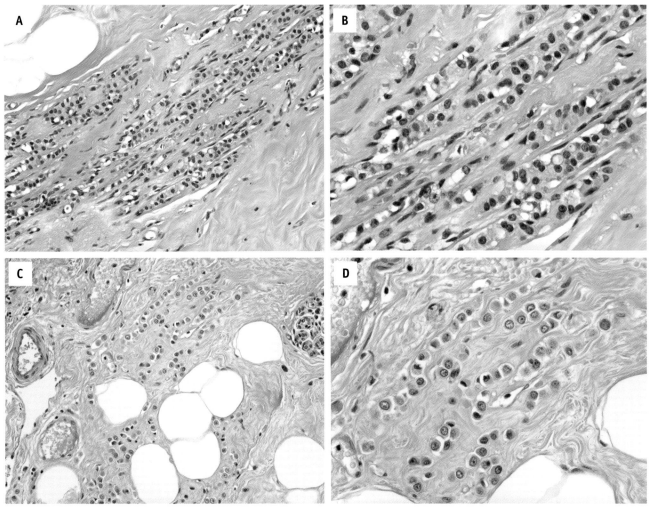

FIGURE 15-12

ALH in a tangentially sectioned TDLU versus infiltrating lobular carcinoma. ALH (A) at low power note the circumscribed normal appearing microanatomy of the TDLU involved by ALH, albeit tangential; (B) higher power shows the characteristic cells in linear array but with surrounding myoepithelial cells. Infiltrating lobular carcinoma (C) at low power showing the haphazard infiltrative pattern of the malignant cells; (D) higher power demonstrating the classic single filing appearance and lack of surrounding myoepithelial cells.

intercellular adhesion is almost always present in at least some acini or ducts, particularly at the luminal/apical aspect of the cells (Figure 15-14). In contrast, the vast majority of ALH cells are dyshesive circumferentially, and if involving a duct in a pagetoid fashion would be interposed between a cohesive luminal epithelial cell layer and a myoepithelial/basement membrane layer.

DCIS

The distinction between LCIS and DCIS has important therapeutic implications (see below). In most cases, the categorization of *in situ* lesions as either LCIS or DCIS does not usually present diagnostic difficulty. Also, the diagnosis of LCIS and DCIS are not necessarily mutually exclusive: DCIS may extend into recognizable lobules and be mistaken for LCIS (also known as 'cancerization of lobules') (Figure 15-15) and LCIS may involve extralobular ducts, mimicking DCIS (Figure 15-

16). It is however important to recognize that LCIS and DCIS may coexist in the same breast and even in the same ductal-lobular unit (Figure 15-17). These situations rarely cause difficulties for the surgical pathologist, particularly when the classic cytologic features and dyshesive growth pattern of LCIS are recognized. However, distinguishing LCIS from DCIS is more problematic in three circumstances:

- *Solid pattern DCIS*: LCIS may be confused with solid low grade DCIS. Several histologic features are useful in distinguishing these lesions. The cells of LCIS are usually at least focally dyshesive, compared to those of DCIS which show cell–cell adhesion circumferentially. Microacini with cells polarized around a central microlumen are found in solid DCIS but not in LCIS. In contrast to DCIS, intracytoplasmic vacuoles are often present in LCIS. A useful feature of solid DCIS is polarization of cells peripherally in the involved space, not found in LCIS (Figure 15-18). Lastly, pagetoid ductal involvement is a feature of LCIS, not

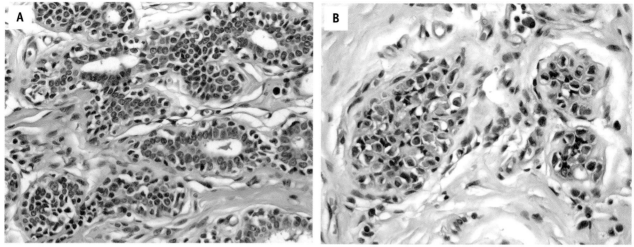

FIGURE 15-13

Myoepithelial cells versus ALH: (A) prominent myoepithelial cells in a TDLU, with clear 'halos' around the small dark pyknotic appearing nuclei, giving an appearance of dyshesion; (B) in contrast, ALH cells in a TDLU have discernible eccentric eosinophilic cytoplasm and both the nucleus and cytoplasm are surrounded by a clear space (i.e. the cell is truly dyshesive).

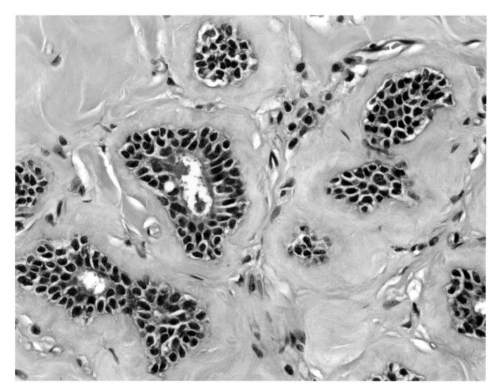

FIGURE 15-14

Pseudodyshesion in TDLU due to fixation artifact. In contrast to ALH, this pseudodyshesion partially involves the epithelial cells with partial cohesion present between cells, particularly at the apical/luminal aspects.

of low grade solid DCIS. E-cadherin immunostaining is often helpful in difficult cases, with the cells of LCIS negative and those of DCIS positive.

- *'Pseudo-acini' in ALH/LCIS*: ALH or LCIS may involve the scaffolding of benign structures in a pagetoid fashion, leading to the appearance of 'acini' in the midst of monomorphic cells, thus mimicking DCIS. For example, collagenous spherulosis may be involved by ALH/LCIS and be confused with cribriform DCIS (Figure 15-5). At low power microscopic

view, both cribriform DCIS and collagenous spherulosis which is involved by ALH/LCIS contain monomorphic cells and appear fenestrated. However, the lumens of collagenous spherulosis contain the characteristic eosinophilic spherules that are hyaline or fibrillar as opposed to cribriform DCIS lumens that may be empty or contain calcifications, debris or necrotic material. Importantly, the spherules of collagenous spherulosis are lined by a layer of myoepithelial cells, whereas the myoepithelial cells

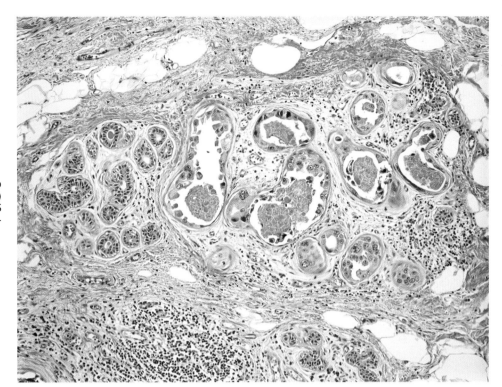

FIGURE 15-15

DCIS extending into lobules (also known as 'cancerization of lobules') should not be mistaken for LCIS merely because of its microanatomical location.

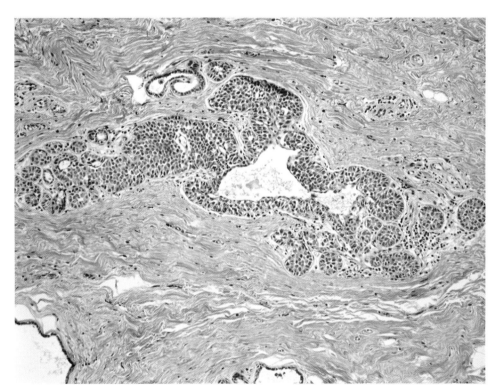

FIGURE 15-16

LCIS involving a duct in a pagetoid fashion should not be misdiagnosed as DCIS; note the small, uniform, dyshesive cells characteristic of LCIS.

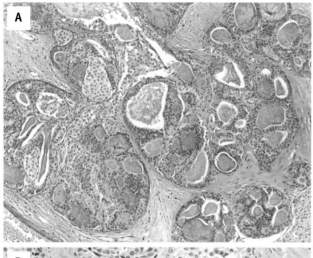

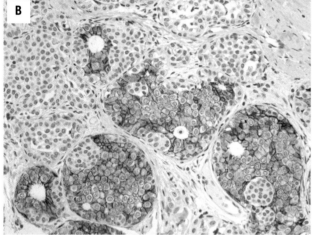

FIGURE 15-17

LCIS and DCIS co-existing in the same ducto-lobular spaces: (A) the LCIS cells are dyshesive, while the DCIS is cohesive and has a cribriform architecture; (B) the LCIS cells are E-cadherin negative and the DCIS cells are E-cadherin positive by immunohistochemistry.

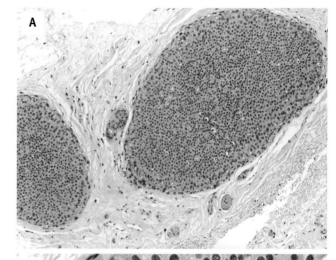

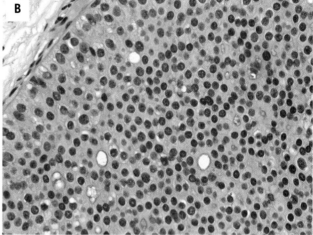

FIGURE 15-18

Solid pattern DCIS mimicking LCIS: (A) low power, showing a solid proliferation of uniform small cells; (B) at higher power, microacini around which cells are polarized and polarization of cells at the periphery of the involved space are useful features of DCIS rather than LCIS.

associated with DCIS surround the lesion. Immunostains for E-cadherin are useful in this situation, as are stains for myoepithelial markers. More commonly, benign TDLUs involved by ALH or LCIS may contain residual lobular acini leading to a false impression of cribriforming spaces as in DCIS. By E-cadherin immunohistochemistry, the epithelium of the residual acini will be positive while the ALH/LCIS cells will be negative.

- Carcinomas *in situ* with indeterminate features: Some *in situ* carcinomas display cytologic and/or architectural features which deviate from the usual patterns, making it difficult to determine if these proliferations are LCIS or DCIS. These histologically ambiguous *in situ* lesions provide both diagnostic and management challenges (see below). There has been much discussion regarding the classification and treatment of such equivocal *in situ* carcinomas, with some authors proposing a combined or mixed ductal and lobular category and others favoring categorization as one type or the other. Analysis of genetic and immunophenotypic characteristics of these histologically ambiguous *in*

situ carcinomas, in comparison to unambiguous cases of LCIS and DCIS should provide useful information toward defining their biologic nature and assisting in their categorization. One marker which has shown recent promise in this regard is E-cadherin (see Ancillary Studies section). Based on histologic features and E-cadherin immunostaining patterns, these variant in situ carcinomas may be divided into three groups for conceptual purposes.

PLEOMORPHIC LCIS

One histologically ambiguous type of *in situ* carcinoma is PLCIS (described above). PLCIS presents both diagnostic and therapeutic dilemmas because the cytologic features are quite similar to those found in the individual cells of high grade DCIS. The distinction may be particularly challenging if necrosis is present in association with PLCIS. In addition, high grade DCIS may occasionally appear dyshesive, in part due to single cell necrosis and/or tissue fixation. All PLCIS cases reported to date have been negative for E-cadherin by IHC, in contrast to high grade DCIS which is E-cadherin positive. This lack of E-cadherin expression suggests that these *in situ* lesions are closer in phenotype to LCIS than DCIS, although whether they differ in clinical behavior is not entirely known (see below).

Another pattern of *in situ* carcinoma that poses diagnostic difficulty consists of lesions with the cytologic and architectural features typical of LCIS (i.e., distention of lobules by a proliferation of dyshesive small cells, with uniform, round-to-oval, usually eccentric nuclei) but with areas of comedo-type (central) necrosis (Figure 15-19). The exact classification and management of such lesions has been a topic of much debate, with a spectrum of opinions regarding the degree of necrosis that is permissible in LCIS. In ours and in other series, all *in situ* carcinomas which differed from LCIS only by the presence of comedo-type necrosis lacked E-cadherin expression by IHC, analogous to the immunophenotype of classic LCIS. These observations indicate that carcinomas in situ with comedo necrosis in which the cells are characteristic of LCIS are, in fact, morphologic vari-

ants of LCIS. However, it is not known if the natural history of such LCIS lesions with comedo necrosis is similar to that of conventional LCIS without comedo necrosis.

IN SITU CARCINOMA WITH MIXED LCIS/DCIS FEATURES

Lastly, some *in situ* carcinomas have features of both LCIS and DCIS rendering categorization very difficult if not impossible on routine histology. These problematic lesions are usually comprised of small, monomorphic neoplastic cells, with or without cytoplasmic vacuoles, akin to those found in classic LCIS. However, in some cases, these small uniform cells grow in a solid, cohesive, mosaic pattern suggestive of solid pattern DCIS (Figure 5-20). In other cases, the cells may grow in a primarily solid pattern and show microacinar-like structures, features suggestive of DCIS, albeit with evidence of cellular dyshesion, a feature more characteristic of LCIS. In our series of in situ carcinomas, we found this group to be heterogeneous with respect to E-cadherin immunostaining: 30% of cases were E-cadherin positive (more akin to DCIS), 35% were E-cadherin negative (akin to LCIS), and 35% had both E-cadherin positive as well as E-cadherin negative tumor cells within the same ductal-lobular space, suggesting a mixed DCIS and LCIS phenotype. E-cadherin-positive cases probably represent true cases of DCIS with morphologic 'artifacts' on routine hematoxylin and eosin (H&E) staining, mimicking LCIS (Figure 15-21). Those *in situ* cases in which the neoplastic cells are negative for E-cadherin most likely represent true cases of LCIS (Figure 15-20). In fact, in several cases in our series, foci of residual benign epithelial and/or myoepithelial structures within the involved lobule stained positive for E-cadherin but were not clearly discernible on routine H&E staining. Therefore, this phenomenon may produce the illusion of DCIS-like architectural structures formed by the neoplastic cells seen on routine stains. Also, loss of cohesion in cases of LCIS might not readily be apparent in lobules distended by cells that are packed together, giving the illusion of a solid proliferation. Histologically indeterminate *in situ* carcinomas which show both E-cadherin-positive tumor cells and E-cadherin-negative tumor cells probably represent true cases with both DCIS and LCIS in the same lobule or duct (Figure 15-22). As alluded to above, the diagnoses of LCIS and DCIS are not mutually exclusive. It should be emphasized that this mixed pattern of immunostaining refers to an intermingling of E-cadherin positive and E-cadherin negative neoplastic cells present in the same space, rather than incomplete or partial immunoreactivity of individual cells. To date, 'transitional' type lesions with individual cells showing partial or incomplete E-cadherin immunoreactivity have not been found.

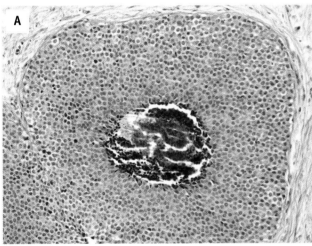

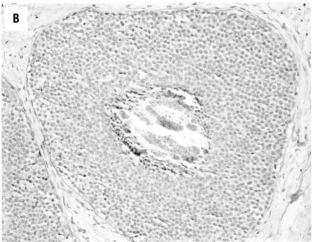

FIGURE 15-19

(A) An *in situ* carcinoma with cytoarchitectural features typical of LCIS, composed of small, uniform, dyshesive cells distending the involved space, but with central (comedo-type) necrosis more commonly found in DCIS. (B) By immunohistochemistry for E-cadherin, all cells are negative, suggestive of an LCIS phenotype.

THERAPEUTIC CONSIDERATIONS

The management of LCIS and DCIS differs, and underscores the importance of the above discussion regarding

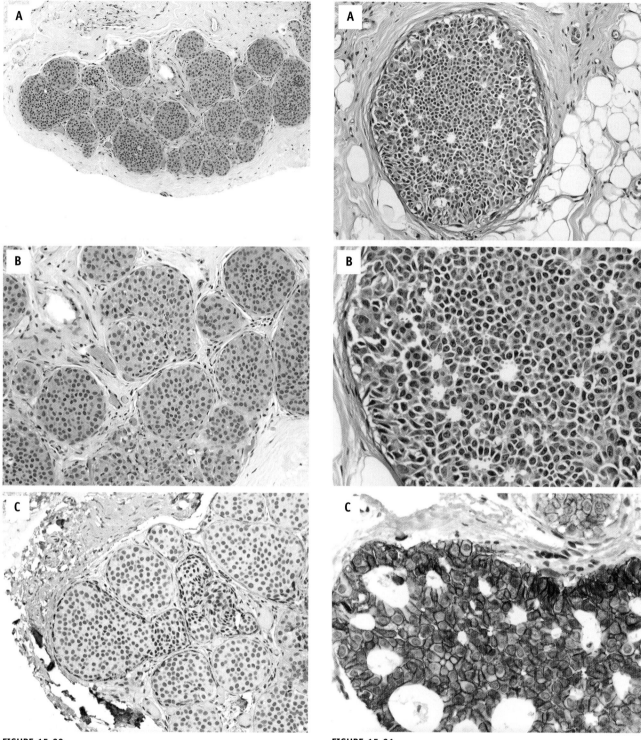

FIGURE 15-20

(A, B) An *in situ* carcinoma composed of small uniform cells in a solid, cohesive, mosaic pattern. Note occasional intracytoplasmic mucin vacuoles. (C) Corresponding E-cadherin immunostain is negative, akin to LCIS.

FIGURE 15-21

DCIS with artifactual dyshesion should not be confused with LCIS. Note the well formed microacini with true polarization of cells, low power (A) and higher power (B). E-cadherin immunostain is positive, consistent with the diagnosis of DCIS (C).

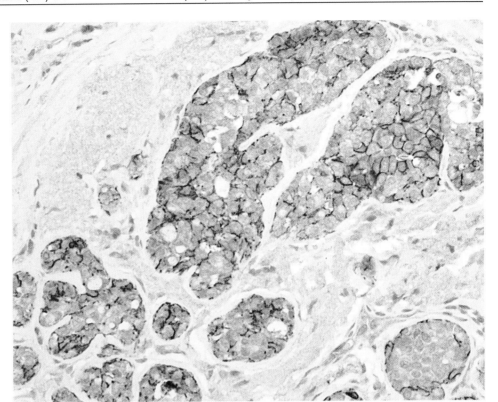

FIGURE 15-22

In situ carcinoma with both E-cadherin positive and E-cadherin negative neoplastic cells, suggestive of a mixed phenotype of both DCIS and LCIS in the same ductolobular unit.

their differential diagnosis. Unlike DCIS, which is a precursor lesion to invasive carcinoma, LCIS is considered a generalized risk factor and currently it is not clear which specific lesions will behave as obligate precursors. Therefore, patients with LCIS are most often managed by careful observation (and more recently with the addition of selective estrogen receptor modulators, such as Tamoxifen), while the treatment of DCIS is aimed at eradication of the lesion (with wide local excision, excision and radiation therapy, or mastectomy). Furthermore, assessment of the microscopic margin status is clinically important in DCIS but not in LCIS. Lastly, how best to manage patients whose core needle biopsy shows LCIS is currently an area of intense debate (see below), whereas the management of DCIS on core biopsy is more clear cut, with all patients requiring further surgical intervention.

Variant *in situ* lesions, such as PLCIS present particular management issues. Even though all PLCIS are negative for E-cadherin expression, suggesting a lobular phenotype, the natural history of these and other E-cadherin negative but histologically ambiguous lesions is not known. In particular it is not known if the level and laterality of breast cancer risk associated with these lesions is more similar to conventional LCIS or to DCIS. Certainly, the morphologic kinship of the individual cells of PLCIS to high grade DCIS, as well as their more 'aggressive' marker profile (higher proliferation and p53 positivity) are cause for concern. Although the follow-up was short (mean 17 months) in a study of Sneige and coworkers from M.D. Anderson Cancer Center, it is interesting to note that the only case of isolated PLCIS

to recur was one which was not adequately surgically excised initially. Meantime, in the absence of larger clinical outcome studies with longer follow-up, it would be prudent to follow a conservative approach with regard to the management of these lesions, such as re-excision of close/positive surgical margins if clinically feasible. Similarly, histologically indeterminate cases that show both E-cadherin positive and negative cells in the same ductal-lobular space, would probably best be as for DCIS rather than LCIS. Further clinical outcome studies in conjunction with immunophenotypic and molecular data are clearly needed to understand the biologic nature of these ambiguous lesions and to guide management.

How best to manage patients whose core needle biopsy (CNB) shows ALH, LCIS or an LCIS-like lesion (such as PLCIS) is currently a matter of intense debate. It seems logical to conclude that since classic LCIS is multicentric and bilateral and considered a marker of a generalized increase in cancer risk which is approximately equal in both breasts, surgical excision is not necessary, just as further surgery is not recommended for patients when LCIS is diagnosed on an open surgical biopsy. Unfortunately, there is little available information regarding the findings in subsequent surgical excision specimens from patients who have had ALH or LCIS identified on CNB, in large part due to the low prevalence of these lesions. In addition, data are extremely limited regarding the outcome of LCIS variants (such as PLCIS) found on CNB, particularly in relation to E-cadherin expression. The few studies that have attempted to address the appropriate management of

LCIS when identified on CNB, are limited by relatively small patient numbers and all studies to date have been retrospective, raising the possibility of selection bias with regard to which patients underwent surgical excision. (We have recently reviewed the literature on this subject; see Suggested Reading list.) Amongst studies to date of lobular neoplasia on CNB, certainly the model study is one in which Liberman and coworkers carefully correlated both the core biopsy histopathology as well as breast imaging findings with subsequent surgical follow-up. Carcinoma at excision was only found in cases where the CNB specimen contained another 'high risk' lesion (such as atypical ductal hyperplasia) in addition to LCIS, or LCIS had ambiguous histologic features overlapping with DCIS or the targeted lesion was not accounted for by the CNB pathology (such as a mass lesion).

In contrast, amongst cases with unambiguous ALH or LCIS alone on CNB, none had carcinoma on excision. To date only one study has addressed E-cadherin expression of *in situ* lesions on core biopsy with a significant proportion (60%) of E-cadherin negative histologically ambiguous *in situ* lesions resulting in carcinoma at excision. It is difficult to draw firm conclusions regarding the most appropriate management of patients with lobular neoplasia (LCIS, ALH or variants) on CNB due to small patient numbers and selection bias with regard to excision in the available studies. Nonetheless, at our institution we believe it most prudent to utilize a multidisciplinary approach with careful radiologic pathologic correlation, similar to that initially proposed by Liberman and co-workers. An incidental diagnosis of histologically unambiguous ALH or LCIS on CNB does not need surgical excision, provided the imaging findings of the targeted lesion correlate with the CNB pathology. Patients with ALH or LCIS should however undergo surgical excision in the following circumstances:

- If there is radiologic–pathologic discordance, suggesting that the targeted lesion was not represented in the CNB specimen (e.g., if the imaging studies show suspicious microcalcifications, a spiculated mass, or other soft tissue density)
- If another lesion which by itself would be an indication for surgical excision is also present on the core biopsy (such as ADH)

- If the ALH or LCIS has ambiguous histologic features which create problems in distinguishing the lesion from DCIS (e.g, PLCIS, LCIS with comedo-type necrosis, etc.). Although immunostaining for E-cadherin may be useful in determining whether the cells have a lobular or ductal phenotype, until additional data are available regarding the biologic behavior of such lesions it is prudent to recommend excision even if the neoplastic cells are negative for E-cadherin by immunohistochemistry (suggesting a lobular phenotype) if the features on routine histologic staining are ambiguous. However, additional, prospective clinical outcome studies are required, with larger numbers of patients while encompassing newer biologic markers (including E-cadherin) to further define the management of *in situ* lobular lesions on core needle biopsy.

SUGGESTED READING

Jacobs TW, Connolly JL, Schnitt SJ. Nonmalignant lesions in breast core needle biopsies: to excise or not to excise? Am J Surg Pathol 2002;26:1095–1110.

Jacobs TW, Pliss N, Kouria G, et al. Carcinomas in situ of the breast with indeterminate features: role of E-cadherin staining in categorization. Am J Surg Pathol 2001;25:229–236.

Lakhani SR. In-situ lobular neoplasia: time for an awakening. Lancet 2003;361:96.

Liberman L, Sama M, Susnik B, et al. Lobular carcinoma in situ at percutaneous breast biopsy: surgical biopsy findings. AJR Am J Roentgenol 1999;173:291–299.

Marshall LM, Hunter DJ, Connolly JL, et al. Risk of breast cancer associated with atypical hyperplasia of lobular and ductal types. Cancer Epidemiol Biomarkers Prev 1997;6:297–301.

Middleton LP, Grant S, Stephens T, et al. Lobular carcinoma in situ diagnosed by core needle biopsy: when should it be excised? Mod Pathol 2003;16:120–129.

Page DL, Schuyler PA, Dupont WD, et al. Atypical lobular hyperplasia as a unilateral predictor of breast cancer risk: a retrospective cohort study. Lancet 2003;361:125–129.

Schnitt SJ, Morrow M. Lobular carcinoma in situ: current concepts and controversies. Semin Diagn Pathol 1999;16:209–223.

Shelley Hwang E, Nyante SJ, Chen YY, et al. Clonality of lobular carcinoma in situ and synchronous invasive lobular carcinoma. Cancer 2004;100:2562–2572.

Sneige N, Wang J, Baker BA, et al. Clinical, histopathologic, and biologic features of pleomorphic lobular (ductal-lobular) carcinoma in situ of the breast: a report of 24 cases. Mod Pathol 2002;15:1044–1050.

Vos CB, Cleton-Jansen AM, Berx G, et al. E-cadherin inactivation in lobular carcinoma in situ of the breast: an early event in tumorigenesis. Br J Cancer 1997;76:1131–1133.

16 Molecular Genetics of ADH/DCIS and ALH/LCIS

Jorge S Reis-Filho · Sunil R Lakhani

INTRODUCTION

Molecular genetic analysis has revolutionized our understanding of preinvasive breast lesions. The multistep model of breast carcinogenesis proposing a transition from normal epithelium to invasive carcinoma via non-atypical and atypical hyperplasia and *in situ* carcinoma is currently deemed oversimplistic and conceptually flawed. In the past few years, advances in molecular pathology have allowed laser capture microdissection and molecular methods to be applied to formalin-fixed paraffin embedded tissue samples. Studies correlating the morphologic and genetic features of breast cancer precursors have been performed using loss of heterozygosity (LOH), comparative genomic hybridization (CGH), fluorescent and chromogenic *in situ* hybridization (FISH/CISH) and cDNA microarrays. While most of the conclusions drawn from early pathologic and epidemiologic studies still hold true, molecular evidence would suggest that risk indicators, such as atypical ductal hyperplasia and atypical lobular hyperplasia/lobular carcinoma *in situ* may behave as true non-obligate precursors.

DUCTAL CARCINOMA *IN SITU*

The term ductal carcinoma *in situ* (DCIS) comprises a heterogeneous group of proliferations with overlapping cytologic and architectural features, originating from the terminal duct-lobular unit. Although the non-obligate precursor nature of DCIS is undisputed, it seems clear that a group of these lesions more frequently progress to invasive carcinoma.

Molecular genetic analyses have helped to unravel the complexities of DCIS. It is now accepted that high nuclear grade (poorly differentiated) DCIS is a genetically advanced lesion, usually harboring complex karyotypic changes. Genome-wide molecular techniques have played an important role in the understanding of these lesions, demonstrating that there are differences in number and type of unbalanced chromosomal

changes in well, intermediate and poorly differentiated DCIS. Although there is a stepwise increase in the number of gross chromosomal abnormalities from low, to intermediate and high grade DCIS, distinct patterns of chromosomal gains and losses are quite specific to each grade. Whilst loss of 16q is the most frequent genetic abnormality in low grade DCIS, it is rarely found in high-grade DCIS. Conversely, high grade DCIS usually harbors gains of 17q, 8q, and 5p, losses of 11q, 14q, 8p, 13q and amplifications on 17q12, 17q22–24, 6q22, 8q22, and 11q13. In addition, most well-differentiated DCIS are near diploid, whereas poorly differentiated lesions are severely aneuploid. As expected, intermediately differentiated DCIS shows similarities to both well and poorly differentiated DCIS, including gain of 1q and loss of 8p, 11q, 16q and 17p. Although loss of 16q is the single most frequent genetic event observed in intermediately and well-differentiated DCIS, the target gene remains elusive.

With the introduction of conservative surgery (wide local excision) as a curative treatment for DCIS, recurrent DCIS has become part of the routine of diagnostic pathologists. It did not take long for pathologists to realize that recurrent and primary lesions are morphologically similar and almost invariably of the same grade. Interestingly, molecular analysis of matching primary and recurrent DCIS has underpinned their clonal genetic relationship and showed that morphologic similarities between paired index and recurrent DCIS are also mirrored at the genetic level.

Taken together, these data militate against the idea of one multistep model of breast carcinogenesis, in which poorly differentiated carcinomas would arise through 'dedifferentiation' of 'better differentiated' lesions. Instead, several lines of evidence suggest that there may be multiple pathways of breast carcinogenesis and progression towards malignancy (Figure 16-1). This idea has been corroborated by molecular studies, using LOH and CGH analysis, and mirrors what is observed in terms of unbalanced chromosomal changes in invasive breast carcinomas. Grade I and II invasive ductal carcinomas (IDC) theoretically arise from low or moderately differentiated DCIS, whereas grade III IDC arise from poorly differentiated DCIS.

Pathologists have always recognized the morphologic similarities between DCIS and matching invasive carcinomas. In addition, well-differentiated DCIS is usually found in the surrounding tissues of grade I invasive ductal (IDC) and tubular carcinomas, whereas

DCIS
Differentiation

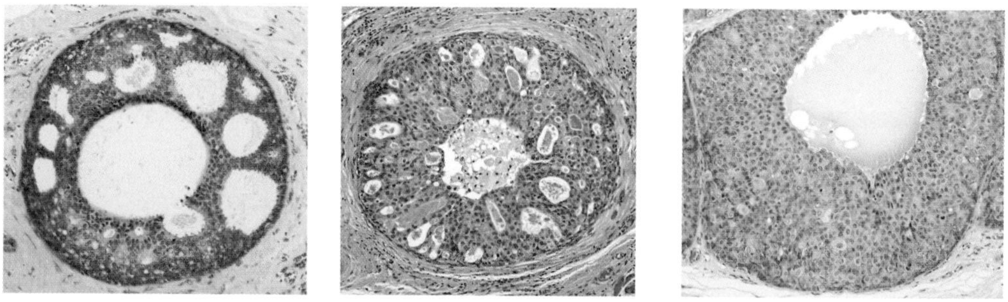

DCIS:	Well	Intermediate	Poorly
ER	+	+/−	−/+
PgR	+	+/−	−/+
Her2/neu	−	−/+	+/−
p53	−	−/+	+/−
Cyclin D1	+	+/−	−/+
Number of changes	Low	Intermediate	High
Ploidy	Near diploid	Aneuploid (~40–50%)	Frequently aneuploid
Recurrent changes	1q+, 16q−	1q+, 8p−, 11q−, 16q−, 17p−	1q+, 3q+, 17q+, 8q+, 11q−, 14q−, 8p−, 13q−
Amplifications	No	11q13	17q12, 6q22, 8q22, 11q13

FIGURE 16-1

DCIS: summary of morphologic, immunohistochemical and molecular genetic features. Note: +: frequently positive; +/−: fairly frequent positivity; −/+: frequently negative.

poorly-differentiated DCIS are usually observed at the vicinities of grade III IDCs. Therefore, it came as no surprise when molecular studies proved the genetic similarities and clonal evolution between DCIS and IDC of similar grades.

Recent data combining pathologic grading, laser-capture microdissection and expression (cDNA) microarrays have supported the idea that DCIS is a biologically advanced lesion, with expression profiles remarkably similar to those of invasive carcinomas. Most importantly DCIS gene expression signatures are associated with distinct grades rather than evolutionary stages.

The genes associated with the transition from *in situ* to invasive carcinoma have proven elusive. Several candidates have been put forward, including HER2/*neu* (c-*erb*-B2) and TP53. c-erb-B2 protein has been identified in a high proportion (60–80 %) of DCIS of poorly differentiated-comedo-type but is not common in the low/well-differentiated forms. This is not surprising as amplifications on 17q12 (HER2/neu loci) are almost restricted to poorly differentiated lesions. Although c-*erb*-B2 is important in the transition from a 'benign' to

'malignant' phenotype, this protein is less frequently overexpressed in grade III IDCs when compared to matching DCIS. The different frequency of expression in *in situ* and invasive carcinoma remains a mystery. Either expression is switched off during invasion or many c-*erb*-B2 positive DCIS do not transform to invasive malignancy. p53 protein expression has been demonstrated using immunohistochemistry in comedo type, poorly differentiated DCIS. The mechanism may be TP53 gene mutation associated with loss of the second allele, but this has only been confirmed in some cases. Recent data have implicated c-myc as a gene that may play a role in the evolution towards invasive malignancy. Comparisons between paired DCIS and IDC have shown a stark increase in c-myc copy numbers in the latter. Moreover, c-myc driven genes, such as H-TERT and FBL, showed higher levels of expression in the invasive counterpart. In addition, several genes associated with poorly differentiated DCIS have also been implicated in the transition to the invasive stages, including RAD51, S100 calcium-binding protein A10 (S100A10), ribonucleotide reductase M2 (RRM2), topoisomerase II alpha (TOP2A), polo-like kinase (PLK), cyclin-dependent kinase inhibitor 3 (CDKN3), BUB1, survivin and CDC28 protein kinase 2.

ATYPICAL DUCTAL HYPERPLASIA (ADH)

ADH is defined as an intraductal lesion characterized by proliferation of evenly distributed, monomorphic cells, which bears a remarkable morphologic resemblance to low-grade forms of DCIS. Despite the controversy in terms of the histopathologic criteria for diagnosing ADH raised by some authorites, molecular genetic analysis has highlighted the similarities between ADH and well-differentiated DCIS and positioned ADH as a non-obligate precursor in the multistep model of breast carcinogenesis.

Whilst a third to half of all ADH show no genetic changes when studied by CGH, the others show profiles that overlap with those of well-differentiated DCIS, including loss of 16q and gains of 17p. These data corroborate previous LOH studies in which loss at 16q and 17p were concurrently observed in paired ADH and DCIS, and give support to the non-obligate precursor nature of ADH.

These data highlight that morphologic similarities between ADH and low-grade DCIS are mirrored at the genetic level (Table 16-1), casting some doubts about the validity of separating ADH and DCIS. On the other hand, as there are morphologic and prognostic differences between ADH and DCIS, the data give support for the concept of ADH being either part of the spectrum of or a precursor to low-grade DCIS and hence of grade I invasive carcinoma.

ATYPICAL LOBULAR HYPERPLASIA AND LOBULAR CARCINOMA IN SITU

Lobular carcinoma *in situ* (LCIS) is a fairly uncommon breast lesion. It is usually not visible on mammography and an incidental finding, identified in up to 3.8 % of all specimens excised for invasive breast carcinoma and from 0.5-4.0 % of otherwise benign breast biopsies. Like DCIS, LCIS also originates from the terminal duct-lobular units with pagetoid involvement of the terminal ducts in three-quarters of cases.

The neoplastic cells of LCIS typically show a discohesive pattern, however they can vary in terms of nuclear morphology and cytoplasmic appearance. Different types of cells are on record: type A, the *bona fide* lobular carcinoma cells, are small, have round-to-ovoid nuclei, uniform chromatin, inconspicuous nucleoli and scant cytoplasm; type B cells are bigger, have a more abundant and clearer cytoplasm, slightly more pleomorphic nuclei, with clumped chromatin and conspicuous nucleoli. The recently described pleomorphic variant is composed of cells that are similar to those seen in apocrine carcinomas, but more discohesive; they have abundant finely granular pinkish cytoplasm, pleomorphic nuclei, with prominent macronucleoli.

The similarities between atypical lobular hyperplasia (ALH), LCIS and their invasive counterparts are overwhelming (see Chapter 15) and are not restricted to the morphologic and immunohistochemical levels. In fact, molecular genetic data confirm the similarities and have also proven the clonality between LCIS and associated invasive lobular carcinomas. Morever, CGH analysis on ALH and LCIS has shown losses of 16p, 16q, 17p and

TABLE 16-1

ADH, ALH/LCIS and pleomorphic LCIS: summary of immunohistochemical and molecular genetic features

	ADH	ALH/LCIS	Pleomorphic LCIS
E-Cadherin	+ (membrane)	–/cytoplasmic	–/cytoplasmic
ER	+	+	+
PgR	+	+	+
Her-2/neu overexpression	–	–	+/–
Her-2/neu amplification	–	–	–/+
Ki-67	Low	Low	Low/Moderate
p53	–/+	–	+/–
Cyclin D1	–/+	–/+	NA
Number of changes (CGH)	Low	Low	NA
Recurrent genetic changes (CGH and LOH)	Loss of 16q and 17 p	Loss of 16q22.1(CDH1), 17 p, 8p and 17q Gain of 1q and 6q	LOH 17p13.1 (TP53), 17q21 (BRCA1) and 16q22–24 (CDH1 and ESR)

Note: +: frequently positive; +/–: fairly frequent positivity; –/+: frequently negative. NA: data not available. Number of changes (CGH): number of unbalanced chromosomal aberrations as defined by comparative genomic hybridization (CGH). Recurrent genetic changes (CGH and LOH): recurrent genetic abnormalities as defined by CGH and loss of heterozygosity (LOH).

22q and gain of material from 1q and 6q, highlighting the overlapping molecular cytogenetic features of these lesions. Although limited, LOH data in ALH, LCIS and associated invasive lobular carcinomas also confirm the similarities between these lesions.

The target gene of 16q loss in ALH and LCIS is CDH1, which maps to 16q22.1 and encodes E-cadherin, a protein involved in cell–cell adhesion and in cell cycle regulation through the β-catenin/Wnt pathway. Although this gene was first reported as an invasion/metastasis associated gene, several lines of evidence suggest that it may also have tumor suppressor properties. CDH1 germline mutations, which are classically associated with familial diffuse gastric carcinoma, have recently been linked to some forms of familial lobular carcinoma.

E-cadherin is reduced or absent in the vast majority of LCIS, whereas it is reported to be expressed in normal or only slightly reduced levels in DCIS and other types of invasive breast carcinomas. Based upon these findings, immunohistochemistry with antibodies for E-cadherin has been advocated as an invaluable ancillary method for differentiating solid low grade DCIS from LCIS. The mechanisms of CDH1 inactivation in ALH, LCIS and invasive lobular carcinoma are not restricted to physical loss of 16q. Actually, truncating and missense mutations, and gene promoter methylation have also been described in these lesions.

Recent array CGH data of paired LCIS and invasive lobular carcinomas have demonstrated loss of the CDH1 locus in 100 % of cases. Other frequently identified losses involved 1p13–p22, 1p33–36 (E2F2 locus), 8p11.1–p11.2, 11q14-qter and 17p13.1 (TP53). The most frequent gains encompassed not only specific regions such as 7p11.2 (EGFR locus), 11q13 (CCND1, FGF19, FGF3 and FGF4 locus), 12q15 (MDM2 locus), but also whole chromosomal arms, including 1q and 16p. Using this approach it was shown that synchronous LCIS and invasive lobular carcinomas are exceedingly similar, thus supporting the non-obligate precursor role of LCIS.

Epidemiologic studies show that the behavior of LCIS and ALH is quite different from that of DCIS. LCIS is multifocal and bilateral in a high proportion of cases and approximately one fifth of the cases will progress to invasive cancer over a 20–25 year follow up period. When an invasive carcinoma is found associated with or following a diagnosis of LCIS, it usually shows lobular morphology. Invasive ductal carcinomas, especially of low-grade/tubular type, can also be found but at a lower frequency. It has been reported that the risk is similar in both breasts, however, several lines of evidence suggest that the risk is skewed in favor of the ipsilateral breast. In addition, concurrent identical truncating CDH1 mutations in LCIS and adjacent invasive lobular carcinoma have been demonstrated, providing strong evidence for the role of E-cadherin gene in the pathogenesis of lobular lesions as well as positioning LCIS as precursor of invasive lobular carcinoma. Therefore, ALH and LCIS should not only be considered risk indicators, but also non-obligate precursors of invasive carcinoma.

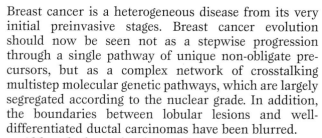

CONCLUSION

Breast cancer is a heterogeneous disease from its very initial preinvasive stages. Breast cancer evolution should now be seen not as a stepwise progression through a single pathway of unique non-obligate precursors, but as a complex network of crosstalking multistep molecular genetic pathways, which are largely segregated according to the nuclear grade. In addition, the boundaries between lobular lesions and well-differentiated ductal carcinomas have been blurred.

Although the molecular revolution in breast cancer taxonomy is still in its early days, it has proven instrumental in confirming several hypotheses generated by morphologic and epidemiologic studies. Instead of dwarfing the pathologist's role, molecular methods have emphasized the importance of proper pathologic analysis, not only for diagnostic and management purposes, but also in the research setting. The identification of genotypic–phenotypic correlations and the untangling of multiple molecular pathways in breast cancer evolution hold the promise of future progress towards tailored therapies not only for invasive disease but even for preinvasive lesions.

The development of novel molecular genetic techniques, such as array based CGH and cDNA microarrays from nucleic acids extracted from paraffin embedded tissue sections may increase the accuracy of identifying target genes to unprecedented levels.

ACKNOWLEDGMENT

Dr Jean-Yves Pierga, Dr Charlotte Westbury and Dr Pete T Simpson are acknowledged for critical comments and discussions.

SUGGESTED READINGS

Molecular Pathology of Pre-invasive Lesions

Cleton-Jansen AM. E-cadherin and loss of heterozygosity at chromosome 16 in breast carcinogenesis: different genetic pathways in ductal and lobular breast cancer? Breast Cancer Res 2002;4:5–8.

Jeffrey SS, Pollack JR. The diagnosis and management of pre-invasive breast disease: promise of new technologies in understanding pre-invasive breast lesions. Breast Cancer Res 2003;5:320–328.

O'Connell P. Genetic and cytogenetic analyses of breast cancer yield different perspectives of a complex disease. Breast Cancer Res Treat 2003;78:347–357.

Reis-Filho JS, Lakhani SR. The diagnosis and management of pre-invasive breast disease: genetic alterations in pre-invasive lesions. Breast Cancer Res 2003;5:313–319.

Shackney SE, Silverman JF. Molecular evolutionary patterns in breast cancer. Adv Anat Pathol 2003;10:278–290.

Simpson PT, Reis-Filho JS, Gale T, Lakhani SR. Molecular evolution of breast cancer. J Pathol 2005;205:248–254.

Molecular Pathology of Atypical Ductal Hyperplasia and Ductal Carcinoma *in situ*

Buerger H, Otterbach F, Simon R, et al. Comparative genomic hybridization of ductal carcinoma in situ of the breast – evidence of multiple genetic pathways. J Pathol 1999;187:396–402.

Cleton-Jansen AM, Buerger H, Haar N, *et al*. Different mechanisms of chromosome 16 loss of heterozygosity in well- versus poorly differentiated ductal breast cancer. Genes Chromosomes Cancer 2004;41:109–116.

Hwang ES, DeVries S, Chew KL, *et al*. Patterns of chromosomal alterations in breast ductal carcinoma in situ. Clin Cancer Res 2004;10:5160–5167.

Lakhani SR, Collins N, Stratton MR, Sloane JP. Atypical ductal hyperplasia of the breast: clonal proliferation with loss of heterozygosity on chromosomes 16q and 17p. J Clin Pathol 1995;48:611–615.

Ma XJ, Salunga R, Tuggle JT, *et al*. Gene expression profiles of human breast cancer progression. Proc Natl Acad Sci USA 2003;100:5974–5979.

Robanus-Maandag EC, Bosch CA, Kristel PM, *et al*. Association of C-MYC amplification with progression from the in situ to the invasive stage in C-MYC-amplified breast carcinomas. J Pathol 2003;201:75–82.

Roylance R, Gorman P, Hanby A, Tomlinson I. Allelic imbalance analysis of chromosome 16q shows that grade I and grade III invasive ductal breast cancers follow different genetic pathways. J Pathol 2002;196:32–36.

Roylance R, Gorman P, Harris W, *et al*. Comparative genomic hybridization of breast tumors stratified by histological grade reveals new insights into the biological progression of breast cancer. Cancer Res 1999;59:1433–1436.

Stratton MR, Collins N, Lakhani SR, Sloane JP. Loss of heterozygosity in ductal carcinoma in situ of the breast. J Pathol 1995;175:195–201.

Waldman FM, DeVries S, Chew KL, Moore DH 2nd, *et al*. Chromosomal alterations in ductal carcinomas in situ and their in situ recurrences. J Natl Cancer Inst 2000;92:313–320.

Molecular Pathology of Atypical Lobular Hyperplasia and Lobular Carcinoma *in situ*

Droufakou S, Deshmane V, Roylance R, *et al*. Multiple ways of silencing E-cadherin gene expression in lobular carcinoma of the breast. Int J Cancer 2001;92:404–408.

Etzell JE, DeVries S, Chew K, *et al*. Loss of chromosome 16q in lobular carcinoma in situ. Hum Pathol 2001;32:292–296.

Lakhani S, Collins N, Sloane J, Stratton M. Loss of heterozygosity in lobular carcinoma in situ of the breast. J Clin Pathol: Mol Pathol 1995;48:M74–M78.

Lishman SC, Lakhani SR. Atypical lobular hyperplasia and lobular carcinoma in situ: surgical and molecular pathology. Histopathology 1999;35:195–200.

Lu YJ, Osin P, Lakhani SR, *et al*. Comparative genomic hybridization analysis of lobular carcinoma in situ and atypical lobular hyperplasia and potential roles for gains and losses of genetic material in breast neoplasia. Cancer Res 1998;58:4721–4727.

Middleton LP, Palacios DM, Bryant BR, *et al*. Pleomorphic lobular carcinoma: morphology, immunohistochemistry, and molecular analysis. Am J Surg Pathol 2000;24:1650–1656.

Palacios J, Sarrio D, Garcia-Macias MC, Bryant B, *et al*. Frequent E-cadherin gene inactivation by loss of heterozygosity in pleomorphic lobular carcinoma of the breast. Mod Pathol 2003;16:674–678.

Reis-Filho JS, Simpson PT, Jones C, *et al*. Pleomorphic lobular carcinama of the breast: role of comprehensive molecular pathology in characterization of an entity. J Pathol 2005;207:1–13.

Sarrio D, Moreno-Bueno G, Hardisson D, *et al*. Epigenetic and genetic alterations of APC and CDH1 genes in lobular breast cancer: relationships with abnormal E-cadherin and catenin expression and microsatellite instability. Int J Cancer 2003;106:208–215.

Simpson PT, Gale T, Fulford LG, *et al*. The diagnosis and management of pre-invasive breast disease: pathology of atypical lobular hyperplasia and lobular carcinoma in situ. Breast Cancer Res 2003;5:258–262.

17 Morphology of Ductal Carcinoma *in situ*

Sarah E Pinder · Frances P O'Malley

INTRODUCTION

Ductal carcinoma *in situ* (DCIS) is a malignant, clonal proliferation of cells within the parenchymal structures of the breast and with no evidence of invasion. As described in Chapter 16, there is emerging evidence that DCIS is a heterogeneous group of lesions genetically. This is reflected in the morphology, biology and clinical behavior of the spectrum of disease which we at present group under the title of DCIS.

CLINICAL AND RADIOLOGIC FEATURES

DCIS is a unicentric neoplastic epithelial proliferation which is generally accepted to be a true precursor of, although not inevitably progressing to, invasive carcinoma. DCIS was infrequently seen prior to the widespread use of breast screening; only approximately 5% of breast cancer cases were DCIS prior to the use of mammography. Using this modality, DCIS is most commonly identified as microcalcifications (see Chapter 5). Approximately 25% of breast cancers in the screen-detected group are seen as DCIS. However, some women will, less commonly, present with a breast mass or with Paget's disease of the nipple or nipple discharge. Paget's disease will not be addressed here as this is covered in Chapter 12. The apparent (but not real) increase in incidence of DCIS as a result of increased detection, has clearly demonstrated deficiencies in our knowledge of the biology, classification and, indeed, behavior of DCIS; a number of methods for categorizing the process have been proposed.

PATHOLOGIC FEATURES

GROSS FINDINGS

Typically there may be no overt macroscopic findings in a surgical excision specimen bearing DCIS. There may be prominence of the fibrous component around the ducts or, on slicing, small specks representing comedo necrosis in the cut ends of the ducts may be seen. This lack of gross findings may make specimen handling difficult and slicing and radiograph of each specimen slice may be required to target the microcalcification present, as no gross features can be seen (see also Chapter 2 on specimen handling). Papillary carcinoma *in situ* is seen as a well-defined circumscribed mass of variable size but other forms of DCIS may also, albeit rarely, present as a mass lesion.

MICROSCOPIC FINDINGS

As described above, DCIS is a malignant epithelial proliferation within the breast parenchyma that most predominantly involves the ducts, although high grade DCIS may extend into the lobules as so-called 'cancerization'. The cells forming the *in situ* proliferation may show a range of histologic features and DCIS has previously been classified on various histologic grounds and using a variety of different systems.

Historically, DCIS was classified based on the architectural pattern of the epithelial proliferation and was categorized as: comedo, cribriform, micropapillary, solid or mixed subtype. However the reproducibility of this is problematic as individual lesions frequently show a mixture of architectures; for example, cribriform and solid or cribriform and micropapillary DCIS very often co-exist. Newer systems of categorization most often utilize nuclear grade, some also incorporating the presence or absence of 'comedo-type' necrosis. DCIS is most commonly classified as being of high, intermediate or low nuclear grade and the architectural pattern recorded separately.

High grade DCIS is formed from pleomorphic, large cells exhibiting marked variation in size and shape with coarse chromatin and often prominent nucleoli (Figure 17-1). Mitoses are frequent. It is often of solid architecture with calcified central ('comedo') necrosis present (Figure 17-2). Comedo necrosis may also, however, be seen in association with other architectural patterns (e.g. cribriform DCIS) and the term comedo does not specify an architecture. The term 'comedo DCIS' is widely used but is not to be encouraged as it specifies neither a grade, nor an architecture and there is no consensus regarding the amount of central necrosis required for diagnosis of this so-called 'type'. High grade DCIS is very often screen-detected, as a result of calcification of the necrotic debris. Even if micropapillary or cribriform arrangements are seen in high grade disease, there is little or no polarization of cells covering the micropapillae or lining the cribriform spaces.

At the opposite end of the spectrum to high grade DCIS, low grade DCIS is formed from evenly-spaced usually small, regular cells with round nuclei. The cells are usually ordered, in micropapillae and/or cribriform patterns and have well-defined cell boundaries. The cells covering the micropapillae or lining the lumina usually show polarization. Uncommonly, low grade DCIS has a solid architecture (Figure 17-3). Mitoses are sparse.

If utilizing the system of grading based entirely on cytonuclear grade, intermediate grade DCIS should be diagnosed when the lesion cannot be assigned to the high or low nuclear grade categories. The nuclei show moderate pleomorphism, less than that seen in high grade disease but lack the monotony and regularity of size and spacing of the low grade form (Figure 17-4). One or two nucleoli may be identified in the nuclei. The growth pattern is most often solid or cribriform and there is usually a degree of polarization.

An advantage of classifying DCIS according to nuclear grade is that there is less commonly a variation in grade which is often the case with the architecture of the disease. However, rarely DCIS may be of mixed grades; the highest grade should be recorded.

This system of grading DCIS according to cytonuclear features has been shown to be related to clinical behavior and to be relatively reproducible, but other systems have also been described. One widely used alternative method of grading DCIS has been described by the Van Nuys group. The Van Nuys grade utilizes a combination of cytonuclear grade and the presence of 'comedo-type' necrosis. Within this system, high grade DCIS is recognized by cytonuclear grade but other cases are sub-classified according to the presence or absence of necrosis; thus the 3 groups are: high grade; non-high grade with necrosis; non-high grade without necrosis. This technique has some advantages with respect to reproducibility. However, there is no agreement on the optimum, globally accepted system for grading DCIS.

In addition to reporting nuclear grade, presence/absence of necrosis and architectural pattern(s), other pathologic features that should be included in a pathology report of DCIS are an estimation of the size/extent of DCIS and the margin status. These topics are addressed in Chapter 2. Use of a synoptic report is invaluable in ensuring that all relevant features are included and allows for standardization of reporting of

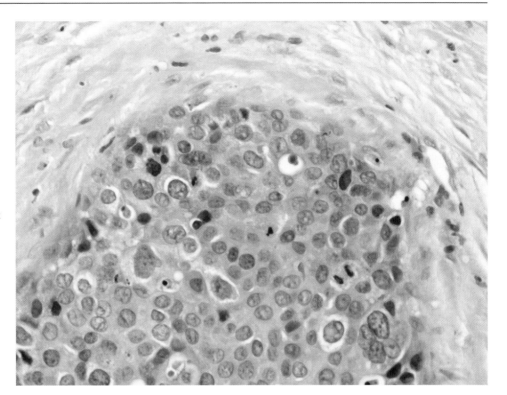

FIGURE 17-1

High grade DCIS. Pleomorphic malignant cells are seen within an eosinophilic boundary of basement membrane.

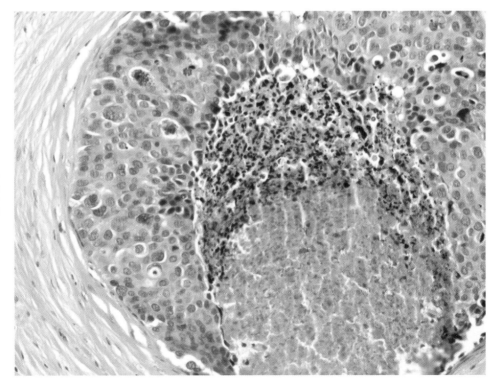

FIGURE 17-2

High grade DCIS with central necrosis of comedo type. The malignant epithelial population is highly pleomorphic with abnormal mitoses also present.

DCIS lesions. One such standardized protocol which highlights features to be included in reporting of both invasive carcinoma and DCIS has been produced by the College of American Pathologists and can be found at http://www.cap.org/apps/docs/cancer_protocols/2005/breast05_pw.pdf; see also Table 17-1.

A number of rare but distinct subtypes of DCIS can be seen which have specific features and which are difficult to categorize by grade alone. In apocrine DCIS, the *in situ* carcinoma cells have features of apocrine cells, including abundant granular cytoplasm and large nuclei with prominent nucleoli.

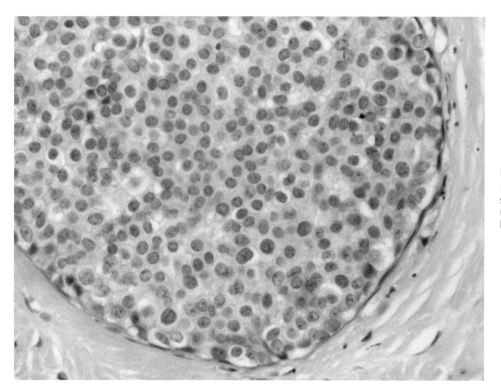

FIGURE 17-3
Low grade solid DCIS. The cells are small and relatively uniform with mitoses absent. Cell boundaries can be clearly seen.

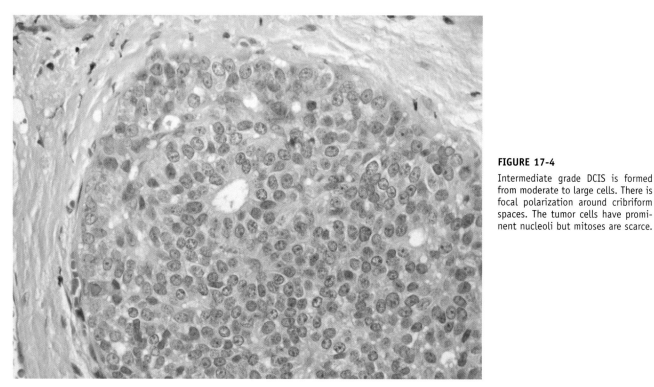

FIGURE 17-4
Intermediate grade DCIS is formed from moderate to large cells. There is focal polarization around cribriform spaces. The tumor cells have prominent nucleoli but mitoses are scarce.

The architecture is often cribriform. There is often moderate to severe cytologic atypia. Central necrosis is often present in high grade apocrine DCIS, indeed the diagnosis of apocrine DCIS should be made with caution in the absence of comedo type necrosis but occasionally the cells may be highly atypical but no necrosis may be evident. Low or intermediate grade apocrine DCIS may be more difficult to diagnose, as benign apocrine cells may show some degree of pleomorphism; caution is advised in the diagnosis of small foci of low grade apocrine DCIS in particular.

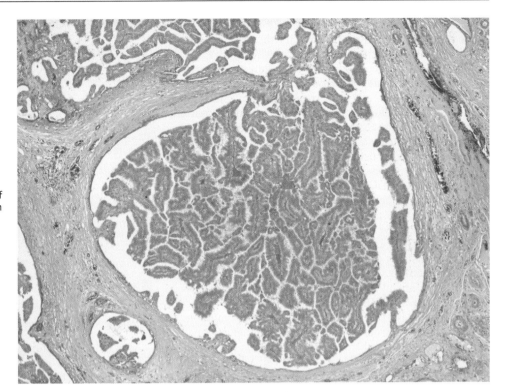

FIGURE 17-5

Low power of H&E stained section of papillary carcinoma *in situ* within expanded duct spaces.

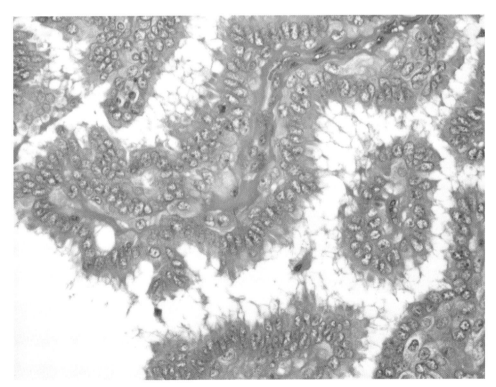

FIGURE 17-6

H&E stained section of papillary carcinoma *in situ* showing fine fibrovascular fronds with overlying columnar carcinoma cells. The absence of a myoepithelial layer could be confirmed with immunohistochemistry.

Intracystic/encysted papillary carcinoma *in situ* is an uncommon but distinctive form of DCIS often seen in older women (Figure 17-5 and 17-6 and see Chapter 9). It is usually circumscribed and accompanied by a hyalinized fibrous wall giving an encysted appearance. There is frequently hemosiderin (or hematoidin) pigment in this tissue. The DCIS has a papillary structure with fine fibrovascular cores, which may be absent in at least part of the lesion. The key feature is the absence of a myoepithelial cell layer surrounding the fibrovascular spaces which can be confirmed with immunohistochemistry for smooth muscle myosin heavy chain or smooth muscle actin. Papillary carcinoma *in situ* may be accompanied by other forms of DCIS in the surrounding tissue, usually of micropapillary or cribriform type.

The cells of neuroendocrine DCIS often have granular cytoplasm and may be either polygonal or spindled cell in morphology and may resemble the cells of a carcinoid tumor. There may be a solid or pseudo-rosette architecture, although very often there are papillary areas. The spindled-shape of the cells may mimic the 'streaming' seen in usual epithelial hyperplasia; fortunately it frequently is seen admixed with more classical papillary or solid DCIS. Estrogen receptor staining, as well as neuroendocrine markers, can be invaluable, as this type of DCIS is frequently strongly and homogeneously ER positive.

Clear cell DCIS is formed from cells with clear cytoplasm and distinct cell margins. These form cribriform or solid structures with central necrosis. Care should be taken not to mistake poor fixation for a clear cell morphology, both in DCIS and invasive carcinoma; assessment of the adjacent breast fixation can be valuable. Other very rare forms of DCIS include signet ring cell DCIS which is formed from signet ring cells often in a solid pattern. The cytoplasm stains positively with D-PAS or alcian blue. So-called 'clinging DCIS' is characterized by a population of tumor cells lining the duct. It is now widely believed that the low grade form of the disease should be regarded as a risk factor rather than true DCIS. The high grade form of the disease is equivalent to flat high grade DCIS. Because of this variation in the morphologic features and the clinical behavior, the term is not widely accepted and categorization by nuclear grade is preferred.

MICROINVASIVE CARCINOMA

This is defined as a DCIS lesion in which there are one, or more, separate foci of invasion none of which measures more than 1 mm in diameter. This is rare, even in high grade DCIS and is particularly unusual in low grade disease; if there is doubt the lesion should be classified as pure DCIS. Stains for myoepithelium (smooth muscle myosin, smooth muscle actin, p63) and basement membrane markers (laminin, type IV collagen) may be valuable but additional deeper level examination of the block is also helpful; often microinvasion is an overdiagnosis and the lesion represents 'cancerization' of lobules, which is clearly identified on deeper sections.

ANCILLARY STUDIES

IMMUNOHISTOCHEMISTRY

As a clonal proliferation, DCIS shows homogeneity of staining with a variety of markers, which can occasionally be valuable in diagnosis. Usual epithelial hyperplasia, conversely, commonly shows heterogeneity of expression, for example of estrogen receptor and basal and luminal cytokeratins (Figure 17-7). No markers are of assistance in distinguishing low grade DCIS from ADH, which requires an assessment of the extent of the process; many authorities believe that these are in fact the same processes as shown by the genetic and immunophenotypic similarities. High grade DCIS

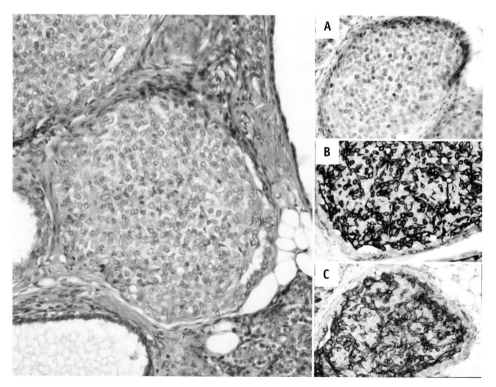

FIGURE 17-7

A solid epithelial proliferation within ducts. There are 'slit-like' peripheral spaces present to the right of the process in the H&E stained section (left). The estrogen receptor (A), cytokeratin 14 (B) and cytokeratin 5/6 (C) stained sections (right) confirm that this is not a clonal proliferation with heterogeneity of expression and admixed positive and negative cells.

expresses estrogen receptor less frequently than low grade disease (but overall a similar proportion of cases are ER positive as seen in invasive disease i.e., 70–80 %). The converse is true of HER2; high grade DCIS frequently expresses this oncoprotein (50–60 % of cases) which is present more often than is seen in invasive breast carcinomas.

Ancillary studies may be helpful in distinguishing DCIS from invasive disease. By definition, DCIS bears a surrounding myoepithelial layer which can be demonstrated by myoepithelial markers (e.g. smooth muscle myosin heavy chain (Figure 17-8) as well as basement membrane stains (laminin and type IV collagen). Deeper levels with routine hematoxylin and eosin stains may, however, be more helpful in avoiding misdiagnosis of 'cancerization of lobules' as invasive tumor. High grade DCIS frequently bears an associated chronic inflammatory cell infiltrate around the ducts with consequent fibrosis, thus smooth muscle actin which stains myofibroblasts may be thus more difficult to interpret.

FINE NEEDLE ASPIRATION CYTOLOGY

Fine needle aspiration cytology (FNAC) cannot be used to distinguish DCIS from invasive carcinoma, although if examined in combination with the clinical and radiologic features, a 'best guess' that the lesion is DCIS rather than invasive carcinoma can be made. Cytology samples from DCIS lesions are frequently less cellular than from invasive lesions and the positive predictive value for FNAC from DCIS is therefore lower than for invasive cancer and inadequate samples are more often received. Core biopsy is therefore strongly recommended for the investigation of microcalcifications, rather than FNAC.

OTHERS

LOH and CGH studies of DCIS confirm the clonal nature of the process (see Chapter 16 for details).

DIFFERENTIAL DIAGNOSIS

Atypical ductal hyperplasia (ADH) is a lesion showing 'some but not all of the features of ductal carcinoma *in situ*' (see Chapter 14 for more details on diagnosis of ADH). In essence, if cellular changes typical of low grade DCIS occupy two or more duct spaces, this is regarded as low grade DCIS; if less, then the process is classified as ADH. It will be re-iterated here that high grade proliferations represent high grade DCIS, regardless of size or number of duct spaces involved and a high grade process should not be regarded as ADH.

As described above, microinvasive carcinoma is frequently overdiagnosed and may be mimicked by lobular

FIGURE 17-8

High power image of high grade solid DCIS with smooth muscle myosin heavy chain (SMMHC) immunohistochemistry. This demonstrates the myoepithelial layer around the well-defined island of malignant cells, confirming the *in situ* nature of the process.

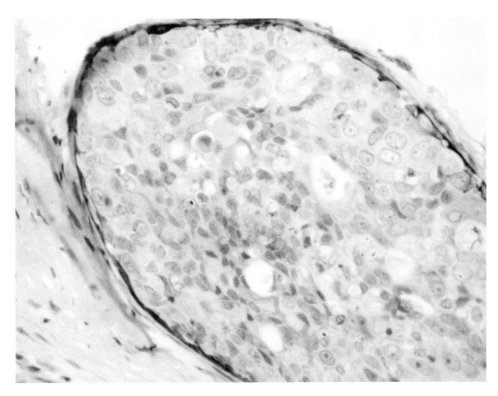

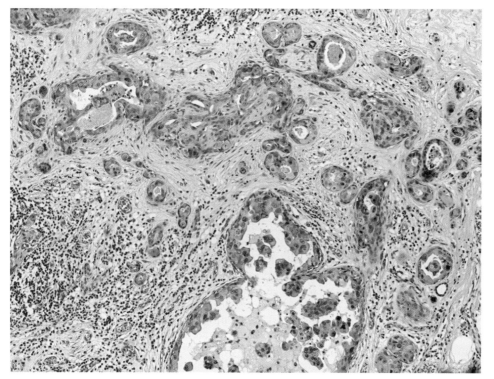

FIGURES 17-9

H&E stained section of high grade micropapillary DCIS. Smaller scattered islands are noted in association with a moderate chronic inflammatory cell infiltrate.

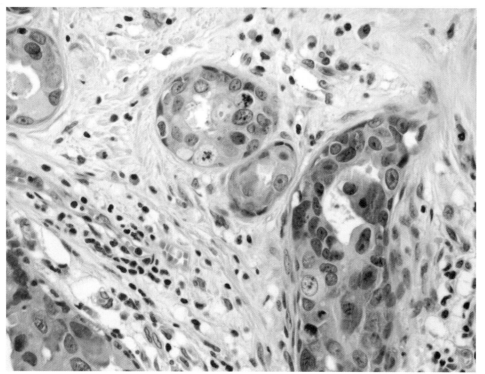

FIGURE 17-10

H&E stained section of high grade micropapillary DCIS. High power view shows that the smaller islands shown in Figure 17-9 have well-defined edges. This is cancerization of lobules/sclerosing adenosis by DCIS.

'cancerization' (Figures 17-9 and 17-10). Examination of the block at deeper levels is helpful in recognizing the lobular architecture and avoiding this pitfall but associated chronic inflammatory reaction may also make interpretation difficult. In particular, 'cancerization' of sclerosing adenosis may mimic invasion and immunohis-tochemistry can be helpful in the identification of a myoepithelial layer around such islands of cells (Figure 17-11).

It can be difficult on occasions to distinguish low grade solid DCIS from lobular carcinoma *in situ* (LCIS). Features in favor of DCIS are the slightly greater cellular cohesion with more evident cell borders, larger cell

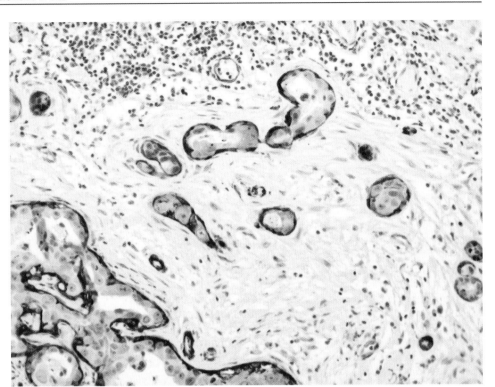

FIGURE 17-11

The same lesion shown in Figures 17-9 and 17-10, stained with SMMHC confirms the presence of surrounding myoepithelial cells.

TABLE 17-1

Pathology checklist: ductal carcinoma *in situ* of the breast

Surgical #:	Patient's Name:
Procedure:	Wire localization biopsy ☐ Lumpectomy/wide local excision ☐ Re-excision ☐ Mastectomy ☐
Side	Right ☐ Left ☐
Nuclear grade:	I ☐ II ☐ III ☐
Necrosis:	Absent ☐ Punctate ☐ Comedo ☐
Architectural type(s) (specify all that apply):	Cribriform ☐ Solid ☐ Micropapillary ☐ Papillary ☐
Extent of DCIS	Size _____ cm

Calcifications	Absent ☐ Present ☐
	    – In DCIS ☐
	    – In association with benign epithelium ☐
	    – In stroma ☐

Resection margins:	Negative (not at margin) ☐ Positive (at margin) ☐ Distance to closest (relevant) margin: _____mm Relevant margin is (e.g. inferior, medial etc)
Microinvasion (invasion ≤ 1 mm):	Present ☐ Absent ☐
Associated benign changes:	
Comment:	
Diagnosis:	Breast, left ☐/right ☐, _____ (procedure): Ductal carcinoma in situ, nuclear grade _____ (I–III)
AJCC (6th Edition) Classification	Tis ☐ T1 mic ☐
Resident/Pathologist reporting case	

size and lack of intracytoplasmic lumina. As described in Chapter 15, E-cadherin immunohistochemistry can be helpful, but it should also be noted that combinations of both processes may exist and also that morphologically unequivocal LCIS may, rarely, express E-cadherin.

PROGNOSIS AND THERAPY

The mainstay for the treatment of DCIS is surgical excision. For large lesions this may require mastectomy but for many smaller screen-detected lesions, a good cosmetic result can be obtained by wide local excision. Recurrence of DCIS occurs invariably at the site of previous excision and represents residual disease. Several studies have, however, shown that approximately half of the recurrences after excision and radiation for DCIS are as in the form of invasive cancer; this alarming fact highlights the need for complete surgical excision and thorough pathologic examination, particularly of the specimen margins. There is, however, no widely agreed specific distance/margin of clearance at which the DCIS is deemed 'completely excised'; some groups require a 10 mm margin or more of surrounding benign tissue, others accept a few millimetres.

There are, similarly, no globally agreed adjuvant therapies for all cases of DCIS. It is widely accepted that irradiation reduces the local recurrence rate of DCIS and is commonly utilized. Many groups believe, however, that not all cases of DCIS require radiotherapy after wide local excision. The role of hormone therapies in the management of DCIS is even more controversial; some authorities believe that data support the use, for example, of tamoxifen, whilst other studies and other experts do not routinely recommend this therapy for the treatment of excised DCIS.

If axillary lymph nodes are found to be involved in a case of DCIS, clearly an invasive focus, albeit small, has been missed and thorough re-examination of the specimen should be undertaken. Lymph node involvement has been reported in less than 1% of cases of pure DCIS, thus axillary dissection is not required for these patients. Studies are underway to assess the value of sentinel lymph node biopsy in cases of extensive DCIS; this technique would obviate the need for a second procedure in cases believed pre-operatively to represent pure DCIS, but which on histologic examination were found to have an invasive focus.

SELECTED READINGS

Bijker N, Peterse JL, Fentiman IS, et al. Effects of patient selection on the applicability of results from a randomised clinical trial (EORTC 10853) investigating breast-conserving therapy for DCIS. Br J Cancer 2002 ;87:615–620.

DCIS Classification Overview. Poller DN, Pinder SE, Ellis IO. In: Ductal Carcinoma in situ of the Breast. Ed Silverstein MJ. Baltimore: Williams and Wilkins; 1997.

Fisher ER, Dignam J, Tan-Chiu E, et al. Pathologic findings from the National Surgical Adjuvant Breast Project (NSABP) eight-year update of Protocol B-17: intraductal carcinoma. Cancer 1999;86:429–438. http://www.cap.org/apps/docs/cancer_protocols/2005/breast05_pw.pdf

Jensen RA, Page DL. Ductal carcinoma in situ of the breast: impact of pathology on therapeutic decisions. Am J Surg Pathol 2003;27:828–831

Pinder SE, Ellis IO. The diagnosis and management of pre-invasive breast disease: ductal carcinoma in situ (DCIS) and atypical ductal hyperplasia (ADH) – current definitions and classification. Breast Cancer Res 2003;5:254–257.

Schwartz GF, Lagios MD, Silverstein MJ. Trends in the treatment of ductal carcinoma in situ of the breast. J Natl Cancer Inst 2004;96:1258–1259

Silverstein MJ, Buchanan C. Ductal carcinoma in situ: USC/Van Nuys Prognostic Index and the impact of margin status. Breast 2003;12:457–471.

18 Invasive Carcinoma: Special Types

Gavin C Harris · Sarah E Pinder · Frances P O'Malley

INTRODUCTION

The main purpose of the identification of specific types of invasive breast carcinoma is to refine the prediction of likely behavior and response to treatment offered by the other major prognostic factors of lymph node stage, histologic grade, tumor size and lymphovascular invasion. In addition, different histologic types of breast carcinoma have different biologies. Given the difficulties of tumor typing, it is a tribute to the diagnostic abilities of previous generations of pathologists that, using purely morphology alone, they were able to identify tumor types with prognostic implications. It is highly likely in the next few years that we will see additional technologies supplement the purely morphologic classification of breast carcinomas in routine practice. This will enable us to identify well-defined, reproducible pathologic and biologic profiles of discrete disease entities with the promise of the corresponding development of more tailor-made therapies. This is concordant with the growing belief that unlike the adenoma–carcinoma sequence in the large bowel, breast carcinomas are a group of different disease entities showing parallel progression pathways from *in situ* to invasive disease. As pathologists we need to ensure that we use robust classification systems to assist in the accurate identification of a patient's disease.

INVASIVE DUCTAL CARCINOMA/NO SPECIFIC TYPE OR NOT OTHERWISE SPECIFIED

It should be understood that this is not a particular tumor type and now many pathologists prefer the term invasive ductal carcinoma/no specific type (NST) to 'ductal' carcinoma. It is merely an acknowledgment that a carcinoma has not been able to be classified as a particular special type and consequently has been placed in this 'holding area' until further classification strategies become available. It is this group which, in the first instance, is likely to benefit from the new technologies, which will be alluded to further below.

CLINICAL FEATURES

The proportion of cases of invasive breast carcinoma classified as being of NST varies to up to 70 % but the Nottingham series had a frequency of 47 %. NST lesions make up a lower proportion of small, screen-detected invasive tumors (40 %). On average, the size of these carcinomas is 2 cm. There appears to be a slightly increased frequency of NST tumors below the age of 35 years (67 %) compared with older patients (53 %) who have an increased proportion of lobular and other special type carcinomas.

Tumors associated with germ-line BRCA1 mutations are more often characterized by a continuous pushing margin, higher mitotic counts and more lymphocytic infiltration relative to sporadic tumors. Cancers associated with germ-line BRCA2 mutations may show less tubule formation, and a pushing margin. Thus, although tumors in patients with BRCA1 mutations have some medullary features (see below), the majority of tumors associated with both the BRCA1 and 2 germ-line mutations are NST, although the rates of this tumor 'type' is similar to the general population. BRCA-associated breast tumors are further discussed in Chapter 21.

PATHOLOGIC FEATURES

GROSS FINDINGS

The tumors are in general moderately or ill-defined with a nodular or stellate configuration. The cut-surface is gray/white and firm.

MICROSCOPIC FINDINGS

The WHO classification requires a non-specialized pattern in over 50 % of the tumor area to be classified as NST. If the NST pattern is noted in 10–49 % of the area, the tumor is classified as mixed NST and special type. NST tumors show variable combinations of morphology which prevent allocation to a special type. Typically combinations of pushing and infiltrative margins are seen in tumors formed from trabecular, sheet-like,

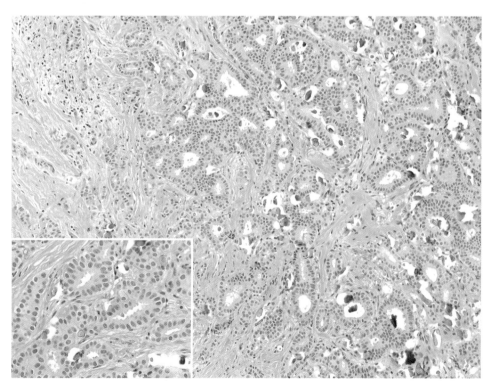

FIGURE 18-1
Invasive ductal carcinoma of no special type, Nottingham grade 1, score 4/9. There is at least 75% tubule formation (score 1), 0 mitosis in 10 HPF (score 1) and moderate nuclear pleomorphism (score 2).

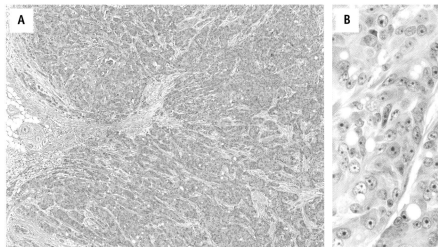

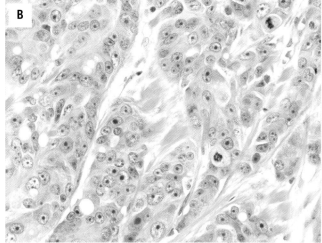

FIGURE 18-2

Invasive ductal carcinoma of no special type, Nottingham grade 3, score 8/9. (A) Low power shows complete absence of tubule formation (score 3). (B) High power shows marked nuclear pleomorphism (score 3); there were 15 mitoses per 10 HPF (field diameter 0.55 mm; score 2).

acinar and nesting morphologies. (Figures 18-1 and 18-2). The cells show variable atypia, often focal necrosis and associated chronic inflammation. Associated ductal carcinoma *in situ* (DCIS) is commonly identified and is usually intermediate or high grade. The stroma can be desmoplastic, collagenous or may be minimal.

Increasingly there is evidence, within the group of grade 3 ductal NST tumors, of a distinct subset showing evidence of myoepithelial/basaloid differentiation. The constituent cells may be round or polygonal and there is frequently necrosis and an inflammatory infiltrate.

ANCILLARY STUDIES

IMMUNOHISTOCHEMISTRY AND MOLECULAR TECHNIQUES

Overall 70–80 % of NST tumors show estrogen receptor positivity and 15–30 % are HER2 positive. There is some evidence that the use of cDNA micro-arrays and comparative genomic hybridization (CGH) can supplement the morphologic classification of invasive carcinoma types. cDNA microarrays have been shown to identify at least five different broad categories (basal-like, HER2 positive, normal breast-like and at least two subclasses of luminal/ER+ tumors). This has been correlated with prognosis in these early studies, with the basal-like and HER2 positive groups showing a reduced relapse-free and overall survival. Increasingly there is also immunophenotypic evidence supporting the basaloid/luminal subdivision of NST tumors; 2–18 % of NST lesions are reported to express cytokeratin 14, a marker of basal cell/myoepithelial differentiation. These latter tumors often also express other myoepithelial markers such as smooth muscle actin and S100.

They tend to be estrogen and progesterone receptor negative and HER2 negative and show a lower number of mean DNA copy number changes.

DIFFERENTIAL DIAGNOSIS

Diagnosis/classification of NST carcinoma is, as noted above, made on exclusion of other tumor type morphologic features which should be seen in <50 % of the lesion. Non-epithelial carcinomas may, rarely, mimic invasive breast carcinoma and can be excluded by the use of immunohistochemical markers for cytokeratins.

PROGNOSIS AND TREATMENT

Overall, NST tumors show a 35–50 % 10-year survival with prognosis dependent on the traditional prognostic factors of grade, lymph node stage, size and lymphovascular invasion.

There is some evidence that the grade 3 NST tumors with evidence of basaloid/myoepithelial differentiation are more likely to develop brain and lung metastases and patients have an increased risk of dying of their disease.

INVASIVE LOBULAR CARCINOMA

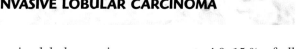

Invasive lobular carcinoma represents 4.9–15 % of all invasive breast carcinomas. Over 90 % of the carcinoma should have a lobular morphology to be classified in this group. For a carcinoma to be classified as a specific subtype of lobular carcinoma (see below) it should be present in at least 80 % of the tumor.

CLINICAL FEATURES

Age at presentation with invasive lobular carcinoma is 54–67 years (mean 63 years). There is some evidence of an increased risk of lobular carcinoma to patients receiving post-menopausal combined hormone therapy and also that the incidence of this carcinoma subtype is increasing. Presentation is often as an area of poorly defined thickening. Whether invasive lobular carcinoma is more frequently multicentric than other types is still debated, but reports vary between 9–31 % depending on whether clinical or histologic assessments have been used.

RADIOLOGIC FEATURES

This tumor has a lower density mammographically and may be occult. It is less likely to be associated with microcalcifications than tumors of NST morphology.

PATHOLOGIC FEATURES

GROSS FINDINGS

Average size at presentation is 2.4 cm. The macroscopic appearance is variable from gray, firm and circumscribed, to poorly defined.

MICROSCOPIC FINDINGS

There are a number of different histologic subtypes of invasive lobular carcinoma. The frequencies of the various subtypes are: mixed, 45.6 %; classical, 30.4 %; tubulo-lobular, 13.5 %; solid, 6.4 %; and alveolar, 4.1 %. Tubulo-lobular carcinomas tend to be grade 1 (Elston-Ellis Nottingham grading), with the remaining variants tending to be grade 2 (scoring 3 for tubules, 2 for pleomorphism and 1 for mitoses), but grades 1 and 3 invasive lobular carcinomas can also be recognized (Figures 18-3 and 18-4).

INVASIVE LOBULAR CARCINOMA – PATHOLOGIC FEATURES

Gross Findings
▶ Firm, gray, well to poorly defined.
▶ Average size 2.4 cm

Microscopic Findings
▶ Subtypes include classical, tubulo-lobular, solid, alveolar and mixed
▶ Cells show discohesive pattern of infiltration with oval nuclei, small amount of cytoplasm and intracytoplasmic lumina
▶ Usually histologic grade 2 (tubulo-lobular tend to be grade 1)
▶ LCIS present in 66 % of cases

Immunohistochemical Studies
▶ Negative or reduced staining for E-cadherin
▶ Usually positive for estrogen and progesterone receptors
▶ Usually negative for HER2 (except pleomorphic variant; grade 3)

Differential Diagnosis
▶ Lymphoid population, either benign or lymphomatous infiltrates

---

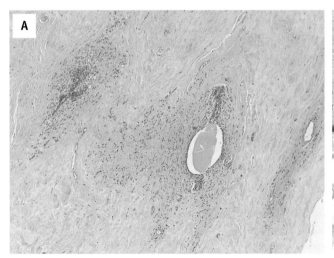 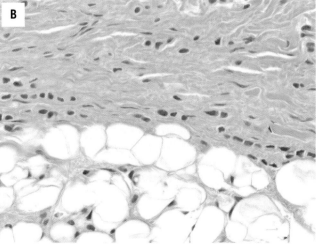

FIGURE 18-3

Invaive lobular carcinoma, Nottingham grade 1, score 5/9. (A) Low power shows the classical targetoid growth pattern of an invasive lobular carcinoma. (B) High power shows the bland nuclear features of a low grade (grade 1) lobular carcinoma. These nuclear features are rare; the majority of lobular carcinomas show nuclear grade 2 features.

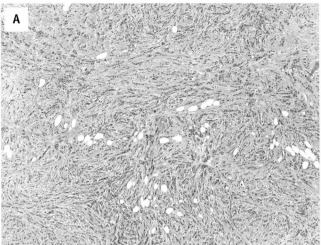
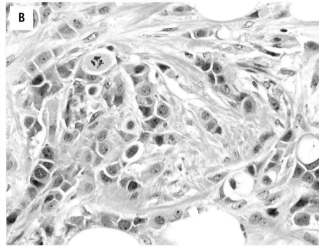

FIGURE 18-4

Invasive lobular carcinoma, Nottingham grade 3, score 8/9. (A) The single file growth pattern typical of a lobular carcinoma is evident. (B) The marked nuclear pleomorphism (score 3) and increased mitoses (score 2) are readily apparent at high power.

The cell type characteristic of invasive lobular carcinoma is non-cohesive, with relatively regular, round or oval, eccentrically placed nuclei with small nucleoli. There is a small amount of cytoplasm in which intra-cytoplasmic lumina may be identified. The classical variant is characterized by single-file (or 'single filing') and a targetoid periductal arrangement. The solid variant is composed of sheets or irregularly shaped nests and the alveolar variant composed of well-defined, circumscribed cell groups of 20 cells or more. LCIS is associated in 66 % of cases and DCIS in 14 %. Tubulolobular carcinomas show the characteristic cells arranged in small round microtubules, rather than open angulated tubules as in tubular carcinoma (see below) admixed with more classical lobular features and with an infiltrative pattern similar to the classical variant; in one series 29 % of these lesions were multifocal.

ANCILLARY STUDIES

IMMUNOHISTOCHEMISTRY

Estrogen receptor positivity is seen in 67–92 %. Lobular carcinomas are in general more likely to be estrogen receptor positive than non-lobular types. Progesterone receptor expression is present in approximately 63 %. E-cadherin immunopositivity is absent or reduced in all subtypes in the vast majority of cases.

MOLECULAR STUDIES

Fifty-four per cent of tumors are diploid. Invasive lobular carcinomas show a high frequency of increased copy numbers of 1q (79 %) and loss of 16q (63 %). Relative to invasive NST tumors, there appears to be a lower number of chromosomal changes (6.4 versus 10.1) and a lower frequency of 8q gain, in addition to increased 16q loss. The E-cadherin gene on 16q22 has been shown to be inactivated in invasive lobular carcinomas in a number of ways including loss, methylation (potentially reversible) and mutation. There is increasing genomic evidence that LCIS may be a precursor lesion for some infiltrating lobular carcinomas.

DIFFERENTIAL DIAGNOSIS

Lobular carcinoma is rarely misdiagnosed as another process, in core biopsies in particular, but rarely, chronic inflammation may mimic invasive lobular carcinoma, and vice versa. Consideration of the correct diagnosis and, as appropriate, immunohistochemical assessment with lymphoid and cytokeratin markers easily allows the correct diagnosis to be made.

PROGNOSIS AND TREATMENT

Thirty-two to 43 % of patients with infiltrating lobular carcinoma have associated axillary nodal metastases and 8 % distant metastases. Histologic subtype of invasive lobular carcinoma is a predictor of prognosis; the tubulolobular variant has a significantly lower risk of regional (17 %) and distant (13 %) recurrence relative to the other subtypes, whereas the solid variant has significantly higher risk of recurrence (82 and 54 %, respectively). The remaining subtypes do not show a significant difference in these rates. These trends are also, however, reflected in disease-free intervals and likelihood of nodal positivity in tumors less than 2 cm in diameter. The 12-year actuarial survival of 100 % for the tubulo-lobular variant contrasts with 47 % for the solid variant. The classical variant has the second best disease-free and overall survival.

There is controversy as to whether patients with invasive lobular carcinoma have a better prognosis relative to those with ductal NST carcinoma. One series, with very long follow-up, showed 5 and 30 year corrected survival rates of 78 and 50 %, respectively for invasive lobular carcinoma, whereas the corresponding figures for ductal NST cancers were 63 and 37 %. However, a more recent series failed to demonstrate a significant difference between overall survival, local or distant recurrence rates relative to non-lobular type carcinomas.

Contralateral invasive carcinoma is reported to be more frequent in patients with a history of invasive lobular carcinoma. Fifty per cent of these also have a lobular morphology. Of particular interest, there is also an increased risk of metastases to serosal (i.e., gynecologic, gastrointestinal) areas, bone and the leptomeninges (15 %), with reduced incidence of pleural and pulmonary metastases.

INVASIVE TUBULAR CARCINOMA – PATHOLOGIC FEATURES

Gross Findings
▶ Moderately well defined, with stellate/gray cut surface.
▶ Average size 1.2–1.6 cm

Microscopic Findings
▶ Angulated tubules with single layer of epithelial cells
▶ Apical snouts often visible
▶ Desmoplastic stroma often present
▶ 20 % multifocal

Immunohistochemical Studies
▶ Usually estrogen and progesterone receptor positive
▶ Usually HER2 negative
▶ Markers for myoepithelial cells, e.g., p63 are negative

Differential Diagnosis
▶ Radial scar/complex sclerosing lesion
▶ Microglandular adenosis
▶ Sclerosing adenosis

TUBULAR CARCINOMA

This tumor type constitutes 0.8–2.3 % of invasive breast carcinomas. Classification requires discrete tubule formation in over 90 % of the lesion. Associated stromal changes, usually desmoplasia, are present. Tumors with a 50–90 % tubular morphology are categorized as mixed NST and tubular carcinomas.

CLINICAL FEATURES

The mean patient age at presentation with tubular carcinoma is 58–64 years. A larger proportion of screen-detected carcinomas are of tubular type than is seen in symptomatic practice.

RADIOLOGIC FEATURES

The characteristic mammographic appearance is of an irregular, spiculated mass usually lacking microcalcification.

PATHOLOGIC FEATURES

GROSS FINDINGS

Mean size at presentation is 1.2–1.6 cm, with 48 % of tumors 1.1–2 cm in diameter. On slicing, these tumors are often moderately defined with a stellate appearance and gray color.

MICROSCOPIC FINDINGS

Early descriptions of tubular carcinoma as a distinctive subtype of invasive carcinoma identified two different histologic types: the sclerosing and the pure types. The former showed irregular infiltrative tubules and the latter a central hyalinized zone with a paucity of tubules with an increased abundance at the periphery. The tubules in both patterns are angulated with a single layer of epithelial cells showing apical 'snouts'. Twenty per cent of cases are reported to show multifocality.

By definition more than 90 % of the lesion must be forming these angulated tubules to be classified as pure tubular carcinoma. In addition, the tubular structures in pure tubular carcinoma are formed from only mild to moderately pleomorphic cells (score for pleomorphism of 1 or 2); if marked pleomorphism (score 3) is seen, the lesion is not regarded as being of pure tubular type. By definition therefore pure tubular carcinoma is of histologic grade 1 (Figure 18-5).

A range of atypical epithelial processes may be associated with tubular carcinoma, including DCIS, LCIS or columnar cell change/hyperplasia often with atypia (flat epithelial atypia) (see Figure 18-5).

ANCILLARY STUDIES

IMMUNOHISTOCHEMISTRY

Tubular carcinomas tend (>95 %) to be HER2 negative and EGFR negative. Ninety-one per cent are

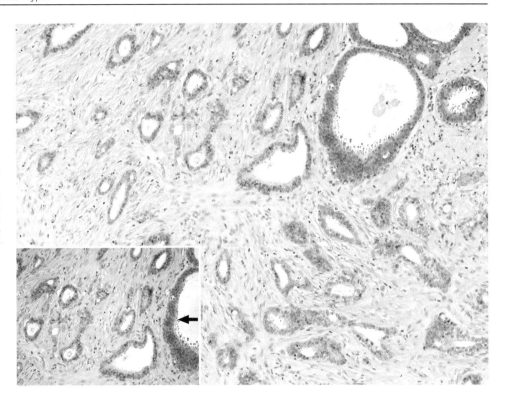

FIGURE 18-5

Invasive tubular carcinoma. Note the open angulated tubules and desmoplastic stroma that are characteristic of this special type carcinoma. There is adjacent flat epithelial atypia (see arrow in inset), a finding commonly associated with tubular carcinomas.

estrogen receptor positive and 75 % are progesterone receptor positive.

MOLECULAR STUDIES

This tumor type tends to be diploid with a low S-phase (89 %) fraction. Seventy-eight percent of cases show loss of 16q (compared with 34 % of invasive NST carcinomas) and 50 % demonstrated a gain of 1q, with 17p loss in only 6 % (38 % of invasive NST carcinoma) with an average of 3.6 chromosomal changes per case.

DIFFERENTIAL DIAGNOSIS

Tubular carcinoma may mimic sclerosing lesions and vice versa, in particular radial scars may occasionally pose diagnostic problems, but sclerosing adenosis and microglandular adenosis may also resemble tubular carcinoma. The absence of a myoepithelial layer in the malignant lesion can be confirmed with appropriate markers such as p63, smooth muscle myosin heavy chain or smooth muscle actin. The angulated appearance of the tubules in tubular carcinoma should be sought as a useful feature to distinguish this invasive carcinoma from microglandular adenosis where the tubular structures are rounded in shape. Assessment of the stroma associated with the tubules can be invaluable; in tubular carcinoma there is frequently a desmoplastic stromal reaction which is not seen around the

entrapped tubular structure in the centre of a radial scar or in other sclerosing processes.

PROGNOSIS AND TREATMENT

Nodal metastases are present in only 12–19 % of cases, most frequently, if involved, only low numbers (1–3) of metastases are seen. The 5-year and overall survival rates for patients with tubular carcinoma of the breast are 94 % and 88 %, respectively, which compare favorably with an age-matched control population; death is thus more likely to be from unrelated causes. The rate of local and systemic recurrence is lower in tubular carcinomas than in patients with grade 1 invasive NST carcinomas. Local recurrence rates have been identified in 1–10 % of pure tubular carcinomas.

CRIBRIFORM CARCINOMA

CLINICAL FEATURES

This is an uncommon (0.8–3.5 %) morphologic type of invasive carcinoma which is closely related to tubular

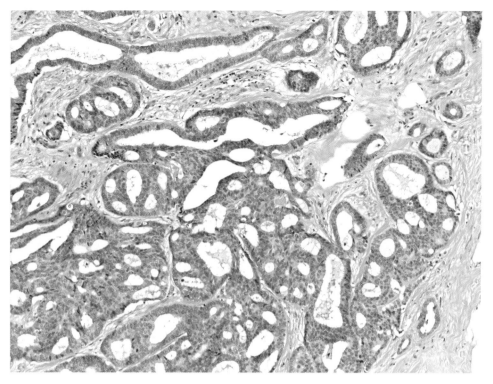

FIGURE 18-6
Invasive cribriform carcinoma. The infiltrating nests show a prominent cribriform morphology.

carcinoma. More than 90 % of the tumor must have a cribriform morphology, unless the non-cribriform areas present in <50 % of the tumor *and* have a tubular morphology. Average age at presentation is 53–58 years.

RADIOLOGIC FEATURES

These tumors often show evidence of microcalcification radiologically, with a spiculated appearance.

PATHOLOGIC FEATURES

GROSS FINDINGS

Average size at presentation is 2.6–3.1 cm. There are no particular gross findings distinguishing this form from other types of invasive breast carcinoma.

MICROSCOPIC FINDINGS

The infiltrating islands of tumor cells have a cribriform morphology with constituent cells showing amphophilic cytoplasm with low to intermediate grade nuclei (Figure 18-6). Occasionally, a giant cell reaction may be seen in the stroma. Cribriform DCIS is often present (80 % of cases).

ANCILLARY STUDIES

IMMUNOHISTOCHEMISTRY

Estrogen receptor positivity is seen in virtually 100 % of cases and progesterone positivity in 69 %. As in tubular carcinoma, HER2 is usually negative.

INVASIVE CRIBRIFORM CARCINOMA – PATHOLOGIC FEATURES

Gross Findings
▶ Moderately well defined with stellate/gray cut surface
▶ Average size 2.6–3.1 cm

Microscopic Findings
▶ Islands of tumor cells forming cribriform structures
▶ Tumor cells only mild to moderately pleomorphic
▶ Often desmoplastic stromal reaction, occasionally with giant cells

Immunohistochemical Studies
▶ Usually estrogen and progesterone receptor positive
▶ Usually HER2 negative

Differential Diagnosis
▶ Adenoid cystic carcinoma
▶ Cribriform DCIS
▶ Neuroendocrine carcinoma

DIFFERENTIAL DIAGNOSIS

Adenoid cystic carcinoma may be excluded by an absence of Alcian blue/Periodic Acid Schiff (AB/PAS) staining in cribriform carcinoma. In addition, whilst almost 100 % of invasive cribriform carcinomas express estrogen receptors, adenoid cystic carcinomas do not. Invasive neuroendocrine tumors of the breast can also be excluded by appropriate histochemical and immunostaining (grimelius, synaptophysin, chromogranin, S100 etc). It is sometimes difficult to distinguish cribriform DCIS from invasive cribriform carcinoma; the invasive nature of the tumor islands can be confirmed by the absence of surrounding myo-epithelial immunostaining (using the myoepithelial marker of choice e.g., alpha smooth muscle actin, smooth muscle myosin heavy chain, p63, calponin, etc) (Figure 18-8).

PROGNOSIS AND TREATMENT

Nodal metastases are seen in 14–37 % of cases, tending to involve low numbers (1–3) of nodes, as in the pure tubular variant with which this type has much in common. In Page et al's original series, with follow-up of 14.5 years, none of the patients died from cribriform carcinoma of the breast. A 100 % 5-year survival rate was also confirmed in a subsequent study.

MUCINOUS CARCINOMA

CLINICAL FEATURES

This tumor type is characterized by a mucinous morphology in over 90 % of the tumor with cases composed of 50–90 % falling into the mixed NST and mucinous category. The incidence ranges from 0.8–6 %, probably reflecting the strictness of applied diagnostic criteria. Patients tend to be post-menopausal women with a mean age of 59–71 years who present with a palpable mass.

RADIOLOGIC FEATURES

Mammography usually shows a well-circumscribed mass lesion with microcalcification also reported in 18 % of cases.

PATHOLOGIC FEATURES

GROSS FINDINGS

The mean size is 1.8–2 cm (range 0.3–12 cm). The tumor is well-circumscribed and a gelatinous appearance is noted on slicing.

MICROSCOPIC FINDINGS

The characteristic histologic features are nests, trabeculae, acini or sheets of epithelial cells, usually with some glandular lumen formation, within pools of extracellular mucin (Figure 18-7). The cells have granular eosinophilic and hyaline cytoplasm. Some, although not all, authorities regard a low nuclear grade (score 1 for pleomorphism) as a prerequisite for the diagnosis of pure mucinous carcinoma. Intracellular mucin may also be present.

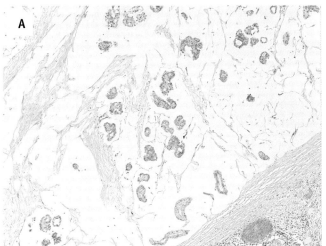
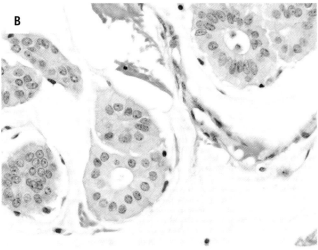

FIGURE 18-7

Invasive mucinous carcinoma. (A) Small glandular structures are noted within pools of mucin. (B) High power shows mild to moderate nuclear atypia and no evidence of mitoses.

INVASIVE MUCINOUS CARCINOMA – PATHOLOGIC FEATURES

Gross Findings

▸ Well-defined mass with a gelatinous cut surface
▸ Average size approximately 2 cm

Microscopic Findings

▸ Nests or trabeculae of tumor cells within lakes of mucin
▸ Tumor cells show mild to moderate nuclear pleomorphism

Immunohistochemical Studies

▸ Usually estrogen and progesterone receptor positive
▸ Usually HER2 negative
▸ Neuroendocrine features may be seen

Differential Diagnosis

▸ Mucocele-like lesion

ANCILLARY STUDIES

IMMUNOHISTOCHEMISTRY

Neuroendocrine differentiation can be identified in invasive mucinous carcinoma using both tinctorial (argyrophilia) stains and immunohistochemistry. Estrogen receptor positivity is seen in 73–95 % and progesterone receptor positivity in 79–84 %. Mucinous carcinomas tend to be negative for HER2 and for EGFR.

MOLECULAR INVESTIGATIONS

Mucinous carcinomas are likely to be diploid and have a low S-phase fraction. In a recent case report comparing the genetic profile of synchronous invasive mucinous and NST carcinomas, the former showed overexpression of 342 genes relative to the latter. Many of these were immunologically related (e.g., leukocyte cell adhesion molecules and MHC antigens) and others related to extracellular matrix components and enzymes, including matrix metalloproteinases.

DIFFERENTIAL DIAGNOSIS

Mucinous carcinomas should be distinguished from mucocele-like lesions. The latter are usually smaller lesions, have an absence of epithelial elements in the mucin pools and show dissection of collagen bundles in connective tissue, rather than the lobulated, circumscribed mucin collections present in invasive mucinous carcinoma. It is helpful to search for associated DCIS and cytonuclear atypia which may be seen in mucinous carcinomas but are absent in mucocele-like lesions.

PROGNOSIS AND TREATMENT

In two recent series only 14 % of cases had evidence of axillary nodal metastases and 96 % of invasive mucinous tumors present as either stage I or stage II disease. The 5-year disease free survival rates range between 81–90 % (94 % if node negative), with the corresponding disease-specific survival rate as 95.3 % and overall 5-year survival of 80 % (86 % if node-negative). The latter corresponds favorably with age-matched patients from the general population. The effect of the finding of neuroendocrine differentiation on survival is uncertain, although a very recent series suggests a positive correlation with favorable histologic/prognostic parameters (including nuclear grade, lymph node stage, progesterone receptor and HER2 status), with increasing significance associated with the increasing number of positive immunomarkers.

MEDULLARY CARCINOMA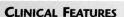

CLINICAL FEATURES

Medullary carcinoma represents 1–7 % of all invasive breast carcinomas, depending on the strictness of the diagnostic criteria (see below). Average age at presentation is 52 years, but 49 % of patients are less than 50 years in age. In multifactorial analysis, a continuous pushing margin, a high mitotic count and prominent lymphocytic infiltrate were found to be statistically significantly more commonly found in BRCA1-related tumors. Thus it has been recorded that medullary/atypical medullary carcinomas are found more commonly in carriers of BRCA1 mutations. However, conversely, by no means all BRCA1-mutation related-tumors will be identified as being of medullary or atypical medullary morphology. Nevertheless, the finding of a medullary type carcinoma, i.e., with grade 3 morphology, lymphocytic infiltrate and pushing margin, particularly in a young patient should prompt the search for a family history/possibility of a genetic predisposition. This is discussed in Chapter 21.

RADIOLOGIC FEATURES

Radiologically, medullary carcinoma appears as a circumscribed mass, reflecting the gross and histologic appearance.

PATHOLOGIC FEATURES

GROSS FINDINGS

The average size of medullary carcinoma of the breast in a non-screening population is 2.5–2.9 cm. Grossly the tumor is usually circumscribed with a pale gray/tan cut surface. Foci of hemorrhage or cystic change may be seen.

MICROSCOPIC FINDINGS

The histologic features defining medullary carcinoma (MC) of the breast have been debated for many years in the pathology literature. In Ridolfi's comprehensive description, typical medullary carcinoma required grade 2–3 nuclei, circumscribed margins, >75 % syncytial growth pattern, a moderate to marked lymphoplasmacytic infiltrate and an absence of glandular differentiation. In an effort to unify the diagnosis, the recent WHO blue book described five classical traits of medullary carcinoma, namely: syncytial growth pattern in >75 %; absence of glandular structures; diffuse moderate-marked lymphoplasmacytic infiltrate; grade 2–3 nuclear pleomorphism and histologic circumscription (Figure 18-8).

MEDULLARY CARCINOMA – PATHOLOGIC FEATURES

Gross Findings
▸ Usually well defined and circumscribed with gray/tan cut surface
▸ Average size 2.5–2.9 cm

Microscopic Findings
▸ Syncytial growth pattern in >75 %
▸ Absence of glandular structures
▸ Moderate/marked lymphoplasmacytic infiltrate
▸ Histologic circumscription
▸ Marked (score 3) nuclear pleomorphism

Immunohistochemical Studies
▸ Estrogen receptor negative
▸ Her2 negative
▸ p53 positive

Differential Diagnosis
▸ NST carcinoma
▸ Chronic inflammation, lymphoma or lymph node

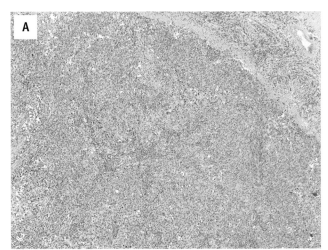

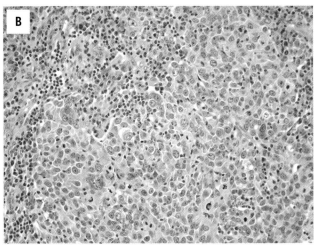

FIGURE 18-8
Medullary carcinoma. (A) The low power view emphasizes the circumscribed margin typical of this tumor. (B) High power shows the syncytial growth pattern, the vesicular nuclei, increased mitoses and the inflammatory infiltrate.

The syncytial growth pattern is composed of vesicular cells with prominent nucleoli and indistinct cell borders. They are organized into sheets, which should be distinguished from trabecular (usually less than 4 cells thick) or aggregated growth (similar to trabecular but nested islands of cells). Squamous metaplasia, necrosis and a giant cell reaction are all consistent with a diagnosis of medullary carcinoma. The presence of an intraductal component does not exclude a diagnosis of medullary carcinoma but is relatively rarely seen.

Ridolfi used the combination of a syncytial growth pattern in >75 % with either focal or prominent margin infiltration, mild-minimal inflammatory infiltrate, low nuclear-grade or glandular differentiation to define atypical medullary carcinoma. However, Ridolfi's group, together with further more recent publications, have suggested abolishing this category in order to ensure the maintenance of the prognostically significant medullary type.

ANCILLARY STUDIES

IMMUNOHISTOCHEMISTRY

The lymphocytes are predominantly peripheral T-cells similar to those which are sometimes associated with infiltrating NST carcinoma; immunohistochemistry to assess the lymphoid nature of the infiltrate is unhelpful, unless lymphoma is considered in the differential diagnosis (see below).

Medullary carcinomas tend to be estrogen receptor negative but do not tend to overexpress HER2. p53 overexpression occurs at an increased level in medullary carcinoma and has been indicated to be a biologic marker for this tumor type.

DIFFERENTIAL DIAGNOSIS

Identification of a lesion as a medullary carcinoma requires strict adherence to the criteria defined. On occasions it can be difficult to decide whether the lesion shows sufficient features; the most important is generally regarded to be the syncytial growth pattern which is a prerequisite for diagnosis. Rarely, particularly on core biopsy, a chronic inflammatory process or lymphoma may be considered in the diagnosis, or indeed the process mistaken for a lymph node. Immunohistochemistry for cytokeratins will confirm the epithelial nature of the lesion whilst lymphoid markers, except in the reactive surrounding cells, will be negative.

PROGNOSIS AND TREATMENT

In Ridolfi's study, 23 % of patients with typical medullary (30 % of those with atypical medullary) carcinoma developed regional lymph node metastases. Node negative patients with medullary carcinoma have a 10 year survival rate of 84 % (92 % 5 year survival). The majority of the deaths occur within the first 5 years after diagnosis, as might be expected with these grade 3 carcinomas.

MICROPAPILLARY CARCINOMA

CLINICAL FEATURES

Invasive micropapillary carcinoma of the breast accounts for 1.2–2.3 % of all invasive breast carcinomas in the pure form, but is much more frequently (7 %) present as a component of a mixed lesion often in combination with NST carcinoma. The average age of presentation is 52.5–58.8 years, with a range of 28–92 years. The characteristic prognostic feature of this particular tumor type is its high incidence of lymphatic invasion and axillary lymph node involvement. It is extremely important that even a minor component of this tumor type be identified, given the associated lymphotropism and likelihood of advanced nodal stage.

PATHOLOGIC FEATURES

GROSS FINDINGS

The tumors have an average size of 2–4 cm (reported range 0.1–10 cm), with up to 23 % being 1 cm or less in

diameter. The gross appearance is not characteristic, with a gray-white, stellate and firm cut surface.

MICROSCOPIC FINDINGS

The characteristic histologic appearance is of solid/tubular epithelial nests composed of eosinophilic cuboidal/columnar cells surrounded by a clear space (Figure 18-9A and B). This appears to be artefactual tissue shrinkage as the spaces are absent in frozen section. The nests lack a true fibrovascular core. This carcinoma has been described as having an 'inside-out' appearance as the polarity of the cells is reversed with luminal marker expression (e.g., epithelial membrane antigen) on the peripheral aspect of the cell islands. As noted above, this pattern is most commonly seen in a mixed lesion or as a small area within a tumor of otherwise no special type. In the majority of cases it comprises less than 20 % of the tumor volume.

The tumors are predominantly of histologic grade 3 (58–82 %). In particular, lymphovascular invasion is frequently seen (63–76 %) (Figure 18-9C). Multifocality is often noted (31 % of cases) in association with foci of lymphatic invasion. Lymph node positivity rates have been recorded in between 69–95 % of cases and even T1b and T1a tumors are associated with a high incidence of axillary nodal metastases (64 % and 75 %, respectively).

INVASIVE MICROPAPILLARY CARCINOMA – PATHOLOGIC FEATURES

Gross Findings
▸ Gray/white, stellate cut surface
▸ Average size 2.4 cm

Microscopic Findings
▸ Solid/tubular nests within a clear space
▸ Usually a component of mixed tumor
▸ Lymphovascular invasion common and a high rate of axillary nodal metastases

Immunohistochemical Studies
▸ EMA – 'inside out' pattern
▸ Estrogen receptor positivity in 60–90 %
▸ Progesterone receptor positivity in 60–70 %
▸ HER2: 45 % positive by FISH analysis

Differential Diagnosis
▸ Retraction artefact
▸ Ductal NST carcinoma (i.e., missed as a tumor type) or invasive papillary carcinoma
▸ Metastatic carcinoma from other primary site

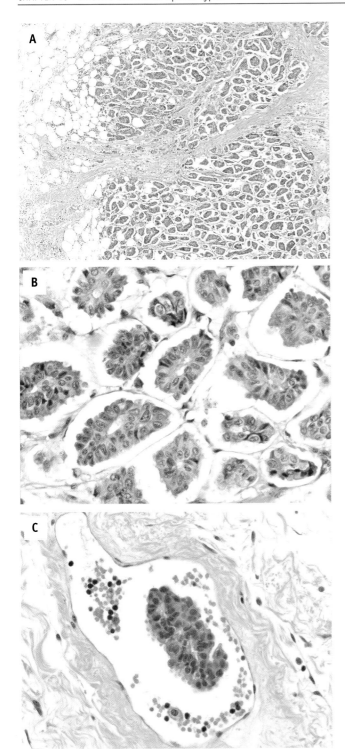

FIGURE 18-9

Invasive micropapillary carcinoma. (A) The low power illustrates the typical growth pattern showing epithelial nests surrounded by clear spaces. (B) At high power one can appreciate the 'inside-out' appearance of the cells within the nests. (C) Lymphovascular invasion is often associated with this special type carcinoma.

ANCILLARY STUDIES

IMMUNOHISTOCHEMISTRY

Immunostaining with epithelial membrane antigen shows a characteristic 'inside out pattern' with positivity noted on the external aspect of the cell clusters (see Figure 18-10B). Reports of estrogen receptor positivity range from 61–90%, and for progesterone receptor 61–70%. HER2 positivity rates are difficult to assess, due to cases scoring 2+ being included as positive in some series, but rates as high as 54% have been reported.

MOLECULAR STUDIES

A recent study employing comparative genomic hybridization (CGH) documented an average of 7.4 chromosomal alterations per case, which was lower than seen in NST tumors. All of the 16 cases demonstrated varying loss of 8p with 88% of cases showing gains of 8q.

DIFFERENTIAL DIAGNOSIS

Invasive papillary carcinoma is excluded if fibrovascular cores are present and there is an absence of clear spaces around the tumor islands. Metastatic micropapillary carcinomas, e.g. bladder and lung and ovarian serous carcinoma should be considered; the presence of DCIS should be sought and supports a primary breast origin. Estrogen receptor positivity may be seen in ovarian carcinomas and cannot be used to distinguish a primary breast carcinoma from an ovarian metastasis.

PROGNOSIS AND TREATMENT

One series with follow-up reported that compared to invasive NST carcinoma, invasive micropapillary carcinoma had a local recurrence rate of 22% (versus 12% for NST) but a similar frequency of distant metastases (25% versus 23% for NST). Ten of 36 patients died within 9 years (28% versus 18% for NST). An additional study reported a 46% mortality rate with a long follow-up (143 months). Although 42–52% of cases of invasive micropapillary carcinoma of the breast present with 4 or more positive lymph nodes, i.e., at a later stage, overall survival is similar to other carcinoma types when matched stage for stage. Skin involvement has been reported to be strongly correlated with a poor prognosis.

METAPLASTIC CARCINOMA

Overall these tumors represent approximately 1 % of all invasive breast carcinomas. The 2003 WHO publication 'Tumors of the Breast and Female Genital Organs' defines metaplastic carcinomas of the breast as a 'heterogeneous group of neoplasms generally characterized by an intimate admixture of adenocarcinoma with dominant areas of spindle cell, squamous, and/or mesenchymal differentiation' and clarifies that, 'the metaplastic spindle cell and squamous cell carcinomas may present in a pure form without any recognizable adenocarcinoma'. They provide a classification of purely epithelial (squamous cell carcinoma, adenocarcinoma with spindle differentiation and adenosquamous carcinoma (including mucoepidermoid carcinoma)) and mixed epithelial and mesenchymal (carcinoma with chondroid or osseous metaplasia and carcinosarcoma). This classification will be followed here.

EPITHELIAL TUMORS

SQUAMOUS CELL CARCINOMA

CLINICAL FEATURES

Average age at presentation is 53 years with patients tending to present with an ill-defined mass, usually present for less than 3 months.

METAPLASTIC CARCINOMA – PATHOLOGIC FEATURES

Gross Findings
- Gray/white, ill-defined cut surface
- May have cystic areas of foci of necrosis macroscopically
- Wide range of sizes reported, often larger than other special types

Microscopic Findings
- Squamous or spindled cell (or mixed) infiltrating islands of cells
- Spindled component may range from low to high grade
- May have heterologous elements, e.g., osteocartilaginous differentiation

Immunohistochemical Studies
- Express cytokeratins, at least focally
- Often estrogen receptor negative

Differential Diagnosis
- Metastatic carcinoma (squamous) or metastatic or primary sarcoma
- Fibromatosis (low grade variants)
- Phyllodes tumor

PATHOLOGIC FEATURES

GROSS FINDINGS

Average size at presentation is 3.9 cm. The tumor is often apparently cystic on slicing with a tan/white coloration. Hemorrhage and necrosis can be seen.

MICROSCOPIC FINDINGS

One of the most comprehensive studies to date of this tumor type included only tumors showing exclusively squamous cell carcinoma that did not appear to involve the overlying skin. The majority were moderately differentiated and appeared to show cystic degeneration, correlating with the macroscopic appearance and an infiltrating margin. There may be associated DCIS confirming the primary nature of the lesion. A small (<25 %) spindle cell component may be present. Axillary metastases have been recorded in 10.5 %.

IMMUNOHISTOCHEMISTRY

Estrogen receptor (ER) assays have been variable and no reliable conclusion can be drawn regarding ER positivity in this tumor type in the breast. Focal immunostaining for S100 and smooth muscle actin has been reported. Mucin stains can be performed to exclude a mucoepidermoid carcinoma which rarely metastasizes.

DIFFERENTIAL DIAGNOSIS

Diagnosis rests on the recognition of the squamous nature of the lesion and on the exclusion of a metastatic origin (e.g., from lung or elsewhere) or an origin from the overlying skin. This may prove difficult and requires clinico-pathologic correlation. Mucin stains can be undertaken to exclude a mucoepidermoid carcinoma.

PROGNOSIS AND TREATMENT

The 5-year disease specific survival rate is reported to be 63 %. As with other forms of metaplastic carcinoma of the breast, there is a risk of metastases developing at other sites despite negative axillary nodes. Mean survival following the development of metastases is 2 years.

LOW-GRADE ADENOSQUAMOUS CARCINOMA (SEE ALSO ADENOSQUAMOUS CARCINOMA)

CLINICAL FEATURES

Average age at presentation is 54–57 years with patients presenting with a palpable mass.

PATHOLOGIC FEATURES

GROSS FINDINGS

Mean size at diagnosis is 2.5–2.8 cm, the tumor appearing as a tan/pale yellow irregular mass which is often poorly circumscribed.

MICROSCOPIC FINDINGS

This tumor type is characterized by a stellate morphology composed of infiltrating compressed glands which may be round or have a comma-shaped outline. The lumina may contain eosinophilic material and keratin may be identified associated with squamous differentiation (which ranges from 5–80%). Mitoses are infrequent with an absence of significant nuclear atypia and little or no necrosis. The stroma is cellular and collagenous or may have an edematous appearance and often bears a mild lymphocytic infiltrate. An association with papillary and sclerosing lesions and adenomyoepithelioma has been reported.

IMMUNOHISTOCHEMISTRY

These tumors tend to show no estrogen or progesterone receptor immunoreactivity.

DIFFERENTIAL DIAGNOSIS

The histology closely resembles syringomatous adenoma of the nipple, but the intramammary site of the tumor should alert the pathologist to the likely diagnosis and risk of recurrence if the lesion is incompletely excised.

PROGNOSIS AND TREATMENT

In one series 20% of women treated by local excision had subsequent local recurrence but there is a low rate of metastases. Complete excision is thus important for local control.

ADENOSQUAMOUS CARCINOMA

This category excludes cases that would be placed in the low grade adenosquamous carcinoma group above. These tumors are histologically identified by the presence of invasive adenocarcinoma with areas of variable but malignant-appearing squamous epithelium.

Prognosis correlates with increasing tumor size and lymph node stage and is similar to comparable NST tumors of the breast. Under the WHO classification, mucoepidermoid carcinomas are included in this category. The low grade type of this lesion is characterized by nests of cells with basaloid/intermediate appearance at the periphery with central epidermoid and mucous secreting cells. There may be a cystic component. The high grade form shows poor differentiation/high histologic grade, with a predominance of squamous and intermediate cells, but with glandular cells intermixed. In one series of nine patients only one developed axillary metastases with no distant metastases or deaths recorded. The high grade form, however, tends to show an aggressive course.

ADENOCARCINOMA WITH SPINDLE-CELL METAPLASIA AND MONOPHASIC SPINDLE CELL CARCINOMA

CLINICAL FEATURES

Mean-age at presentation is 57–63 years with a palpable mass.

PATHOLOGIC FEATURES

GROSS FINDINGS

A mean size of 4.4 cm has been recorded with a nodular or irregular, well-defined appearance. Foci of necrosis can be identified and the cut surface is gritty with a white/gray/tan cut surface.

MICROSCOPIC FINDINGS

In a study by Wargotz et al., the majority of tumors showed an infiltrative border to some degree. The tumor cells were composed predominantly of bland, plump, spindle-cells arranged in interlacing fascicles, possibly with a storiform pattern. The stroma was collagenous or focally myxoid. DCIS was identified in 7%, together with a component of invasive ductal NST (48%) or squamous cell-carcinoma (11%), which merged with the atypical spindle cell component. Monophasic spindle-cell tumors were also seen. Seventy percent of the spindle-cell tumors showed low-grade nuclear characteristics. Three percent showed vascular space invasion and six percent showed evidence of axillary metastases. There tended to be an associated lymphoplasmacytic infiltrate. Focal necrosis and osseous and chondroid metaplasia were occasionally seen.

IMMUNOHISTOCHEMISTRY

Particularly in low-grade cases, the vast majority (98–100%) show evidence of cytokeratin immunopositivity in the spindle-cell component including luminal cytokeratins (cytokeratin 7, 19 and cam 5.2) and myoepithelial/basaloid cytokeratins (34βE12, cytokeratin 5, 14), with a greater degree of immunostaining of the latter. Smooth muscle actin (SMA) positivity may also be seen. Together with S100 immunopositivity in some cases, this has been taken as evidence of myoepithelial differentiation. The new WHO classification actually limits immunostaining of the spindle cell component to cytokeratin 7 in 'adenocarcinoma with spindle cell metaplasia'. EMA and vimentin staining may also be seen. Data is limited on estrogen and progesterone receptor expression but there is a tendency to negativity and low-grade tumors are most often HER2 negative.

DIFFERENTIAL DIAGNOSIS

The main differential diagnoses are fibromatosis and stroma-rich areas of phyllodes tumors. Extensive sampling of resection specimens is essential to search for the epithelial component of the latter, in addition to DCIS or an associated adenocarcinomatous component. Immunostaining for a wide panel of cytokeratins is essential. In one very recent series, a minimum of four cytokeratins including 34βE12 (which was the cytokeratin most likely to be positive) and CK 14 or 5, was proposed due to the heterogeneity of cyto-keratin immunostaining. The stroma of phyllodes tumors is more likely to be CD34, and possibly bcl2, positive but cytokeratin negative. Fibromatoses tend to show SMA positivity but no reactivity for cytokeratins, S100 and EMA.

PROGNOSIS AND TREATMENT

In Wargotz et al.'s series, size was reported to correlate with risk of recurrence as did an absence of histologic circumscription. With an average of 5.4 years follow-up, 17 % of patients suffered local recurrence alone and 15 % either local recurrence and metastasis or metastasis alone. In the same study, 29 of 30 patients with metastasis subsequently died, whereas 71 % with local recurrence only, survived. The cumulative 5-year survival rate, with adjustment for death from other causes was 64 %. In a further series there was a 29 % local recurrence rate in patients treated by local excision with low-grade (fibromatosis-like) spindle cell carcinoma, and two patients developed distant metastatic disease.

MIXED EPITHELIAL AND MESENCHYMAL

Under the WHO classification this group includes tumors composed of invasive adenocarcinoma with heterologous elements. The heterologous elements appear to be of myoepithelial/epithelial derivation.

CLINICAL FEATURES

Average age at presentation is 56 years and patients present with a palpable mass.

PATHOLOGIC FEATURES

GROSS FINDINGS

The mean size of the tumors is 3.9 cm and they tend to be well circumscribed. The cut surface has a variable appearance with hemorrhage and necrosis seen, occasionally with myxoid foci.

MICROSCOPIC FINDINGS

The defining histologic characteristic is the presence of adenocarcinoma (usually NST carcinoma, often grade 3) with associated mesenchymal heterologous elements. The commonest of these latter are bone and cartilage. DCIS, if present (reported in 28 % of cases), is often high grade. The heterologous elements can show a benign or atypical morphology and, in cases where the mesenchymal component is malignant, the term carcinosarcoma could be applied. The heterologous elements in the latter include osteosarcoma, chondrosarcoma, rhabdomyosarcoma, liposarcoma or fibrosarcoma. Some also apply the term when the spindle cell component is very atypical and cellular.

IMMUNOHISTOCHEMISTRY

Tumors showing osteocartilaginous differentiation have shown no reactivity for estrogen or progesterone receptor. The majority of cases show evidence of immunopositivity for 34βE12 (i.e., high molecular weight cytokeratins).

DIFFERENTIAL DIAGNOSIS

The presence of 'more typical' invasive breast carcinoma and DCIS and cytokeratin immunopositivity support the diagnosis of a metaplastic carcinoma with heterologous elements over a primary sarcoma of the breast, which is very uncommon, particularly if not associated with a phyllodes tumor.

PROGNOSIS AND TREATMENT

Axillary nodal metastases have been identified in 23 % of cases with osteocartilaginous elements and the overall survival of patients with an osteocartilaginous component to the lesion has been reported to be approximately 60 %. A wide range of 5-year survival (38–65 %) has been recorded. The prognosis, however, appears to compare favorably with invasive NST carcinoma when adjusted for other prognostic parameters.

APOCRINE CARCINOMA

CLINICAL FEATURES

More than 90 % of the tumor should show cytologic and immunohistochemical evidence of apocrine differentiation to be classified as being of apocrine type; focal apocrine differentiation is not uncommon in invasive breast carcinoma and strictness of criteria is required. The reported incidence of pure invasive apocrine carcinoma is 0.3–4 %.

The tumors present as a mass but there are no characteristic clinical or radiologic features.

PATHOLOGIC FEATURES

The tumors have an overall growth pattern of NST carcinomas, but the constituent cells show either eosinophilic granular cytoplasm with enlarged nuclei and prominent nucleoli or occasionally have foamy cytoplasm. The eosinophilic cytoplasmic granules show DPAS positivity. Other special types of carcinoma, e.g., medullary, tubular and lobular cancers may show focal apocrine differentiation.

APOCRINE CARCINOMA – PATHOLOGIC FEATURES

Gross Findings
▸ As for tumors of no special type

Microscopic Findings
▸ Must be 90 % apocrine morphology
▸ Cells have abundant eosinophilic granular cytoplasm
▸ Large nuclei with prominent nucleoli
▸ May be admixed with other special types

Immunohistochemical Studies
▸ GCDFP-15 positive
▸ Estrogen and progesterone receptor negative
▸ Androgen receptor positive

Differential Diagnosis
▸ Atypical apocrine proliferation in a sclerormg lesion

ANCILLARY STUDIES

ULTRASTRUCTURAL

With the electron microscope, two types of cells are identified, one with electron dense cytoplasmic granules 303–722 nm in diameter and another with empty vesicles, corresponding to the granular and foamy cell types identified histologically, respectively.

IMMUNOHISTOCHEMISTRY

Gross cystic disease fluid protein-15 (GCDFP-15) stains the cytoplasm diffusely in these tumors with strong positivity seen in the majority of the cells. Invasive apocrine carcinomas fail to stain with estrogen or progesterone receptor but are reported to show strong androgen receptor positivity. Recently HER2 status has been reported to be 2+ or 3+ with immunohistochemistry in 66 % of cases; 44 % show HER2 gene amplification with FISH.

MOLECULAR FEATURES

Comparative genomic hybridization reveals an average of 14.8 DNA copy number changes with gains of 1q, 2q, 1p and losses of 1p, 22q, 17q, 12q and 16q. Overlap is seen with DCIS and hyperplastic apocrine lesions.

DIFFERENTIAL DIAGNOSIS

Apocrine carcinomas may rarely be mimicked by benign lesions such as apocrine change, particularly if atypical, in sclerosing adenosis, but myoepithelial markers can be used to confirm the absence of myoepithelium in the former. Apocrine carcinomas may not be recognized if the apocrine nature of the malignant cells is not perceived. GCDFP-15 immunohistochemistry can be undertaken, but the abundant cytoplasm with granules present and large nuclei with prominent nucleoli should enable the correct classification to be made.

PROGNOSIS AND TREATMENT

The distribution of size, grade and lymph node stage are similar to NST carcinomas and when matched with NST carcinoma for these standard prognostic parameters, no difference in the survival rates has been found and the tumor type, at present, has no recognized prognostic significance.

NEUROENDOCRINE CARCINOMA

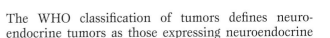

The WHO classification of tumors defines neuroendocrine tumors as those expressing neuroendocrine markers in >50 % of the cell population and identifies three subtypes: solid neuroendocrine, small cell/oat cell and large cell neuroendocrine. A recent study confirmed that 10–18 % of breast carcinomas showed evidence of neuroendocrine differentiation, but none showed >50 % positivity. In this study there was no prognostic impact for this level of neuroendocrine differentiation.

CLINICAL FEATURES

There appears to be an increasing incidence of neuroendocrine carcinomas of the breast with increasing age. Patients with small cell carcinoma tend to present with a mass.

PATHOLOGIC FEATURES

GROSS FINDINGS

The size of small-cell carcinoma of the breast ranges from 1.3–5 cm. The margin is ill-defined and the cut surface tan/gray.

MICROSCOPIC FINDINGS

Solid neuroendocrine carcinoma has an infiltrative morphology with component cells arranged in nests, sheets or trabeculae separated by scant connective tissue. Acinar formation and peripheral palisading of cell groups may be seen around a characteristic collagen core. The cells are relatively uniform with eosinophilic granular cytoplasm and may have a spindle, polygonal

or plasmacytoid appearance. The tumors are histologic grade 1 or 2. Mitotic figures do not exceed 4 mitoses per 10 high power fields (HPF). The appearances are, in essence, similar to a carcinoid tumor. Also included in this group is an alveolar variant which is composed of cells with faintly granular clear cytoplasm. There are 6–12 mitoses per 10 HPF and most are grade 2. The stroma is dense and collagenous.

In large cell neuroendocrine carcinoma, the cells are arranged in clusters with vesicular nuclei and relatively abundant cytoplasm. There are large numbers of mitoses (18–65 per 10 HPF) and focal necrosis can be seen. Most tumors are grade 3.

Small cell carcinoma of the breast is composed of relatively small cells with scant cytoplasm, finely granular chromatin and a high mitotic rate, characteristic of small cell carcinomas at non-mammary sites. The growth pattern can be solid, alveolar, trabecular or single file but is infiltrative. Necrosis, lymphovascular invasion and non-small cell carcinoma components may be present, as may an in situ component which resembles the invasive small cell carcinoma morphologically.

ANCILLARY STUDIES

IMMUNOHISTOCHEMISTRY/SPECIAL STAINS

Neuroendocrine carcinomas show positive staining with Grimelius histochemical stains and for chromogranin, neuron specific enolase, synaptophysin and CD56 immunostaining. Small cell carcinoma shows cytokeratin 7, Cam 5.2 and cytokeratin 19 positivity, but negativity for cytokeratin 20. However, 67 % show estrogen receptor positivity, 56 % progesterone receptor positivity but these lesions do not express HER2. TTF1 reactivity has been reported in 20 % of cases.

DIFFERENTIAL DIAGNOSIS

It is important to exclude metastasis to the breast, particularly from the lung. The presence of an in situ component and absence of a primary elsewhere would favor a mammary origin. Cytokeratin 7 immunopositivity also favors a breast primary as pulmonary small cell carcinoma is frequently negative.

PROGNOSIS AND TREATMENT

Histologic grade and estrogen receptor status influence prognosis, and the presence of mucin may also have a favorable prognostic effect for non-small cell neuroendocrine carcinomas. In the small series of small cell carcinomas published by Shin et al., 2 of 9 patients developed distant metastases; it is highly likely that stage at diagnosis is important in prognosis.

NEUROENDOCRINE CARCINOMA – PATHOLOGIC FEATURES

Gross Findings
▸ Ill-defined mass lesion
▸ Variable in size, from 1.3–5 cm

Microscopic Findings
▸ Infiltrating tumor cells forming nests, trabeculae or acinar groups
▸ Cells may be small and uniform with eosinophilic granular cytoplasm or larger with vesicular nuclei or have a spindled cell morphology

Immunohistochemical Studies
▸ Chromogranin, synaptophysin, CD56 and NSE positive
▸ Cytokeratin 7 positive
▸ Estrogen receptor often positive
▸ HER2 negative

Differential Diagnosis
▸ Metastatic neuroendocrine carcinoma, e.g., from lung

INVASIVE PAPILLARY CARCINOMA

CLINICAL FEATURES

This tumor type accounts for up to 2 % of all invasive breast carcinomas and appears to occur more frequently in non-Caucasian post-menopausal women.

PATHOLOGIC FEATURES

GROSS FINDINGS

Macroscopically the tumor is usually well circumscribed.

MICROSCOPIC FINDINGS

The characteristic histologic feature is a tumor formed from islands of malignant cells centered around fibrovascular cores. Whilst more tubular structures may be seen, these often have papillary structures at the periphery. The constituent cells may show apocrine features and 63 % of cases in the NSABP-04 study had an intermediate nuclear grade. An intraductal component, often also papillary, is frequently (80 %) present. Conversely, invasive carcinomas associated with encysted (in situ) papillary carcinomas are usually invasive ductal of no specific type.

ANCILLARY STUDIES

IMMUNOHISTOCHEMISTRY

Estrogen and progesterone receptor positivity and HER2 negativity have been documented in this tumor type.

PROGNOSIS AND TREATMENT

Nodal metastases have been reported in 32 % of cases, although there is reportedly a relatively favorable prognosis when compared with tubular, mucinous and NST carcinomas. After 5 years follow-up there was only one reported death from invasive papillary carcinoma in the NSABP-04 study and an 18 % death rate in the NSABP-06 series (the latter in contrast to 37 % in a NST group).

SECRETORY CARCINOMA

CLINICAL FEATURES

This is one of the most uncommon types of invasive breast carcinoma and was originally described in children but adult cases are now well recognized. The reported age range is wide (5–87 years). A review of the literature showed 37 % patients with this tumor type were younger than 20 years but 62 % of patients could 'not be regarded as children or juvenile'. Patients usually present with a palpable mass, often near the areola.

PATHOLOGIC FEATURES

GROSS FINDINGS

Mean size of tumors at presentation is 1.6–2.6 cm. On slicing they are often firm to hard with a relatively well-circumscribed margin and gray/white/brown cut-surface.

MICROSCOPIC FINDINGS

These tumors often show a central hyalinized area with a cellular periphery. The tumor architecture is solid, papillary, microcystic, cystic or tubular or combinations thereof. Focal apocrine differentiation may be seen. The component cells have relatively uniform nuclei with nucleoli and abundant clear/vacuolated amphophilic to lightly eosinophilic granular cytoplasm. Numbers of mitoses are variable. Prominent intra- and extracellular amphophilic/weakly eosinophilic secretion is seen. Associated DCIS may be present.

ANCILLARY STUDIES

IMMUNOHISTOCHEMISTRY/SPECIAL STAINS

PAS staining of secretions is seen and alcian blue positivity is also noted. Strong immunostaining for S100, α-lactalbumin and polyclonal carcinoembryonic antigen (CEA) has been identified. Estrogen receptor status has been reported to be negative (5/6 patients in one series) and progesterone receptor positive (3/3 patients) but in a more recent series, 4/13 cases showed estrogen receptor and 2/13 progesterone positivity. HER2 overexpression has been detected in 1/13 cases. The mean MIB1 index appears to be low (11.4 %). GCDFP-15 immunostaining is negative.

MOLECULAR TECHNIQUES

Most tumors are diploid. Tumors show an average of 2.0 genetic alterations per carcinoma using CGH, with apparently characteristic recurrent gains of 8q (37.5 %), 1q (25 %) and losses of 22q (25 %). There is expression of the ETV6-NTRK3 fusion gene (a chimeric tyrosine kinase). Loss of heterozygosity (LOH) studies have suggested that the only significant difference between infiltrating NST and secretory carcinomas is at 17p13 (the p53 gene locus) with 47 % of NST carcinomas showing LOH and 0 % of secretory carcinomas.

PROGNOSIS AND TREATMENT

Axillary metastases may occur but disseminated disease is unusual, consequently the benefit of systemic adjuvant treatment is questionable. Late recurrences are a possibility, but overall this tumor type is considered to have a good prognosis; death from metastatic disease is unusual. Local recurrence is related to incomplete excision but there is some evidence of a more aggressive course in adults.

ADENOID CYSTIC CARCINOMA

CLINICAL FEATURES

This tumor type is analogous to the same morphologic type of carcinoma arising in salivary glands. It represents 0.05–0.1 % of all invasive breast carcinomas. Median age of presentation is 66 years and 96 % of patients are post menopausal. Often the tumor has a peri-areolar location.

PATHOLOGIC FEATURES

GROSS FINDINGS

Average diameter at presentation is 1.9–2.5 cm. The tumors tend to have a well circumscribed margin.

ADENOID CYSTIC CARCINOMA – PATHOLOGIC FEATURES

Gross Findings
▸ Well-defined mass lesion
▸ Average 1.9–2.5 cm

Microscopic Findings
▸ Infiltrating tumor cells forming solid, trabeculae or cribriform groups
▸ Biphasic with majority of cells basaloid, small in size and hyperchromatic lining pseudocysts containing basement membrane material
▸ Epithelial cell component lines true acinar structures and are moderate in size with more abundant eosinophilic cytoplasm

Immunohistochemical Studies
▸ Pseudocysts Alcian blue positive, true acinar/glandular component PAS positive
▸ Basaloid cells express cytokeratin 14, laminin and collagen IV
▸ Glandular cells are positive for cytokeratin 7
▸ Estrogen receptor negative

Differential Diagnosis
▸ Invasive cribriform carcinoma

MICROSCOPIC FINDINGS

The margin is at least focally infiltrative and the morphology of the tumor is tubular, cribriform, solid or mixtures thereof. The component cells are biphasic with the majority of the tumors composed of small hyperchromatic cells with sparse cytoplasm (basaloid cells) (Figure 18-10A). These line the so called 'pseudocysts' which contain amorphous eosinophilic basement membrane material. True glandular lumens are present lined by the epithelial cell component with more abundant eosinophilic cytoplasm and round nuclei (Figure 18-10B). Mitotic counts are usually low. In Ro *et al.*'s series of patients, 6 were grade 1, 6 were grade 2 and 1 was grade 3. This grading system was the same as that used for salivary gland carcinomas, with grade 1 tumors showing a cystic and glandular appearance with no solid components, but grades 2 and 3 were differentiated on lesser and greater solid components, with a 30 % cut off.

An association with microglandular adenosis has been identified and the suggestion raised that atypical microglandular adenosis may represent the precursor component of this tumor.

ANCILLARY STUDIES

ULTRASTRUCTURAL FEATURES

Electron microscopy identifies both epithelial and myoepithelial cells. The former are seen as glandular lumina with microvilli and desmosomes whilst the myoepithelial cells contain myofilaments, pinocytic vesicles and have associated basement membrane material. The pseudocysts contain reduplicated basement-membrane material.

IMMUNOHISTOCHEMISTRY/SPECIAL STAINS

The pseudocysts show positive staining for Alcian Blue and are PAS negative, which contrasts with the PAS positive contents of the true glandular lumens. The basaloid cells show immunopositivity for vimentin and cytokeratin 14, type IV collagen and laminin. Focal staining with S100, smooth muscle actin, calponin and p63 may be seen. The epithelial cells lining the glandular lumens are positive for cytokeratin 7 and E-cadherin.

These tumors are characteristically estrogen and progesterone receptor negative immunohistochemically and this may be valuable in distinguishing these lesions from invasive cribriform carcinoma, which is invariably ER and PR positive.

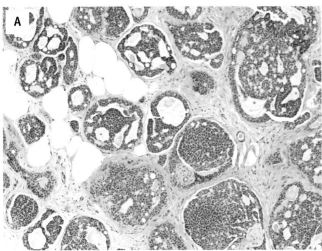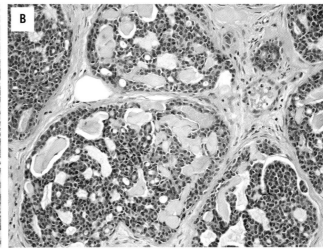

FIGURE 18-10

Adenoid cystic carcinoma. (A) On low power one can appreciate the biphasic nature of the cells comprising the cell nests; central basaloid cells and larger epithelial cells at the periphery. (B) High power demonstrates the true lumina and pseudocysts containing amorphous eosinophilic material.

MOLECULAR TECHNIQUES

These tumors have a low S-phase fraction (90 %) and 92 % are diploid. Abnormalities of 6q have been noted.

DIFFERENTIAL DIAGNOSIS

This tumor type should be distinguished from cribriform carcinoma, as described above.

PROGNOSIS AND TREATMENT

There appears to be a relatively low risk of local recurrence (0–7 %) and distant metastases, thus this tumor type has a very favorable prognosis. Axillary metastases are very rare; Arpino *et al.* documented axillary nodal metastases in only 4 % (1 case) of patients. In Ro *et al.* series no grade 1 tumors recurred but two grade 2 tumors recurred in distant sites, both in the absence of axillary metastases; it thus appears that metastases can rarely occur in the presence of negative axillary nodes. Five year disease-free survival rates of 100 % have been recorded, with 5 year overall survival rates of 85 %. The literature suggests that axillary dissection may not be appropriate in this particular tumor type given the low rate of involvement and the lack of prognostic information provided. Sites of distant metastases include lung, liver, brain and kidney, with the majority occurring in the lungs.

ACINIC CELL CARCINOMA

CLINICAL FEATURES

This very rare lesion tends to present in women in their sixth decade with a palpable mass, 2–5 cm in diameter.

PATHOLOGIC FEATURES

GROSS FINDINGS

Macroscopically the tumor is often solid with poor circumscription and a gray-pink cut surface.

MICROSCOPIC FINDINGS

The component cells have central round nuclei with prominent nucleoli and granular eosinophilic to amphophilic cytoplasm. The granules may be fine or coarse and globular. The cells may have a solid and nested or tubular growth pattern or it may be a mixed pattern. An appearance similar to microglandular adenosis can be seen. Eosinophilic material may be seen within lumina. A clear cell component may be present.

ANCILLARY STUDIES

IMMUNOHISTOCHEMISTRY/SPECIAL STAINS

PAS staining, following diastase digestion, can be used to detect the cytoplasmic granules. The cells can show S100, amylase, lysozyme and EMA immunopositivity. The tumors appear to be negative for estrogen and progesterone receptor staining.

ULTRASTRUCTURAL FEATURES

Electron microscopy reveals electron-dense granules consistent with zymogen granules.

DIFFERENTIAL DIAGNOSIS

The presence of nuclear atypia, frank invasion and the absence of a basement membrane excludes the diagnosis of microglandular adenosis. The possibility of a metastatic process should be excluded by careful clinical work-up. GCDFP-15 immunostaining (negative in acinic cell carcinoma) excludes apocrine carcinoma.

PROGNOSIS AND TREATMENT

Only small numbers of tumors have been recorded to date. In one series of 6 patients, 3 had axillary dissections and 2 had evidence of metastases. Four patients were alive and well with 1 to 5 years of follow-up and a further patient developed a local recurrence. Another report records 3 of 11 patients developing axillary metastases and death in 1 of 10 patients.

CLEAR CELL CARCINOMAS

This group of tumors is composed of glycogen-rich clear cell carcinoma (GRCC) and lipid-rich carcinoma (LRC), which will be considered together. Both types show a clear cell morphology in 90 % of the tumor, in GRCC this is due to glycogen and in LRC due to neutral lipids.

CLINICAL FEATURES

GRCC is extremely rare. Mean age of presentation is 54 years with presentation as a palpable mass. LRC is also exceptionally rare, with a median age of presentation of 60 years, again with a palpable mass as the main presenting complaint.

PATHOLOGIC FEATURES

GROSS FINDINGS

GRCC have an average size of 28 mm. LRC are poorly circumscribed with a firm cut surface. The median size in one series was 3.2 cm.

MICROSCOPIC FINDINGS

GRCC tend to have either an infiltrative or circumscribed margin and are Elston-Ellis (Nottingham) grade 2 or 3. There are sheets or nests of cells and acinar formation is uncommon. Mitoses are numerous and necrosis may be identified. Focal apocrine differentiation may be seen. There is usually associated DCIS, often of solid clear-cell type.

LRC shows an infiltrating margin, with the component cells having clear or bubbly cytoplasm. There is a moderate degree of nuclear pleomorphism and tumors are usually of histologic grade 3. Associated DCIS and/or LCIS may be seen.

ANCILLARY STUDIES

IMMUNOHISTOCHEMISTRY/SPECIAL STAINS

In GRCC the presence of cytoplasmic glycogen is assessed using PAS staining, before and after diastase digestion. Estrogen and progesterone receptor immunostaining is variable. Stains for mucin can be focally positive. LRC shows positive cytoplasmic staining with Oil Red O or Sudan Black.

DIFFERENTIAL DIAGNOSIS

A clear cell morphology of a carcinoma in the breast should be assessed in the light of quality of fixation. This often reflects poor fixation and artefact and examination of the fixation of the adjacent tissue should be undertaken. Metastatic clear cell tumors, e.g., from a renal cell carcinoma should be excluded with appropriate immunostaining. The presence of DCIS should be sought and supports a primary breast origin. Myoepithelial tumors will show immunopositivity, for example, smooth muscle actin, S100 or cytokeratin 14. Mucin staining excludes secretory carcinoma.

PROGNOSIS AND TREATMENT

It is difficult to assess the prognosis of GRCC; 20 % of axillary dissections have been documented to contain metastases. However, in another study 11 of 12 patients had lymph node metastases at the time of diagnosis and

50 % of the patients died within 2 years with a further case of local recurrence and brain metastasis in another. Review suggests that it is likely that, when matched for grade, stage and tumor size, the behavior is similar to other invasive carcinomas types.

The prognosis of LRC is unclear.

MISCELLANEOUS INVASIVE CARCINOMA TYPES

A variety of case reports or small series of other invasive carcinoma types have been identified which do not have a very extensive supporting literature. These include mucinous cystadenocarcinoma, sebaceous carcinoma and oncocytic carcinoma.

SUGGESTED READINGS

Invasive ductal carcinoma of no special type (NST)

Ellis IO, Schnitt SJ, Sastre-Garau X et al. Invasive breast carcinoma. In Tavassoli FA, Devilee P eds. World Health Organization Classification of Tumours. Pathology and Genetics of Tumours of the Breast and Female Genital Organs. Lyon: IARC Press, 2003:13–59.

Pinder SE, Elston CW, Ellis IO. Invasive carcinoma-usual histological types. In Elston CW, Ellis IO eds. The Breast Systemic Pathology Volume 13. Edinburgh: Churchill-Livingstone, 1998:283–337.

Tsuda H, Takarabe T, Hasegawa F, Fukutomi T, Hirohashi S. Large, acellular zones indicating myoepithelial tumour differentiation in high-grade ductal carcinomas as markers of predisposition to lung and brain metastases. Am J Surg Pathol 2000;24:197–202.

Jones C, Nonni AV, Fulford L et al. CGH analysis of ductal carcinoma of the breast with basaloid/myoepithelial cell differentiation. Br J of Cancer 2001;85:422–427.

Invasive Lobular Carcinoma

Bane AL, Tjan S, Parkes RK, Andrulis I, O'Malley FP. Invasive lobular carcinoma; to grade or not to grade. Mod Pathol 2005;18:621–628.

Dixon JM, Anderson TJ, Page DL, Lee D, Duffy SW. Infiltrating lobular carcinoma of the breast. Histopathology 1982;6:149–161.

Droufakou S, Deshmane V, Roylance R, Hanby A, Tomlinson I, Hart IR. Multiple pathways of silencing E-cadherin gene expression in lobular carcinoma of the breast. Int J Cancer 2001;92:404–408.

Sastre-Garau X, Jouve M, Asselain B, et al. Infiltrating lobular carcinoma of the breast: clinicopathologic analysis of 975 cases with reference to data on conservative therapy and metastatic patterns. Cancer 1996;77:113–120.

Mucinous Carcinoma and Tubular Carcinoma

Diab SG, Clark GM, Osborne CK et al. Tumor characteristics and clinical outcome of tubular and mucinous breast carcinomas. J Clin Oncol 1999;17:1442–1448.

Medullary Carcinoma

Ridolfi RL, Rosen PP, Port A, Kinne D, Mike V. Medullary carcinoma of the breast A clinicopathologic study with 10-year follow-up. Cancer 1977;40:1365–1385.

Ellis IO, Schnitt SJ, Sastre-Garau X et al. Invasive breast carcinoma. In Tavassoli FA, Devilee P eds. World Health Organization Classification of Tumours. Pathology and Genetics of Tumours of the Breast and Female Genital Organs. Lyon: IARC Press, 2003:13–59.

Micropapillary Carcinoma

Zekioglu O, Erhan Y, Ciris M et al. Invasive micropapillary carcinoma of the breast: high incidence of lymph node metastasis with extranodal extension and its immunohistochemical profile compared with invasive ductal carcinoma. Histopathology 2004;44:18–23.

Thor AD, Eng C, Devries S et al. Invasive micropapillary carcinoma of the breast is associated with chromosome 8 abnormalities detected by comparative genomic hybridisation. Hum Pathol 2002;33:628–631.

Metaplastic Carcinoma

Ellis IO, Schnitt SJ, Sastre-Garau X et al. Invasive breast carcinoma. In Tavassoli FA, Devilee P eds. World Health Organization Classification of Tumours. Pathology and Genetics of Tumours of the Breast and Female Genital Organs. Lyon: IARC Press, 2003:13–59.

Apocrine Carcinoma

Eusebi V, Milis RR, Cattani MG, Bussolati G, Azzopardi JG. Apocrine carcinoma of the breast – A morphologic and immunocytochemical study. Am J Pathol 1986;123:532–541.

Jones C, Damiani S, Wells D, Chaggar C, Lakhani SR, Eusebi V. Molecular cytogenetic comparison of apocrine hyperplasia and apocrine carcinoma of the breast. Am J Pathol 2001;158:207–214.

O'Malley FP, Bane AL. The spectrum of apocrine lesions of the breast. Adv Anat pathol 2004;11:1–9.

Neuroendocrine Carcinoma

Miremadi A, Pinder SE, Lee AHS et al. Neuroendocrine differentiation and prognosis in breast adenocarcinoma. Histopathology 2002;40:215–222.

Invasive Papillary Carcinoma

Ellis IO, Schnitt SJ, Sastre-Garau X et al. Invasive breast carcinoma. In Tavassoli FA, Devilee P eds. World Health Organization Classification of Tumours. Pathology and Genetics of Tumours of the Breast and Female Genital Organs. Lyon: IARC Press, 2003:••.

19 Histologic Grade

Ian O Ellis · Christopher W Elston

BASIC PRINCIPLES OF GRADING

GRADING REQUIRES HIGH QUALITY TISSUE PRESERVATION AND SECTION PREPARATION

A number of studies have shown that delayed fixation can affect assessment of mitotic frequency. Start and colleagues have shown that as little as a six-hour delay may reduce the number of visible mitoses in a given sample by up to 76 %. Therefore the first prerequisite for accurate histologic grading is good specimen preparation. Ideally the tumor should be sliced in the fresh state to allow good penetration of fixative. It is well established that formalin penetrates tissues poorly. Good liaison with surgical colleagues is required and special arrangements may have to be made. Immersing the whole breast unsliced into a specimen pot containing fixative will lead to poor preservation of morphologic details and cannot be endorsed.

Careful high quality tissue processing is important. Sections should be cut at 3–5 µm; if sections are cut too thick, nuclear detail is obscured. Conventional staining with haematoxylin and eosin (H&E) is sufficient and special stains are not required.

BLOCK SAMPLING IS IMPORTANT

Blocks should be selected to give good representation of the whole tumor and in particular the periphery. The number of blocks taken will depend on the size of the tumor. Ideally, for a tumor of sufficient size, four radiating blocks can be taken to allow assessment in all three dimensions.

WHICH TUMORS SHOULD BE GRADED?

Grading is carried out in invasive carcinomas; this grading system is not suitable for tumors that are completely or predominantly *in situ*. It is our policy to grade all histologic types of invasive carcinoma; our reasoning is discussed later, but assessment is not restricted to tumors of ductal/no special type as recommended by some authorities. The histologic grade is obtained by analysis of the following three features.

FOLLOW THE PROTOCOL

Histologic grading requires commitment and strict adherence to the accepted protocol. The method involves the assessment of three components of tumor morphology, each of which is given a score of 1–3: tubule/acinar/glandular formation, nuclear atypia/pleomorphism and frequency of mitoses. Addition of the scores gives the overall histologic grade.

UNDERSTAND TUMOR HETEROGENEITY

Some degree of variation in appearance from one part of a tumor to another undoubtedly occurs; this is particularly true of tumors of mixed type. Assessment of tubular differentiation is made on the overall appearances of the tumor and so account is taken of any variation. Nuclear appearances including mitotic frequency are evaluated at the periphery and/or the least differentiated area of the tumor, to obviate differences between the growing edge and the less active center.

EXPECTED DISTRIBUTION OF GRADE SCORES

Do not expect equal numbers of cancers to fall in each grade category. Published ratios for grades 1, 2 and 3 are approximately 2:3:5 in symptomatic breast cancer, so about half of all symptomatic cancers are grade 3. If an audit of grade distribution shows substantially fewer grade 3 cases, or a majority of grade 2 cases, the grading protocols should be carefully reviewed although screen detected cancer series are likely to include a smaller proportion of high grade cases.

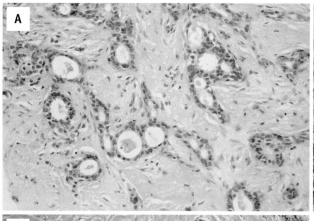
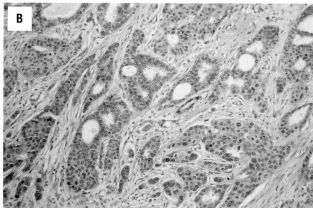
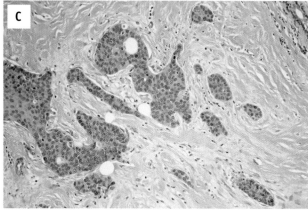

FIGURE 19-1

Glandular (acinar)/tubular diferentiation. Three cases of invasive breast carcinoma illustrating the range of tubular/glandular differentiation seen. (A) A high proportion (>75% of tumour cell groups forming tubules/glands giving a score of one. (B) The tumour has some, but less than 75%, gland formation. In (C) the tumour shows minimal gland formation (<10%).

HISTOLOGIC ASSESSMENT METHODOLOGY

GLANDULAR (ACINAR) / TUBULAR DIFFERENTIATION (Figures 19-1 and 19-2)

Score:
1. >75% of tumor area forming glandular / tubular structures
2. 10–75% of tumor
3. <10% of tumor

All parts of the tumor are scanned and the proportion occupied by tumor islands showing clear acinar or gland formation or defined tubular structures with a central luminal space is assessed semi-quantitatively. This assessment is generally carried out during the initial low power scan of the tumor sections.

In the assessment of glandular differentiation, only structures in which there are clearly defined central lumens, surrounded by polarized tumor cells, should be counted. Care must be taken not to mistake clefts induced by shrinkage artefact for glands / tubules.

In Greenhough's original paper (Table 19-1), he referred to adenomatous (glandular) arrangements and it was Patey and Scarff who introduced the term tubule formation for the recapitulation of the acinar structure of the normal lobule. This has subsequently been mis-

interpreted by some as identification solely of distinct tubular structures, reminiscent of those found in tubular carcinoma of the breast, which is an incorrect interpretation of the methodology. For this reason we prefer to use the term glandular / tubular differentiation rather than just tubular.

NUCLEAR PLEOMORPHISM (Figure 19-3)

Score:
1. Nuclei small with little increase in size in comparison with normal breast epithelial cells, regular outlines, uniform nuclear chromatin, little variation in size.
2. Cells larger than normal with open vesicular nuclei, visible nucleoli and moderate variability in both size and shape.
3. Vesicular nuclei, often with prominent nucleoli, exhibiting marked variation in size and shape, occasionally with very large and bizarre forms.

Assessment of nuclear pleomorphism is the most subjective element of histologic grade. Individual pathologists differ markedly in their approach to nuclear grading, and breast specialists appear to allocate higher grades than non-specialists.

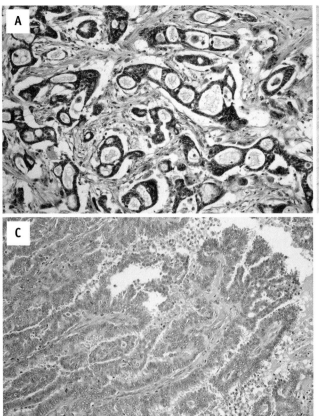

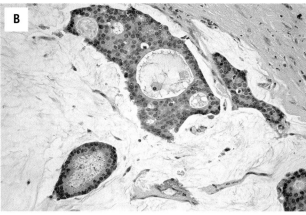

FIGURE 19-2

Glandular (acinar)/tubular differentiation. Although the term tubules is used for grading purposes, this component is regarded as a reflection of glandular differentiation and tumors exhibiting distinct acinar formation other than true 'tubules' should be classified in a similar fashion. The examples show glandular differentiation in an invasive cribriform carcinoma (score 1) (A), mucinous carcinoma (score 1) (B) and a papillary carcinoma (score 2) (C).

FEW CANCERS POSSESS THE VERY BLAND NUCLEI WARRANTING AN ATYPIA/PLEOMORPHISM SCORE 1

In order to introduce a degree of objectivity we use the size and shape of normal epithelial cells present in breast tissue within or adjacent to the tumor as the reference point. If normal epithelial cells cannot be identified, then stromal lymphoid cells may be used as a surrogate, with appropriate adjustment for their relatively smaller size. Tumors in which nuclei are small and regular, showing little variation in size and shape compared with normal nuclei are given 1 point. It should be noted that most tumors exhibit some degree of nuclear enlargement and pleomorphism and it is rare to attribute a score of 1 to the common forms of invasive cancer. Two points are given when the nuclei are larger than normal, have a more open vesicular structure and there is a moderate variation in size and shape. A marked variation in size and shape particularly when very large and bizarre nuclei are present, scores 3 points. In the latter two categories, nucleoli are often present, and multiple nucleoli in a nucleus favor a score of 3.

THE FINDING OF AN OCCASIONAL ENLARGED OR BIZARRE NUCLEUS SHOULD NOT BE USED TO GIVE A SCORE OF 3 RATHER THAN 2

MITOTIC COUNTS (Figure 19-4)

Accurate mitosis counting requires high quality fixation, obtained when fresh specimens are sectioned promptly as well as tumor blocks of optimal thickness (3–4 mm) fixed immediately in neutral buffered formalin. This can be achieved without compromising evaluation of resection margins.

Mitosis score depends on the number of mitoses per 10 high power fields. The size of high power fields is very variable, so it is necessary to standardize the mitotic count. The size of a 'high power field' (HPF) may vary up to six fold from one microscope to another and it has been calculated that the count for the same tumor as assessed by different instruments may range from 3–20 mitoses per 10 HPF. We recommend that the field diameter of the microscope is measured using the

---

TABLE 19-1

Summary of the history of histologic grade in invasive breast carcinoma

---

1880	Recognition that the morphologic appearances of malignant tumors relate to their degree of 'malignancy' by von Hansemann.
1925	First formal analysis in carcinoma of the breast by Greenhough who identified three grades based on eight histologic factors and showed a clear association between grade and 'cure'.
1928	Patey and Scarff re-assessed Greenhough's method and found that tubule formation, variation in size of nuclei and hyperchromatic figures were the most important factors. Mitotic figures were noted but not considered to make a significant contribution to the evaluation of prognosis.
1938	Scarff and Handley using the Patey and Scarff method confirmed a clear correlation between histologic grade and survival.
1950	Bloom favored the Greenhough method and used three factors: the degree of tubule formation; regularity in the size, shape and staining of nuclei; and hyperchromatism with mitotic activity assessed subjectively as absent or present in slight, moderate or marked degree.
1955	Black *et al* assessed tubular structures and nuclear appearances separately and concluded that tubular differentiation did not contribute to the prediction of prognosis, but that the nuclear morphology did. Four 'nuclear grades' were devised, but the numerical order of the grades was reversed so that nuclear grades 0 and I apply to the poorly differentiated tumors and grade IV to the well-differentiated tumors.
1957	Bloom and Richardson refined Bloom's grading method in the form of a numerical scoring system. The previous designation of slight, moderate and marked was replaced by a score of 1–3. This gave a total score of 3–9, and the grades were arbitrarily assigned as follows: grade I – 3, 4 or 5 points, grade II – 6 or 7 points, grade III – 8 or 9 points.
1968	The Patey and Scarff method, with the modifications made by Bloom and Richardson has become known colloquially as the Scarff-Bloom-Richardson (SBR) technique. It was shown conclusively in a substantial number of studies to be both practical and useful in determining prognosis.
1975	Fisher suggested a system combining elements of both SBR histologic grade and nuclear grade. A satisfactory correlation with survival was established and a further modification was introduced later by incorporation of the degree and type of tubule formation. However, approximately two-thirds of cases are placed in their poorly differentiated grade, thus stratification by this method is poor.
1982	Elston modified the SBR method to improve objectivity of assessment of mitotic counts and eliminated the inclusion of 'hyperchromatic' nuclei.
1987	Contesso and colleagues made a further attempt to improve the objectivity of the SBR method by modifying the way in which mitotic figures are assessed. Like Elston et al, they were critical both of the use of hyperchromatic nuclei and the vague numerical counts. They proposed an evaluation of mitoses based on the maximum number of mitoses in a single field at 400× magnification after examination of 20 successive fields.
1989	Le Doussal and colleagues used multivariate analysis to test the prognostic value of SBR grading and confirmed its importance in predicting metastasis-free survival. They found that nuclear pleomorphism and mitotic count were the most predictive elements. Using only these two factors they rearranged the score to produce five modified SBR categories (MSBR) and claimed that this new grading method produced better separation of prognostic groups. A closely similar method has been devised by Schumacher and colleagues (1993) based on studies in node negative breast cancer.
1991	The Nottingham group improved the objectivity of histologic grading by producing a stricter protocol for the assessment of each component factor. The details of this method are described in the text of this chapter. This system has been adopted by the UK National Health Service, European Union, United States Directors of Anatomic and Surgical Pathology, AJCC and WHO.

---

stage graticule or Vernier scale, and the scoring categories are read from the corresponding line of the table (Table 19-2). Field diameter is a function of objective and eyepiece, so if either of these is changed, this exercise should be repeated.

A minimum of 10 fields should be counted at the periphery of the tumor, where it has been demonstrated that proliferative activity is greatest. If there is variation in the number of mitoses in different areas of the tumor the least differentiated area (i.e, with the highest mitotic count) should be assessed. If the mitotic frequency score falls very close to a score cut point then one or more further groups of 10 HPF should be assessed to estab-

lish the correct (highest) score. It is recommended that identification of the most mitotically active or least differentiated part of the tumor forms part of the low magnification preliminary assessment of the histologic section. This area should be used for mitotic count scoring. If there is no evidence of heterogeneity, then mitotic scoring should be carried out at a part of the tumor periphery chosen at random. Fields chosen for scoring are selected during a random meander along the peripheral margin of the selected tumor area. Only fields with a representative tumor burden should be used. The low power scan of the tumor can be used to provide an assessment of the typical tumor to stromal ratio.

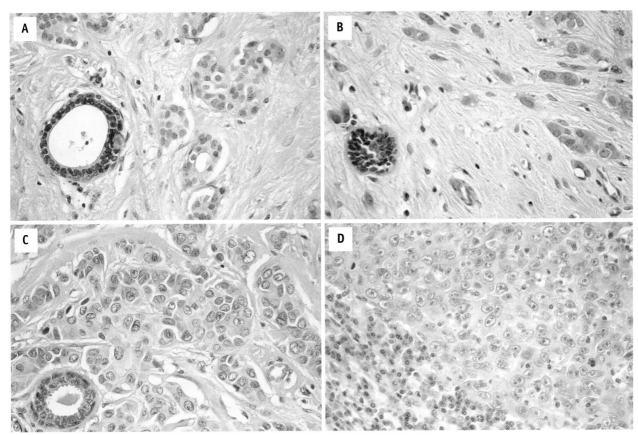

FIGURE 19-3

Nuclear pleomorphism. Examples of four tumors illustrating nuclear pleomorphism scores of (A) 1, (B) 2 and (C,D) 3.

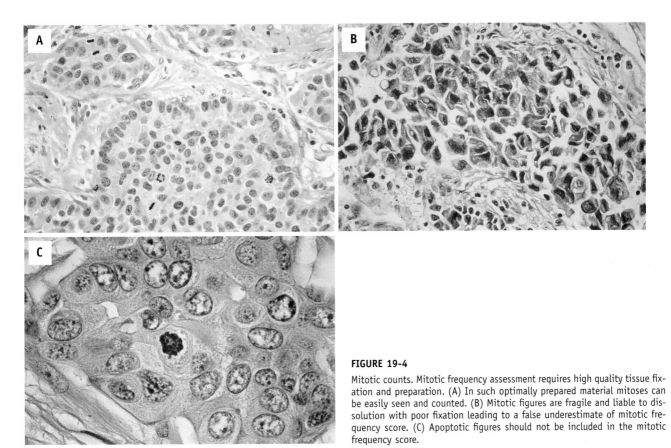

FIGURE 19-4

Mitotic counts. Mitotic frequency assessment requires high quality tissue fixation and preparation. (A) In such optimally prepared material mitoses can be easily seen and counted. (B) Mitotic figures are fragile and liable to dissolution with poor fixation leading to a false underestimate of mitotic frequency score. (C) Apoptotic figures should not be included in the mitotic frequency score.

TABLE 19-2
Scoring categories of mitotic counts.

Field diameter in mm	Number of mitoses corresponding to		
	Score 1	Score 2	Score 3
0.40	up to 4	5 to 8	9 or more
0.41	up to 4	5 to 9	10 or more
0.42	up to 4	5 to 9	10 or more
0.43	up to 4	5 to 10	11 or more
0.44	up to 5	6 to 10	11 or more
0.45	up to 5	6 to 11	12 or more
0.46	up to 5	6 to 11	12 or more
0.47	up to 5	6 to 12	13 or more
0.48	up to 6	7 to 12	13 or more
0.49	up to 6	7 to 13	14 or more
0.50	up to 6	7 to 13	14 or more
0.51	up to 6	7 to 14	15 or more
0.52	up to 7	8 to 14	15 or more
0.53	up to 7	8 to 15	16 or more
0.54	up to 7	8 to 16	17 or more
0.55	up to 8	9 to 16	17 or more
0.56	up to 8	9 to 17	18 or more
0.57	up to 8	9 to 17	18 or more
0.58	up to 9	10 to 18	19 or more
0.59	up to 9	10 to 19	20 or more
0.60	up to 9	10 to 19	20 or more
0.61	up to 9	10 to 20	21 or more
0.62	up to 10	11 to 21	22 or more
0.63	up to 10	11 to 21	22 or more
0.64	up to 11	12 to 22	23 or more
0.65	up to 11	12 to 23	24 or more
0.66	up to 11	12 to 24	25 or more
0.67	up to 12	13 to 25	26 or more
0.68	up to 12	13 to 25	26 or more
0.69	up to 12	13 to 26	27 or more
0.70	up to 13	14 to 27	28 or more

ONLY ACCEPT FIGURES WHICH CLEARLY FULFIL THE MORPHOLOGIC CRITERIA FOR THE VARIOUS STAGES OF MITOSIS

Only definite mitotic figures (in any phase of the growth cycle) should be counted (see Figure 19-4A). Hyperchromatic nuclei and or apoptotic nuclei should not be scored (see Figure 19-4C). Poor quality fixation can result in underscoring of mitotic frequency and optimal fixation is essential (see Figure 19-4B). It is in this category that the present method differs most from those described previously, which concentrated on both hyperchromatic nuclei and mitotic figures. It is now known that hyperchromicity is more likely to indicate individual cell necrosis (apoptosis) than proliferation and such nuclei should be excluded from the counts.

GENERAL PRACTICAL CONSIDERATIONS

- One potential problem with the point scoring system for the assessment of tubules and nuclear pleomorphism lies in the tendency of inexperienced observers, when faced with a choice of 1–3, to 'play safe' and opt for the middle, i.e. a score of 2. This can be obviated by making an initial decision to reduce the available options to two. Thus in a tumor with a large tubular component the score can only be 1 or 2; the score of 3 is eliminated. Similarly, when assessing nuclear pleomorphism the presence of large, irregular nuclei more than twice the size of a normal epithelial cell rules out a score of one; the number of these nuclei then influences the choice between 2 and 3.
- Some degree of variation in appearance from one part of a tumor to another undoubtedly occurs; this is particularly true of tumors of mixed type and is one of the main reasons for examining multiple blocks. Assessment of tubular differentiation is made on the overall appearances of the tumor, and so account is taken of any variation. Nuclear appearances are evaluated at the periphery of the tumor to obviate differences between the growing edge and the less active center.
- To date we have not quantified prospectively the minimum area of a tumor which should show marked nuclear pleomorphism before a score of 3 is allocated; this is a matter of personal judgement for each case, but as a general rule this should be at least one quarter. The finding of an occasional enlarged or bizarre nucleus should certainly not be used to give a score of 3 rather than 2.
- Mitoses are counted at the periphery of the tumor to obviate differences between the growing edge and the less active center.
- In biphasic tumors (e.g, mixed ductal/NST and mucinous carcinoma) the least differentiated area should be counted. In practice we have found that tumor heterogeneity rarely poses a problem in assigning an accurate grade.
- It is recommended that grading is not restricted to invasive carcinoma of ductal/NST, but is undertaken on all histologic sub-types. There are two major reasons for this recommendation:
  1. There are occasionally problems in deciding whether to classify a tumor as NST or some other sub-type.
  2. There may be significant variation in prognosis within certain sub-types, e.g, lobular carcinoma, and grading provides additional information.

OVERALL GRADE

The use of terms such as well differentiated or poorly differentiated in the absence of a numerical grade is considered inappropriate. The scores for tubule formation,

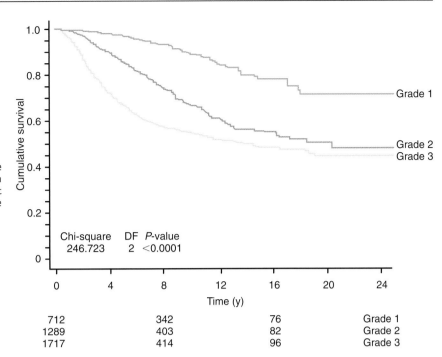

FIGURE 19-5

Clinical significance of histologic grade. Invasive carcinoma, overall survival by histologic grade in the updated Nottingham Tenovus Primary Breast Cancer Study in over 2500 patients with invasive breast carcinoma treated in one unit.

nuclear pleomorphism and mitoses are added together and assigned to grades, as below:

Grade 1 = scores of 3–5
Grade 2 = scores of 6 or 7
Grade 3 = scores of 8 or 9

VALIDATION

Despite the objective improvements which we have made to the grading method, any assessment of morphologic characteristics must retain a subjective element. For this reason it is advisable, where possible, to validate results. To achieve internal consistency in our own department, tumors are graded independently by two experienced histopathologists. In cases where an initial difference in assessment of grade occurs (and this is rarely by more than 1 point) disagreements are resolved by consensus after joint review on a conference microscope. With increasing experience this may become less necessary and for those pathologists working in a single-handed practice it may be sufficient to re-check a sample of cases without knowledge of the previous result.

CLINICAL SIGNIFICANCE AND PROGNOSTIC IMPLICATIONS

The method described above has been evaluated prospectively in the Nottingham Tenovus Primary Breast Carcinoma Series (NTPBCS). The initial results, based on life table analysis of over 1800 patients, confirmed conclusively the highly significant relationship between histologic grade and prognosis. Nineteen per cent of tumors were well differentiated, grade 1 (342 cases), 34% moderately differentiated, grade 2 (632 cases) and 46% poorly differentiated, grade 3 (857). The data has now been re-examined with longer follow-up, ranging from a minimum of eight years to over 20 years, and the correlation is confirmed. Overall survival is significantly better in patients with grade 1 tumors than in those with grade 2 or grade 3 tumors (Figure 19-5).

There can now be no doubt that histologic grading of primary breast carcinomas provides important independent prognostic information. We have made a comprehensive study of the inter-relationships of a large number of potential prognostic factors in the NTPBCS. In multivariate analysis, individual factors are assessed independently whilst taking into account the weight of all the other factors. The only factors found to have a significant correlation with prognosis were pathologic tumor size, lymph node stage (assessed histologically) and histologic grading. Based on the coefficients of significance produced in the multivariate analysis a simple composite prognostic index has been devised as follows: Nottingham Prognostic Index (NPI) = 0.2 × tumor size (cm) + lymph node stage (1–3) + histologic grade (1–3). See Chapter 20 for more details.

HISTOLOGIC GRADE AND TUMOR TYPE

The methods of histologic grading referred to in this chapter were devised before it was fully appreciated that

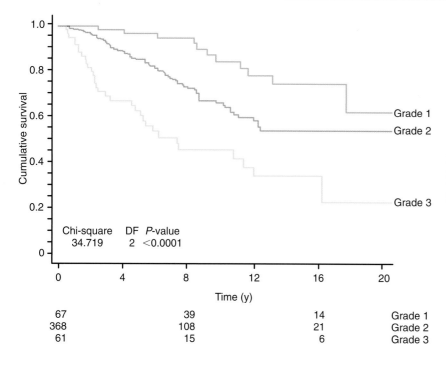

FIGURE 19-6

Histologic grade and tumor type. Nottingham Tenovus Primary Breast Cancer Study – infiltrating lobular carcinoma by grade.

67	39	14	Grade 1
368	108	21	Grade 2
61	15	6	Grade 3

carcinoma of the breast encompasses a variety of morphologic types. It should be noted, however, that when grade is assessed within tumors of particular histologic types it is usually found to be appropriate. For example, by definition the special tumor types such as pure tubular and invasive cribriform carcinoma have a low grade morphology; their prognosis is excellent and in keeping with that of other grade 1 carcinomas. The majority of infiltrating lobular carcinomas, especially those of classical pattern, are designated as grade 2, and it is interesting that the overall survival curve for lobular carcinomas overlies that of grade 2 carcinomas of all other types. However, a minority of lobular carcinomas fall into the grade 1 or grade 3 category and their survival curves show an appropriate and significant separation (Figure 19-6).

Medullary carcinoma might appear to be one subtype in which grading is not appropriate. By definition these tumors are of histologic grade 3, but have been considered by some groups to have a much more favorable prognosis than this degree of differentiation would imply. However, in the NTPBCS, despite the application of very strict diagnostic criteria we have been unable to demonstrate a significant survival advantage for medullary carcinoma when compared with other grade 3 tumors.

It is also important to emphasize that the assessment of histologic type is essentially subjective, as shown by the wide range in the reported frequency of the special types. This is due in part to a lack of agreement on diagnostic criteria but also to the recognition by some, but not all, authorities of mixed or variant types.

We believe these data demonstrate that histologic grading of all invasive breast carcinomas provides valuable prognostic information, irrespective of tumor type. If grading is restricted to the ductal/NST group alone,

then in a symptomatic series at best only 75% and at worst only 53% of cases will be assessed and this prognostic information lost in a substantial proportion of patients. It is therefore recommended that both grading and typing be carried out in all cases of invasive breast carcinoma.

CONSISTENCY AND REPRODUCIBILITY

Histologic grade has only recently become accepted as an important prognostic factor in invasive breast cancer. One of the reasons cited in the past for the reluctance of clinicians to use grading in patient management has been the perceived lack of reproducibility of the method. This is highlighted by the relatively wide variation in the proportion of each grade in published series.

The historical literature on the consistency and reproducibility of histologic grading has been contradictory, but it is interesting that those publications which have claimed that levels of agreement are poor have been the most influential and widely quoted, especially in studies promoting the new molecular markers of prognosis. Three studies have now tested the Elston/Ellis Nottingham method and the results are extremely encouraging. Interestingly Dalton and colleagues used the intermediate system prior to the development of more strictly defined criteria. Nevertheless, greater than 87% agreement on final grade was obtained between 25 pathologists, none of whom was deemed to be an expert in breast pathology. The median weighted kappa value of 0.7 indicated very good inter-observer agreement. The pathologists were expected to have learnt the method but no formal training was carried out. In the study described by Frierson *et al*, six pathologists from four centers tested the updated Nottingham method. Each was provided with a copy of the paper and a clear written protocol. Pairwise kappa values for agreement ranged from moderate to substantial (0.43–0.74) and consensus agreement (four out of six) was 88.5%. A rather different approach was taken by Robbins *et al* who compared the consensus results of three pathologists from Perth, West Australia and two from the City Hospital, Nottingham using the Nottingham method. Complete agreement was reached in 83% of cases in which fixation was considered to be satisfactory, giving a kappa statistic of 0.73. These results represent a considerable improvement over a preliminary study carried out previously in Perth and this was considered to be due to the use of the strict Nottingham protocol. The method has also been shown to maintain validity, despite limitations of technical quality, when retrospective review and grading were undertaken on cases derived from eight different sources, including private laboratories.

The studies described in the paragraph above have all shown that grading can be carried out with satisfactory reproducibility, provided that a strict protocol is followed. As Scarff and Torloni pointed out 30 years ago, experience and dedication are essential requirements for accurate histologic grading. It is, perhaps, self-evident but still worth stressing that the very basis of all histopathology is a professional approach with proper attention to detail.

SUGGESTED READINGS

Connor AJM, Pinder SE, Elston CW et al. Intratumoral heterogeneity of proliferation in invasive breast carcinoma evaluated with MIB1 antibody. The Breast 1997;6:171–176.

Dunne B, Going JJ. Scoring nuclear pleomorphism in breast cancer. Histopathol 2001;39:259–265.

Elston CW, Ellis IO. Pathological prognostic factors in breast cancer. I. The value of histological grade in breast cancer: experience from a large study with longterm follow-up. Histopathol 1991;19:403–410.

Lynch J, Pattekar R, Barnes DM et al. Mitotic counts provide additional prognostic information in grade II mammary carcinoma. J Pathol 2002 Mar;196(3):275–279.

Pereira H, Pinder SE, Sibbering DM et al. Pathological prognostic factors in breast cancer. IV. Should you be a typer or a grader? A comparative study of two histological prognostic features in operable breast carcinoma. Histopathol 1995;27:219–226.

Page DL, Ellis IO, Elston CW. Histologic grading of breast cancer. Let's do it. Am J Clin Pathol 1995;103:123–124.

Verhoeven D, Bourgeois N, Derde MP et al. Comparison of cell growth in different parts of breast cancers. Histopathol 1990;17:505–509.

20

Invasive Carcinoma: Other Histologic Prognostic Factors – Size, Vascular Invasion and Prognostic Index

Michael A Gonzalez · Sarah E Pinder

Most of the prognostic information required for therapeutic decision-making is based on meticulous pathologic examination of the breast cancer specimen. In addition to lymph node stage and histologic grade, tumor size and the presence of vascular invasion are strong, independent factors that determine clinical outcome in patients with invasive breast cancer. Other prognostic and putative prognostic factors are covered elsewhere and those not addressed previously will be covered in this short chapter.

TUMOR SIZE

Increasing tumor size is independently associated with a worsening survival (Figure 20-1). For prognostic purposes, the gross tumor size should be assessed pathologically. Clinical examination is inaccurate with clinicopathologic agreement in only 54 % of cases. Should an estimate of tumor size be required for therapeutic stratification, imaging the breast lesion, by ultrasonography, magnetic resonance imaging or mammography, in order of accuracy respectively, provides a more accurate approximation than can be obtained clinically.

Pathologic tumor size can initially be assessed macroscopically in the fresh state (in three planes) and subsequently confirmed following fixation, when the margins may be more clearly defined. Microscopic assessment using a Vernier scale is required for small tumors, particularly those measuring less than 10 mm in diameter or in cases where a large *in situ* component is present. Since carcinomas are invariably asymmetrical, the greatest dimension is taken as the final tumor size. When two or more distinct invasive tumors are identified, each is measured individually and they are not combined into a single larger measurement. Thus, if there are satellite foci in association with a main carcinoma mass, only the largest, dominant lesion is given as invasive tumor size, for staging purposes or for calculation of the Nottingham Prognostic Index.

On rare occasions, when foci of tumor are seen in close proximity, it can be difficult to distinguish whether histologically one is examining one ill-defined mass of invasive carcinoma, or a smaller lesion with a surrounding satellite focus or foci. As a rule of thumb, if the deposits are separated by normal breast parenchymal structures, the possibility that these represent satellite foci should be considered. It is, however, impossible to provide definitive advice and it should be remembered that a single tumor deposit may appear as multiple foci due to plane of slicing or of histologic sectioning. In these instances a somewhat pragmatic approach to reporting the cancer size is required and common sense applied.

It can also be difficult to assess size accurately if there is abundant *in situ* carcinoma admixed with multiple invasive foci. If one invasive focus, which is clearly the dominant lesion, is seen within an area of ductal carcinoma *in situ* (DCIS), then the maximum dimension of this invasive focus is given as the invasive cancer size, although the whole tumor (DCIS plus invasive) size should also be recorded. If it is not possible to distinguish any one focus as dominant then the whole size of the *in situ* and invasive carcinoma is reported. In such cases our policy has been to report that there are multiple foci of invasion measuring x cm in maximum dimension, admixed with DCIS extending over an area of y cm (whole tumor dimension).

The term minimally invasive carcinoma (MIC) has been used to describe very small tumors with a very good prognosis. It represents a different lesion from microinvasive carcinoma (i.e., carcinoma <1 mm in size seen in association with DCIS) (which is addressed in Chapter 17). Small invasive carcinomas have been detected with increasing frequency following the introduction of population-based mammographic screening for breast cancer but there is no consensus for the definition of MIC and the use of the term is, therefore, not recommended. The American College of Surgeons uses a figure of 10 mm whereas the American Cancer Society limits the maximum diameter to 9 mm.

In general, tumors <15 mm confer a good prognosis. Consistent with a favorable clinical outcome, the frequency of axillary lymph node metastases in small carcinomas is approximately 15–20 % in contrast to >40 % in tumors measuring >15 mm in diameter. In women with small (<15 mm) invasive breast cancer, detected during the prevalent round of breast cancer screening, the frequency of axillary node metastases ranges from 0–15 %.

It is important that histopathologists measure tumor size as accurately as possible for its prognostic value but

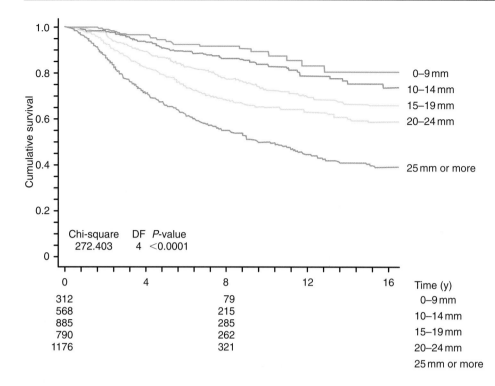

Chi-square   DF   P-value
272.403   4   <0.0001

	0–9 mm
	10–14 mm
	15–19 mm
	20–24 mm
	25 mm or more

FIGURE 20-1

Relationship between pathologic tumor size and overall survival in 3731 patients with primary operable breast cancer in the Nottingham Tenovus Primary Operable Breast Cancer Series.

	Time 0	Time 8	Time (y)
312	79		0–9 mm
568	215		10–14 mm
885	285		15–19 mm
790	262		20–24 mm
1176	321		25 mm or more

lesion size is also important in the assessment of the ability of radiologists in interpreting breast screening mammograms. The aim of breast screening programs to detect impalpable breast cancers when as small as possible can be evaluated by the proportion of small cancers detected, which itself relies on the accuracy of the pathologist's measurement.

VASCULAR INVASION

The presence of tumor emboli in vascular spaces is an important independent prognostic factor that may be present in up to 50 % of invasive breast carcinomas. The proportion of cases reported as showing vascular invasion (VI) in the medical literature shows a great deal of variation, undoubtedly in part due to assessment in different stages of disease but also due to differences in stringency of diagnosis. VI is predominantly seen in thin-walled channels (capillaries or lymphatics) and rarely in muscular blood vessels. It is not possible, on routine hematoxylin and eosin-stained sections to distinguish lymphatics from small blood vessels and the terms vascular invasion or lympho-vascular invasion are used.

Strict criteria for determination of the presence of VI must be used. Assessment should, in general, be concentrated on breast parenchyma adjacent to the primary carcinoma and not within it. Tumor emboli within clear spaces must have an endothelial cell lining (Figure 20-2). Fixation shrinkage artefact may mimic VI, especially

when spaces arise around nests of malignant cells. DCIS, especially if extending outside the invasive tumor, should not be mistaken for VI, the former will bear a surrounding layer of myoepithelial cells (Figure 20-3) and immunohistochemistry for myoepithelium can be undertaken if required to confirm the presence of these. Invasive tumor islands, particularly in some special types of carcinomas such as invasive micropapillary carcinoma, may be seen within clear spaces (in addition to a propensity for vascular invasion in this sub-type) and care must be taken not to overdiagnose VI (Figure 20-3).

The topographical appearances may be helpful and the presence of immediately adjacent small vessels may indicate that the focus of concern is, indeed, likely to be a vascular space. In addition, it can be valuable to consider the shape of the tumor deposit; if the focus has exactly the same outline as the space within which it is identified, then the possibility that this represents retraction artefact should be considered. True emboli frequently do not have the same outline as the surrounding vascular channel. In rare circumstances, when considered important (for example, if at the margin of excision) equivocal cases may be resolved by immunostaining for endothelial markers, such as CD31. In routine practice this is rarely performed.

VI is significantly associated with locoregional lymph node involvement but the absence or presence of VI is also associated with patient survival independent of nodal stage (Figure 20-4). Although not as prognostically informative as lymph node stage, VI may serve as a valuable surrogate in cases where nodes have not been removed for examination. Furthermore, VI is specifically of prognostic value in node-negative disease and predicts for local recurrence following breast

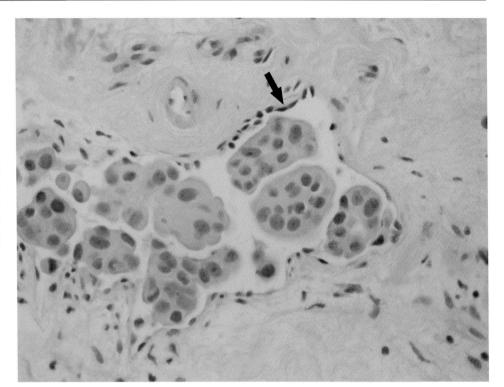

FIGURE 20-2

Definite vascular invasion is seen in this H&E stained section. An unequivocal endothelial lining to the space is identified (arrow). Additional features are the shape of the cell tumor emboli which is different to the surrounding space, thus excluding artefactual shrinkage as a cause.

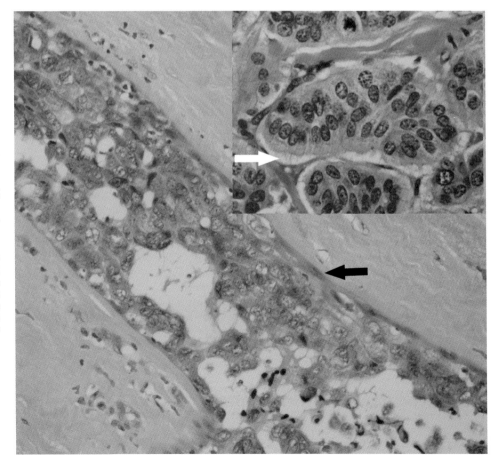

FIGURE 20-3

Mimics of vascular invasion include DCIS (main picture) and artefactual shrinkage around invasive carcinoma islands (inset). Particularly if the sample is poorly fixed, an apparent space may be noted around tumor cells. No endothelial lining will be seen but rather a myoepithelial layer surrounds the DCIS (black arrow). Similarly, with retraction around invasive carcinoma (white arrow), no endothelium is present. Care should be taken, particularly with invasive micropapillary carcinoma as seen in this image, as vascular invasion is also frequently present elsewhere and the section must be thoroughly examined.

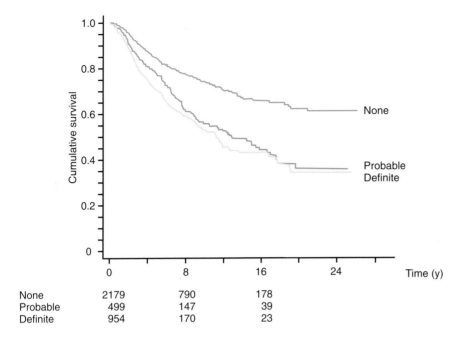

FIGURE 20-4

Relationship between vascular invasion and overall survival in 3632 patients with primary operable carcinoma of the breast in the Nottingham Tenovus Primary Operable Breast Cancer Series.

None	2179	790	178
Probable	499	147	39
Definite	954	170	23

conservation surgery, as well as flap recurrence after mastectomy.

OTHER HISTOLOGIC PROGNOSTIC FACTORS

The prognostic significance of several other pathologic features of breast carcinomas remains inconclusive. Tumor necrosis may confer an adverse clinical outcome and is relatively common, especially in high grade ductal NST carcinomas. Tumor necrosis may be visible, macroscopically, in the center of the specimen as a sharply demarcated area of dullness. Most probably, it reflects a high tumor growth rate that exceeds its vascular supply. An important obstacle in establishing the prognostic value of tumor necrosis has been the lack of reproducible criteria for the definition of necrosis and its relative extent and it is not possible to be certain, in truth, whether this feature is of value prognostically.

Stromal features such as fibrosis and elastosis are also frequent findings in breast carcinoma and some reports raise the possibility that both may be associated with a favorable prognosis. Perineural invasion may be associated with a poor clinical outcome. Further studies are required to clarify the importance of all these features.

THE NOTTINGHAM PROGNOSTIC INDEX

In clinical practice, the only prognostic factor used consistently to assist in therapeutic decision-making following primary breast cancer surgery is lymph node

(LN) stage. The value of prognostic factors in breast cancer lies in their utilization to identify a group of patients who have a very poor prognosis and who will benefit from an aggressive therapeutic approach and a further group of patients who would not significantly benefit (and indeed may suffer morbidity) from adjuvant treatments. LN stage on its own is, however, unable to discriminate a 'cured' group of patients from those at high risk of developing distant metastases and early death from breast cancer. Lymph node negativity alone does not predict for a group of patients with very good outcome and lymph node positivity *per se* does not indicate necessarily that the patient will die of disease unless treated aggressively.

In an attempt to refine prognostication further, the factors which show the strongest, independent associations with overall survival when analyzed alone (in univariate analysis) or when compared to each other (in multivariate analysis) have been combined to formulate several prognostic indices. This approach was used to derive the Nottingham Prognostic Index (NPI) which is based on three factors using the following formula:

NPI score = lymph node stage (1, 2 or 3) + histologic grade (1, 2 or 3) + [tumor size (cm) × 0.2]

LN stage and histologic grade are the strongest prognostic factors in breast cancer and carry equal weighting in the NPI, compared to tumor size which is not as powerful a parameter in the estimation of prognosis (and is therefore adjusted by a factor of 0.2). Vascular invasion and inconclusive histologic prognostic factors such as tumor necrosis and stromal fibrosis or elastosis are not included in the NPI (Figure 20-5). It would be possible to include additional morphologic markers and molecular indicators in the index but it has been maintained as described for simplicity of calculation and ease of use. The higher the value of the NPI score the

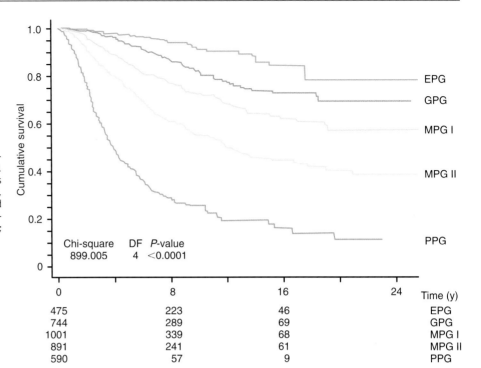

FIGURE 20-5

Relationship between Nottingham Prognostic Index Group and overall survival in 3731 patients in the Nottingham Tenovus Primary Operable Breast Cancer Series. EPG, excellent prognostic group; GPG, good prognostic group; MPGI and MPGII, moderate prognostic groups 1 and 2, respectively; PPG, poor prognostic group.

TABLE 20-1

5-, 10- and 15-year survival by Nottingham Prognostic Index Group Overall Survival (%)

Prognostic group	5 Year	10 Year	15 Year
Excellent (<2.41)	97	91	84
Good (<3.41)	93	82	74
Moderate I (3.41-4.4)	85	73	63
Moderate II (4.41-5.4)	75	55	46
Poor (>5.4)	42	26	18

worse the prognosis. Cut-off points are used to divide patients into five prognostic groups: those in an excellent prognostic group (EPG; NPI score <2.41, 15 year survival 84 %), good prognostic group (GPG; NPI score <3.41, 15-year survival 74 %), moderate prognostic group I (MPGI; NPI score between 3.41 and 4.4, 15-year survival 63 %), moderate prognostic group II (MPGII; NPI score between 4.41 and 5.4, 15-year survival 46 %) and poor prognostic group (PPG; NPI score >5.4, 15-year survival 18 %) (see Table 20-1).

The NPI is unique in having been validated both retrospectively and prospectively in several large series.

New prognostic tools, such as the web-based programme *Adjuvant!* (www.adjuvantonline.com), are continuously emerging. These indices include the traditional pathologic factors and hormonal status, and may additionally incorporate treatment response data derived from large meta-analyses which can be extremely valuable to clinician and patient. However, the majority of these indices remain to be validated prospectively before replacing more established prognostic indices such as the NPI.

USING THE NPI FOR PATIENT MANAGEMENT

Following primary breast cancer surgery, stratification of patients into different prognostic groups may assist the clinician in selecting which patients should receive systemic adjuvant therapy, either chemotherapy or adjuvant hormonal therapy. Adjuvant chemotherapy is not indicated in patients in an EPG or GPG according to the NPI because the survival advantage is small and outweighed by the risk of potentially life-threatening toxicities. In contrast, however, patients in a MPG (I or II) or PPG may benefit significantly from anthracycline-based adjuvant polychemotherapy (in terms of disease-free and overall survival), particularly if the primary invasive carcinoma is hormone receptor negative.

With respect to carcinomas rich in estrogen receptor (ER) or progesterone receptor (PR), the survival advantage gained from five years of adjuvant hormonal therapy is minimal for patients in the EPG or GPG relative to those women with cancers that place their predicted outcome in the MPG (I or II) or PPG, who will obtain significant benefit. In addition, patients in the EPG or GPG may be unnecessarily exposed to hormonal drug side-effects or their complications (e.g., endometrial cancer or thromboembolic disease with a standard dose of tamoxifen 20 mg daily) which argues against recommending any post-operative hormonal treatment to such patients.

SUGGESTED READINGS

Carter GL, Allen C, Henson DR. Relation of tumour size, lymph node status, and survival in 24 740 breast cancer cases. Cancer 1989;63;181–187.

Elston CW, Ellis IO, Goulding H, Pinder SE. Role of pathology in the prognosis and management of breast cancer. In: CW Elston, IO Ellis. The Breast. Churchill Livingstone 1998; p385–433.

Galea MH, Blamey RW, Elston CE, Ellis IO. The Nottingham Prognostic Index in primary breast cancer. Breast Cancer Res Treat 1992;22:207–219.

Haybittle JL, Blamey RW, Elston CW, *et al*. A prognostic index in primary breast cancer. Br J Cancer 1982;45:361–366.

Pinder SE, Ellis IO, Galea M, *et al*. Pathological prognostic factors in breast cancer. III. Vascular invasion: relationship with recurrence and survival in a large series with long-term follow-up. Histopathology 1994;24:41–47.

21

Familial Breast Cancer

Anita Bane · Frances P O'Malley

INTRODUCTION

Hereditary or familial breast cancer accounts for approximately 10 % of all breast cancers and two highly penetrant breast cancer susceptibility genes, BRCA1 and BRCA2 account for approximately 20–50 % of these familial cases. A small number of genetic syndromes caused by other highly penetrant genes such as p53, PTEN, ATM and STK11 together account for only a minority of familial aggregation. In contrast to BRCA1/2 mutation-associated breast tumors, no distinguishing features have been described for the breast cancers associated with these rare genetic syndromes. The gene or genes responsible for the remainder of familial breast cancer remain unknown.

BRCA1 AND BRCA2 CANCER SYNDROMES

The *BRCA1* and *BRCA2* genes are the best characterized breast cancer susceptibility genes and in aggregate they account for approximately 20–50 % of all familial cases. Most families with both breast and ovarian cancer or with six or more cases of early onset breast cancer are attributable to mutations in one of these two highly penetrant genes, with a lifetime risk for the development of breast cancer in mutation carriers being 37–85 % by age 70. Mutation carriers are also at significantly increased risk of other malignancies, most notably ovarian carcinoma. The lifetime risk for developing ovarian cancer for *BRCA1* and *BRCA2* mutation carriers by age 70 is 44 % and 27 %, respectively.

BRCA1 ASSOCIATED BREAST CANCER

INTRODUCTION

BRCA1, a tumor suppressor gene, is located on chromosome 17q21, and encodes a protein 1863 amino acid residues in length. The functions of this protein are myriad and include repair of DNA double strand breaks by homologous recombination, transcriptional regulation, chromatin remodeling and protein ubiquitination. Germline mutations in this gene predispose to the devel-

opment of not only female breast and ovarian cancer, but also carcinomas of the cervix, endometrium, fallopian tube, peritoneum, stomach, liver, and prostate for male carriers. The prevalence of *BRCA1* mutations in the general population is approximately 1 in 1000, with a variable but high penetrance. Certain ethnic or geographically distinct groups such as those of Ashkenazi Jewish decent, French Canadians and Finns have a higher prevalence of disease due to the presence of founder mutations.

CLINICAL FEATURES

Patients may attend genetic counseling clinics due to a family history of breast cancer or alternatively they will present with symptomatic disease. There is, as with all familial cancer syndromes, a propensity for the development of early onset disease and/or multiple primary tumors.

RADIOLOGIC FEATURES

Most BRCA1 associated breast cancers have the same mammographic findings as seen in sporadic cancers. However, there is a significant percentage that can appear mammographically as a well-defined mass. This appearance may mimic a benign lesion, both mammographically and by ultrasound examination.

PATHOLOGIC FEATURES

MACROSCOPIC FINDINGS

BRCA1 associated breast tumors may have circumscribed margins, although the majority are indistinguishable grossly from sporadic breast cancers.

MICROSCOPIC FINDINGS

The histopathologic phenotype of BRCA1 associated breast cancer has been the subject of numerous publications and the consensus opinion is that these tumors are predominantly high-grade invasive ductal carcinomas of no special type. Between 5 % and 19 % of BRCA1

BRCA1 ASSOCIATED BREAST CANCER – FACT SHEET

Definition

▶ Hereditary breast cancer that results from the inheritance of a germline mutation in the *BRCA1* gene, 17q21

Gender, Race and Age Distribution

▶ Mutations in *BRCA1* have been described in all races with a prevalence of approximately 0.1%
▶ Certain ethnic or geographically distinct groups have an increased incidence due to the presence of founder mutations
▶ Young age of disease onset is typical

Clinical Features

▶ Early onset and multiple primary breast tumors
▶ Family history of breast or ovarian carcinoma

Radiologic Features

▶ Mass lesion, which may mimic a benign growth

Prognosis and Treatment

▶ Preventative strategies available to *BRCA1* mutation carriers include intensive surveillance, chemoprophylaxis with tamoxifen (controversial), bilateral mastectomy and salpingo-oophorectomy
▶ Current treatment modalities for incident cases do not differ for age and stage matched sporadic breast tumors.
▶ The prognosis for BRCA1 associated breast cancers has not been clearly established

BRCA1 ASSOCIATED BREAST CANCERS – PATHOLOGIC FEATURES

Gross Findings

▶ Firm tumor mass, typically completely or partially circumscribed

Microscopic Findings

▶ High grade invasive ductal carcinoma of no special type
▶ Higher reported incidence of medullary/atypical medullary features
▶ High mitotic count
▶ Significant nuclear pleomorphism
▶ Absent tubule formation
▶ Prominent host inflammatory response
▶ Pushing tumor margins

Immunohistochemical Features

▶ Majority of tumors are ER negative and PR negative
▶ Negative for HER2/neu protein overexpression /*HER2/neu* gene amplification
▶ Have a high frequency of p53 mutations
▶ Frequently express basal type cytokeratins, CK5/6, CK14

Differential Diagnosis

▶ NA

associated tumors have medullary or atypical medullary features, including pushing (circumscribed) tumor margins, a prominent lymphocytic response, syncytial growth pattern and marked nuclear pleomorphism (Figures 21-1 to 21-4). Another common finding is a high mitotic count; these tumors may have as many as 50–100 mitoses per 10 high power fields (Figure

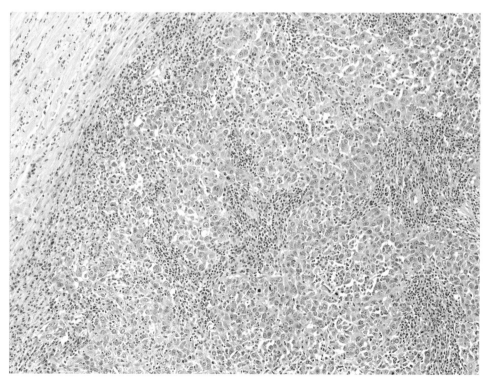

FIGURE 21-1
BRCA1 associated breast cancer. These tumors are typically high-grade invasive ductal carcinoma of no special type with a high prevalence of medullary and atypical medullary features. Low-power view showing a pushing (circumscribed) tumor margin.

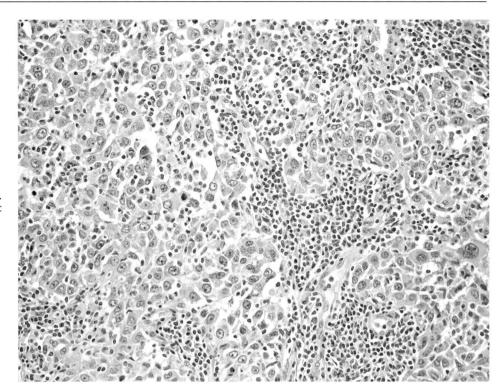

FIGURE 21-2

BRCA1 associated breast cancer. Typically, a prominent lymphocytic response is seen.

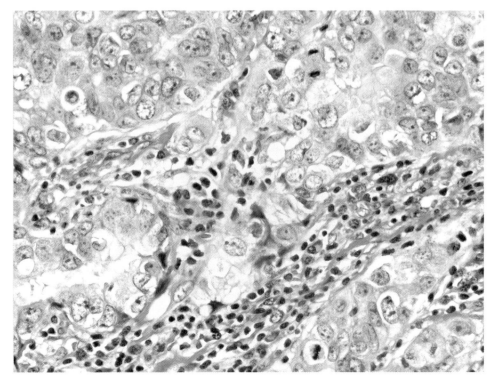

FIGURE 21-3

BRCA1 associated breast cancer. High power showing a syncytial growth pattern with islands of malignant epithelial cells appearing to 'float' in a 'sea' of lymphocytes. Stroma and cellular borders are inconspicuous.

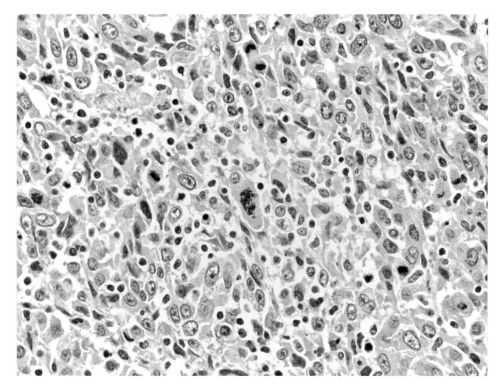

FIGURE 21-4
BRCA1 associated breast cancer. High power view showing marked nuclear pleomorphism and numerous mitoses, some of which are atypical.

21-4). DCIS may be present, within or adjacent to the tumor mass; early reports suggested DCIS rarely occurred in BRCA1 associated tumors, but more recent studies have shown no difference in the rates of associated DCIS in tumors from BRCA1 carriers and controls.

ANCILLARY STUDIES

IMMUNOHISTOCHEMISTRY

These tumors are generally negative for both estrogen (ER) and progesterone receptors (PR) and, despite their high histologic grade are usually negative for HER2/neu protein overexpression.

MOLECULAR STUDIES

cDNA microarray studies, together with confirmatory immunohistochemical studies on BRCA1 associated breast cancer have found that they have a 'basal-type' molecular phenotype characterized by ER negativity, expression of basal cytokeratins (CK5/6, CK14) and frequent p53 mutations. More conventional genetic studies have illustrated the increased incidence and a unique spectrum of p53 mutations in BRCA1 associated tumors relative to sporadic tumors.

HER2/neu protein overexpression is rarely found in BRCA1 associated tumors. The small percentage (generally less than 5%) of tumors that are positive for HER2/neu protein overexpression have been found to have a low level of gene amplification when assessed by fluorescent *in situ* hybridization (FISH). This is speculated to result from the fact that the HER2 gene is located on the long arm of chromosome 17 which is a frequent site of loss of heterozygosity (LOH) in BRCA1 associated tumors.

PROGNOSIS AND TREATMENT

The treatment options for patients with known BRCA1 mutations include:
- Intensive surveillance: Current surveillance strategies in most centers consist of breast self examination, clinical examination and annual mammography, with the use of ultrasound where appropriate, beginning at 25–35 years of age. Preliminary results suggest that MRI, or multimodality screening including MRI may be more beneficial in this high risk cohort.
- Chemoprophylaxis: The role of anti-estrogen agents such as tamoxifen in the prevention of breast cancers in BRCA1 mutation carriers is controversial.
- Surgical prophylaxis: Prophylactic bilateral mastectomy is offered to BRCA1 mutation carriers, particularly if they have previously diagnosed high risk lesions, such as atypical ductal hyperplasia or LCIS. Additionally, bilateral salphingo-oophorectomy upon completion of childbearing has been demonstrated to significantly lower the risk of ovarian and fallopian tube carcinoma and also to reduce the risk of breast cancer.

The prognosis for patients with BRCA1 associated breast tumors is not clearly established, with some studies suggesting a better, others a worse and still

---

BRCA2 ASSOCIATED BREAST CANCER – FACT SHEET

Definition
▶ Familial breast cancer attributable to inheritance of a germline mutation in the tumor suppressor gene located on chromosome 13q12-13

Gender, Race and Age Distribution
▶ Mutations in BRCA2 have been described in all races with a prevalence of approximately 0.1%
▶ Certain ethnic or geographically distinct groups have an increased incidence due to the presence of founder mutations
▶ Young age of disease onset is typical

Clinical Features
▶ Early onset and multiple primary breast tumors
▶ Family history of breast cancer (male and female), ovarian carcinoma, pancreatic, bilary tract and prostatic carcinomas

Radiologic Features
▶ Mass lesion with or without micro-calcifications

Prognosis and Treatment
▶ Preventative strategies available to *BRCA2* mutation carriers include intensive surveillance, chemoprophylaxis with tamoxifen, and bilateral mastectomy
▶ Current treatment modalities for incident cases do not differ for age and stage matched sporadic breast cancer cases.
▶ The prognosis for BRCA2 associated breast cancers has not been clearly established

---

BRCA2 ASSOCIATED BREAST CANCER – PATHOLOGIC FEATURES

Gross Findings
▶ Firm tumor mass in the breast parenchyma

Microscopic Findings
▶ High grade invasive ductal carcinomas of no special type.
▶ Lack of tubule formation
▶ Significant nuclear pleomorphism
▶ Pushing tumor margins
▶ Co-existent DCIS

Immunohistochemical Features
▶ Generally ER and PR positive
▶ Negative for *HER2/neu* overexpression/ gene amplification

Differential Diagnosis
▶ NA

---

others an outcome equivalent to that of age and stage matched sporadic breast cancer controls. Many of these studies have been limited by small sample size and accrual bias. Ongoing large, multicenter population based studies are expected to shed further light on this controversial issue.

BRCA 2 ASSOCIATED BREAST CANCER

INTRODUCTION

BRCA2 is a tumor suppressor gene located on chromosome 13q12. It encodes the BRCA2 protein, which is 3418 amino acid residues in length and has a number of functions ascribed to it, including repair of DNA double strand breaks by homologous recombination, transcriptional regulation and chromatin remodeling. Germline mutations in this gene confer a significantly increased risk for both male and female breast cancer, ovarian cancer, fallopian tube carcinoma, uveal tract and skin melanoma, pancreatic, biliary tract and prostatic carcinomas.

The prevalence of mutations in this gene in the general population is estimated at 1 in 1000. Similar to

BRCA1, certain geographically or ethnically distinct groups, such as Icelanders and those of Ashkenazi Jewish descent, have an increased prevalence due to the presence of founder mutations.

CLINICAL FEATURES

Patients present to genetic counseling clinics due to family history or alternatively to surgical outpatients with symptomatic disease. Both early onset and multiple primaries are characteristic of this genotype.

RADIOLOGIC FEATURES

Radiological findings are usually those of a mass and/or micro-calcifications.

PATHOLOGIC FEATURES

MACROSCOPIC FINDINGS

The gross appearance of BRCA2 tumors has not been reported to be different to that of sporadic controls.

MICROSCOPIC FINDINGS

A number of studies that have assessed the pathologic characteristics of BRCA2 associated tumors have yielded divergent results. Two earlier studies reported a lower histologic grade in BRCA2 associated tumors compared to controls, with an increased incidence of

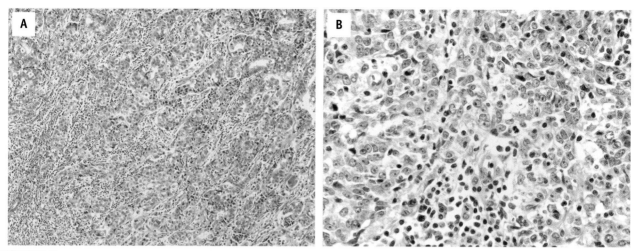

FIGURE 21-5

BRCA2 associated breast cancer. Tumors show an overall higher histologic grade than seen in sporadic breast cancers. (A) Low power view showing minimal tubule formation and a moderate lymphocytic response. (B) High power shows marked nuclear pleomorphism and increased mitoses.

invasive lobular or tubulo-lobular carcinomas. However the growing consensus is that BRCA2 associated tumors are predominantly invasive ductal carcinomas of no special type, with an overall higher histologic grade than sporadic breast cancer controls (Figure 21-5). Pushing tumor margins, as described for the BRCA1 cohort have also been described as part of the BRCA2 histologic phenotype. DCIS within the tumor or in adjacent tissue occurs with high frequency.

ANCILLARY STUDIES

IMMUNOHISTOCHEMISTRY

BRCA2 associated tumors tend to be ER and PR positive. The expression of HER2/neu protein by these tumors has not been extensively studied but preliminary results suggest that their rate of HER2/neu overexpression is similar to that of sporadic controls.

MOLECULAR STUDIES

BRCA2 associated tumors show a higher frequency of p53 mutations than sporadic breast tumors.

cDNA microarray analysis of a limited number of BRCA2 tumors has been performed and the molecular profile of these tumors is distinct from that of BRCA1 associated tumors and appears to cluster with the luminal A subgroup. This group is characterized by ER positivity and the expression of ER regulated genes.

PROGNOSIS AND TREATMENT

Treatment options available to *BRCA2* mutation carriers are similar to those discussed for *BRCA1* mutation carriers. It is not clear whether the prognosis

of *BRCA2* mutation carriers differs from *BRCA1* carriers or from controls. This is being studied in population based cohorts.

LI FRAUMENI SYNDROME

Li Fraumeni syndrome (LFS) is a rare, highly penetrant, autosomal dominant condition caused by germline mutations in the *TP53* gene. The *TP53* gene is located on chromosome 17p13.1 and its product p53, has been called the 'guardian of the genome'; it performs, or directs, many cellular processes involved in cell cycle control and apoptosis. Individuals harboring germline mutations in this gene develop multiple primary tumors in childhood and early adulthood including soft tissue sarcomas, osteosarcomas, breast tumors, brain tumors, leukemia and adrenocortical cancers. Within LFS families, breast cancer accounts for up to one-third of all cancers and occurs at an average age of 36 years. The incidence of breast cancer in women harboring germline mutations in *TP53* is estimated to be as high as 56 % by the age of 45 years. These tumors have not been described to have specific histologic features.

ATAXIA TELANGIECTASIA

Ataxia telangiectasia (ATM) is a rare autosomal recessive condition caused by homozygous germline mutations in the ATM gene. ATM is characterized by progressive cerebellar ataxia, oculocutaneous telengiectasias, immunodeficiency and increased cancer susceptibility including breast cancer. The ATM gene is located on chromosome 11q22-23 and encodes for a serine threonine kinase. This protein plays a central role in sensing and signaling the presence of DNA double strand breaks.

Approximately 0.2–1 % of the general population has been estimated to be a heterozygous carrier of a mutant ATM gene and they have been reported to a have a three- to eightfold increased risk of breast cancer. The risk of ATM carriers developing breast cancer is estimated to be 11 % by the age of 50 years and 30 % by the age of 70 years. No distinguishing clinico-pathologic features are known for ATM heterozygous breast cancer patients apart from early age of onset and frequent bilaterality.

COWDEN SYNDROME

Cowden syndrome is an autosomal dominant disorder characterized by multiple hamartomas in many organ systems including trichilemmomas and a high risk of breast, uterine and non-medullary thyroid carcinomas. It is caused by germline mutations in the *PTEN* gene, a tumor suppressor gene, located on chromosome 10q23.3 which encodes for a dual specificity phosphatase involved in apoptosis. The prevalence of a mutant gene in the general population is estimated to be 1:300 000. Females affected with the syndrome have a 25–50 % life-time risk of developing invasive breast cancer. In addition they have an increased incidence of benign disease such as fibrocystic change, hamartomas and fibroadenomas. Males with the syndrome are also at increased (unquantified) risk of developing breast cancer.

PEUTZ-JEGHERS SYNDROME

Peutz-Jeghers syndrome (PJS) is an autosomal dominant condition characterized by hamartomatous polyps of the gastrointestinal tract (especially the small bowel) and pigmentation of the lips, buccal mucosa and skin. The syndrome is caused by germline mutations in the *STK11/LKB1* gene located on chromosome 19p13.3. The gene encodes a serine/threonine kinase that functions as a tumor suppressor. Individuals harboring germline mutations in this gene are predisposed to malignancies of the stomach, colon, pancreas, small bowel, thyroid, breast, lung, uterus, ovaries and cervix. The most commonly reported malignancies in PJS kindred are those of the colon and breast with a mean age at diagnosis of 45 years.

OTHER GENES

E-cadherin is essential for functional cell–cell adhesion. Germline mutations in E-cadherin (located on chromo-

some 16q22.1) have been suggested to be important in the susceptibility to hereditary gastric cancer and breast cancer is also described in some families.

The *HRAS1* gene is also associated with an increased risk of breast cancer. Other genes, including the *APC* gene, the *TNFalpha* gene, the *N*-acetyl transferases, the glutathione *S*-transferase family and the cytochrome p450 family amongst others, have also been proposed as being related to an increased incidence of breast carcinoma in some families. Thus a number of low penetrance genes are implicated, not only with regard to mutation but also polymorphisms. It is likely that a combination of mutations and polymorphisms in these genes (and others) confers different degrees of breast cancer risk.

BRCAX GENE

Some families with early onset female breast cancer do not show evidence of linkage to any of the above genes. Many therefore believe that at least one other breast cancer gene with high penetrance is as yet undiscovered (called, by some, the BRCAX gene).

SUGGESTED READINGS

Pathology of Familial Breast Cancer

Agnarsson BA, Jonasson JG, Bjornsdottir IB, *et al*. Inherited BRCA2 mutation associated with high grade breast cancer. Breast Cancer Res Treat 1998;47:121–127.

Eisinger F, Jacquemier J, Charpin C, *et al*. Mutations at BRCA1: the medullary breast carcinoma revisited. Cancer Res 1998;58:1588–1592.

Lakhani SR, Jacquemier J, Sloane JP, *et al*. Multifactorial analysis of differences between sporadic breast cancers and cancers involving BRCA1 and BRCA2 mutations. J Natl Cancer Inst 1998;90:1138–1145.

Lidereau R, Eisinger F, Champeme MH, *et al*. Major improvement in the efficacy of BRCA1 mutation screening using morphoclinical features of breast cancer. Cancer Res 2000;60:1206–1210.

Marcus JN, Watson P and Page DL, *et al*. BRCA2 hereditary breast cancer pathophenotype. Breast Cancer Res Treat 1997;44:275–277.

Nielsen TO, Hsu FD, Jensen K, *et al*. Immunohistochemical and clinical characterization of the basal-like subtype of invasive breast carcinoma. Clin Cancer Res 2004;10:5367–5374.

Osin P, Crook T, Powles T, *et al*. Hormone status of in-situ cancer in BRCA1 and BRCA2 mutation carriers. Lancet 1998;351:1487.

Osin PP, Lakhani SR. The pathology of familial breast cancer: Immunohistochemistry and molecular analysis. Breast Cancer Res 1999;1:36–40.

Quenneville LA, Phillips KA and Ozcelik H, *et al*. HER-2/neu status and tumor morphology of invasive breast carcinomas in Ashkenazi women with known BRCA1 mutation status in the Ontario Familial Breast Cancer Registry. Cancer 2002;95:2068–2075.

Turner N, Tutt A, Ashworth A. Hallmarks of 'BRCAness' in sporadic cancers. Nature Rev Cancer 2004;4:814–819.

Molecular Classification of BRCA1/2 associated Breast Cancer

Foulkes WD. BRCA1 functions as a breast stem cell regulator. J Med Genet 2004;41:1–5.

Hedenfalk I, Ringner M, Ben-Dor A, *et al*. Molecular classification of familial non-BRCA1/BRCA2 breast cancer. Proc Natl Acad Sci USA 2003;100:2532–2537.

Sorlie T, Tibshirani R, Parker J, *et al*. Repeated observation of breast tumor subtypes in independent gene expression data sets. Proc Natl Acad Sci USA 2003;100:8418–8423.

Tavassoli FA, Devilee P. Pathology and Genetics of Tumours of the Breast and Female Genital Organs. World Health Organisation of Classification of Tumours. Lyon. IARC Press 2003.

van de Vijver MJ, He YD, van't Veer LJ, *et al.* A gene-expression signature as a predictor of survival in breast cancer. N Engl J Med 2002;347:1999–2009.

Management of BRCA1/2 Breast Cancer

Chung MA, Cady B. Surgical treatment planning in newly diagnosed breast cancer patients at high risk for BRCA-1 or BRCA-2 mutation. Breast J 2004;10:473–474.

Eisinger F, Charafe-Jauffret E, Jacquemier J, *et al.* Tamoxifen and breast cancer risk in women harboring a BRCA1 germline mutation: computed efficacy, effectiveness and impact. Int J Oncol 2001;18:5–10.

Hartmann LC, Sellers TA, Schaid DJ, *et al.* Efficacy of bilateral prophylactic mastectomy in BRCA1 and BRCA2 gene mutation carriers. J Natl Cancer Inst 2001;93:1633–1637.

King MC, Wieand S, Hale K, *et al.* Tamoxifen and breast cancer incidence among women with inherited mutations in BRCA1 and BRCA2: National Surgical Adjuvant Breast and Bowel Project (NSABP-P1) Breast Cancer Prevention Trial. J Am Med Assoc 2001;286:2251–2256

Rebbeck TR, Lynch HT, Neuhausen SL, *et al.* Prophylactic oophorectomy in carriers of BRCA1 or BRCA2 mutations. N Engl J Med 2002;346:1616–1622.

22 Handling and Evaluation of Sentinel Lymph Nodes

Donald L Weaver

This chapter will discuss various aspects of sentinel lymph node biopsy, including performance of the procedure, pathologic handling and microscopic examination of the lymph nodes.

TECHNIQUES FOR PERFORMING SENTINEL LYMPH NODE BIOPSY

Two main techniques are used to identify sentinel nodes. The first emerged from sentinel node research in malignant melanoma. A vital blue dye is injected into the breast around the primary tumor, skin flaps are then raised over the low axilla, blue tinged lymphatics are identified then followed to the sentinel lymph node(s). Vital blue dye is an intra-operative technique as the dye enters lymphatics rapidly then dissipates quickly. The second technique employs an injection of radioactive technetium, attached to a colloid or protein, which drains to the sentinel nodes. The radioactive formulation travels more slowly through the lymphatic channels and accumulates in nodes allowing injection of the tracer hours prior to surgery. A hand-held gamma particle detector, or probe, is used to identify areas of radioactive uptake prior to making a skin incision. The detector is collimated in a manner that allows directional localization of the radio-labeled node(s) during surgical dissection. Precise surgical localization minimizes disruption of surrounding tissue. When used together, both techniques tend to label the same lymph nodes in any particular patient, but nodes labeled only with blue dye or radioactivity are encountered. This may be due to the different fluid dynamics of each labeling technique or due to different dynamic drainage patterns if patients are left lying or allowed to move about after injection.

Ideally, individual lymph nodes are removed from the patient by the surgeon and sent to the pathologist. In some cases, a directed low axillary sampling or packet of lymph nodes is removed that contains several lymph nodes including one or more sentinel nodes. This latter approach may disrupt more axillary tissue and does not allow rank ordering of sentinel nodes but would be expected to have a similar rate of detecting positive axillary nodes. The gamma detectors used in sentinel node biopsy integrate particle detection over time allowing the removed nodes to be identified by their 10-second

gamma particle counts. This is useful to the pathologist as metastases are most likely to be detected in the nodes with the highest levels of radioactivity, corresponding to the node(s) first receiving drainage. Small colloid particle size in the radioactive tracer or long delays between injection and surgical dissection can label more than several lymph nodes as second echelon nodes become

SENTINEL LYMPH NODE BIOPSY – FACT SHEET

Definition
▶ First lymph node receiving lymphatic drainage from a specified anatomic site
▶ The sentinel node may be visually identified using a blue dye or radio-pharmaceutically identified with the aid of a gamma particle detector
▶ The blue dye or radioactive agent is injected into the breast prior to surgery

Location
▶ In the breast, the sentinel node(s) are most often located in the lower axilla but may be located in the upper axilla, on the lateral chest wall, within the breast, the internal mammary chain, or the supraclavicular nodes
▶ The typical number of sentinel nodes identified is one to three.

Morbidity
▶ Morbidity from the sentinel node procedure is predicted to be less than a full axillary dissection due to removal of fewer nodes and less disruption of lymphatic channels
▶ Complications from axillary dissection include seroma formation, decreased range of arm motion, loss of sensation and lymphedema.

Prognosis and Treatment
▶ Sentinel node biopsy may provide prognostic and staging information equivalent to an axillary dissection
▶ Staging information derived from sentinel node biopsy alone may be less accurate than an axillary dissection based on a defined false negative rate
▶ The radiation and chemotherapy received by the majority of breast cancer patients may result in axillary recurrence rates that are clinically acceptable and not substantially different from recurrence rates after axillary dissection
▶ Sentinel node biopsy has increased the rate of micrometastasis detection necessitating changes in the AJCC/UICC TNM Staging System

---

SENTINEL LYMPH NODES – PATHOLOGIC FEATURES

Gross findings

▶ Sentinel nodes are ideally submitted to pathology individually, appropriately labeled and dissected free of adipose tissue
▶ Rank ordering of nodes utilizing intensity of blue dye or radioactive counts is highly desirable
▶ Occasionally, several sentinel nodes are submitted in a packet of adipose tissue
▶ Potentially less desirable and more morbid is one or more sentinel node or nodes within a large packet of adipose tissue representing a limited or directed low axillary sampling that includes sentinel nodes

Microscopic Features and Processing

▶ Sentinel nodes are thinly sliced and entirely submitted for histologic evaluation
▶ Each slice should ideally be no thicker than 2 mm
▶ Systematic strategies that control the amount of unexamined lymph node are the most reliable for reproducibly stratifying patients within the TNM nodal staging classification system

Immunohistochemical Features

▶ The use of immunohistochemical stains greatly enhances the detection of extremely small tumor deposits known as isolated tumor cells or clusters (ITCs)
▶ The clinical significance of ITCs (metastases no larger than 0.2 mm) is unknown at present
▶ Early data suggest no adverse prognostic significance
▶ Immunohistochemical stains can also facilitate identification of bland or histologically indistinct micrometastases (metastases larger than 0.2 mm but no larger than 2.0 mm)
▶ The prognostic significance of micrometastases is less clear than for ITCs; older literature is contradictory
▶ Systematic strategies for pathologic sentinel node evaluation may produce more homogeneous and reliable stratification of patients with metastases less than or equal to 2 mm
▶ There is no recommendation or endorsement for the routine use of immunohistochemistry for evaluation of sentinel nodes although the technique is widely applied
▶ Careful documentation of the size and extent of nodal disease is mandatory, particularly when immunohistochemistry is employed

labeled. Sentinel nodes labeled only with blue dye can also be rank ordered semi-quantitatively by the surgeon using terms such as 'bluest node', and 'next bluest node'. Localization within part of a lymph node has also been demonstrated. When only one part of a node is labeled with blue dye or if a blue lymphatic can be traced to one aspect of the lymph node, the labeled portion of the node is more likely to contain metastases than the unlabeled portion.

PATHOLOGIC FEATURES

GROSS EXAMINATION

In an era when the likelihood of positive axillary lymph nodes was high and the size of the metastases was large, a single section of each lymph node was adequate for identifying metastases. In the current era, due to extensive surveillance screening, nearly three-quarters of women with breast cancer have negative lymph nodes at the time of presentation and, when nodal disease is present, the median size metastasis is now approximately 6 mm. Pathologists do not routinely take all their sections from one area of a solid tumor and, similarly, sections should not be taken exclusively from one area of a lymph node, grossly or microscopically. The guiding principle in examination of lymph nodes is to minimize the chance of missing significant metastases by controlling the amount of unexamined lymph node. Submitting the entire node for histologic examination and thinly slicing the lymph node, prior to embedding in the paraffin tissue block, are the first steps needed to accomplish this task.

Examination of lymph nodes has unarguably become more thorough over time, particularly in the case of sentinel nodes. Nodes that are grossly positive for metastatic disease require only a single section to confirm disease; however, random sampling of clinically negative nodes misses metastatic disease that would otherwise be easily identified. When lymph nodes are grossly bisected then followed by one routine histologic section of each node half, approximately 40 % of positive sentinel nodes are missed if only one half of the node is examined. Furthermore, approximately 20 % of patients will have metastases confined to only one half of a single lymph node and, accordingly, 10 % of patients would be under-staged by chance when the wrong half of a node is chosen for histologic examination. Several organizations recommend, and there is now general acceptance, that lymph nodes be entirely submitted for histologic evaluation.

Current recommendations also include slicing sentinel lymph nodes as close to 2 mm as possible. This can be achieved in most typical nodes with bisection. Small nodes can be submitted intact but large nodes, or nodes largely replaced by adipose tissue, require serial sectioning prior to embedding. By sectioning nodes at the time of gross examination, the pathologist controls the maximum thickness of unexamined node. Two millimeters is close to the physical limit for gross sectioning. Sections much thinner than 2 mm may curl during further fixation and thus be difficult for histologists to embed flat. If some degree of fixation occurs before sectioning, thinner sections can be achieved. However, when intraoperative examination is performed, fixation is not possible prior to sectioning. When a 5–6 mm thick node is bisected, the resulting capsular relaxation after sectioning often produces sections close to 2 mm. Section thickness can be re-evaluated after fixation and prior to submitting for processing and embedding. When a node is multiply sectioned, care should be taken to place each cut surface sequentially into the tissue cassette so that no more than 2 mm of unexamined tissue are present between each histologic section. Histologists are trained to place sections into the paraffin block so that the surface facing downward in the tissue cassette will be the first surface cut in the paraffin block.

Sentinel nodes are often subject to more intense pathologic evaluation than routinely dissected nodes; sentinel nodes are more likely to contain metastases than non-sentinel nodes and the presence of metastatic disease within a sentinel node may determine whether a patient has a completion axillary dissection. The mean number of sentinel nodes removed ranges from 2–4 but occasionally as many as 6 or 10 are identified. Except for large nodes, most sentinel nodes can be totally embedded in a single block. Because sentinel nodes are much more likely to contain small occult metastases, care must be taken to section them, either grossly or microscopically so that no more than 2 mm remains unexamined. There is some debate over whether nodes should be sectioned perpendicular or parallel to the longest axis of the node.

Perpendicular sections are technically easier but produce more total sections. Sectioning parallel to the long axis is more difficult but produces fewer sections, a potential advantage. Metastatic tumor cells have been shown to concentrate at the junctions of the afferent lymphatics and subcapsular sinus. A review of old lymphangiogram literature discloses that afferent lymphatics are more likely to enter the node at the periphery in the plane of the long axis. Sections parallel to this axis may maximize the number of afferent lymphatics in the plane of section and potentially maximize the number of metastases detected with initial sections from the paraffin block.

A particular problem that should be conscientiously avoided while evaluating sentinel nodes is over counting positive nodes. The prosector must carefully document how the nodes were sectioned and submitted and the pathologist responsible for reporting the findings must correlate the histologic findings for each grossly identified node with the submission key. The total number of positive nodes influences the overall stage in the sixth edition staging manuals. It is possible for a tri-sected or multiply sectioned node that contains metastatic disease to be counted as more than one positive node and this would unfairly prejudice the patient's prognosis. In our institution, we place each bisected or sectioned node identified in a single cassette or multiple cassettes. Only intact, small nodes are placed more than one to a cassette. In the less likely event that smaller sectioned nodes are placed in a single cassette, one is marked with colored ink to avoid over counting. We follow a similar practice of using the gross examination for determining the total number of nodes examined. Bisected or sectioned nodes may produce more than the expected number of sections as an artifact of embedding and histologic sectioning. For this reason, we record the number of nodes placed in each cassette based on gross identification and discount those tissue fragments that exhibit no nodal tissue on histologic sections or obtain deeper sections when the number of tissue fragments is less than expected.

MICROSCOPIC EVALUATION

There is virtually no agreement on a method for microscopic evaluation of sentinel nodes and hence this aspect of assessment has created the greatest heterogeneity in classification of nodes with the least amount of tumor. This is due to several factors including:
- A body of conflicting literature on the clinical significance of occult micrometastases in axillary lymph nodes, as discussed in Chapter 23;
- A lack of data on the distribution of micrometastases within nodes; and
- Confusion between enhancing sensitivity of detection on histologic sections and systematic screening of an entire node.

An environment has been created that places far too much emphasis on the dichotomous presence or absence of nodal metastases and too little emphasis on exploring semi-quantitative nodal tumor burden. A better understanding of these issues, if applied to clinical practice, should contribute to developing more uniform approaches to evaluation of sentinel nodes and more reproducible nodal classifications within the AJCC/UICC staging system.

MICROMETASTASIS DISTRIBUTION AND DETECTION

Incomplete data on the distribution of metastases within lymph nodes is a major issue contributing to a lack of standardization in sentinel node analysis. Micrometastases are not randomly distributed within the microanatomy of the lymph nodes. They are much more likely to be in the subcapsular sinus, clustering near the entry points of the afferent lymphatics. We know something about the anatomy of afferent lymphatics but we cannot determine reliably in each lymph node the best place to look for metastases. In that respect, the distribution of metastases can be considered random. Metastases have been preferentially identified in some sentinel nodes in a region or half of the node that contains more blue dye or increased radioactive uptake; these studies support the observation that tumor cells congregate at the afferent lymphatic junction but the technique is unable to exclude metastases in the unlabeled regions of the node. This inability to precisely predict the location of metastases should encourage a systematic rather than overly weighted approach to sentinel node analysis.

The likelihood of identifying micrometastases and isolated tumor cells (ITCs) is directly proportional to the size of the metastasis and the number of sections examined from each lymph node block. Compared to a single section from the surface of the lymph node, when one or two additional cytokeratin–immunohistochemistry (CK-IHC) stained sections are examined, 10–14 % of nodes will have micrometastases or ITCs identified. If a more comprehensive strategy with additional sections is utilized, the rate increases to 25–30 %. Assuming that a metastasis is randomly distributed within the three dimensional space of a lymph node, mathematical models confirm the relationship between section interval, or the number of sections examined, and the likelihood of identifying a metastasis. The initial method of node examination also influences the likelihood of identifying metastases on deeper sections. Interestingly, the overall node positive rate, when the findings from initial hematoyxlin and eosin stained (H&E) sections and deeper CK-IHC stained sections are combined, is similar (38–42 %) for several sentinel node series even though the rates for initial (17–32 %) and occult metastases (10–30 %) are different and demonstrate wider variation. This observation underscores the fact that, if sentinel nodes are thinly sliced prior to initial examination, there is a higher likelihood that the largest and most clinically significant metastases will be detected without resorting to exhaustive examination of the paraffin tissue blocks. This is an important practical consideration. In breast cancer, ITCs in the subcapsular lymph node sinus are approximately 10 microns (0.01 mm) in diameter and an exhaustive search for every cancer cell in the sentinel nodes is prohibitively expensive and time consuming. Each 2 mm of lymph node tissue would require 200 sections spaced at 10 microns to exclude the presence of single occult tumor cells. Even with this level of scrutiny, partial tumor cells or poorly stained cells are missed. Ultimately, the threshold size of the metastases to be identified must be a prospective decision.

If a pathologist slices a node at 2 mm intervals and examines a single section from the surface of each embedded tissue slice, then at the end of the analysis, the patient and oncologist can be reassured that it is unlikely that there are any residual occult metastases in the lymph node blocks larger than 2 mm. On the other hand, if a 0.2 mm metastasis is identified there is a very good chance that this patient's metastasis was incidentally identified and it would not be possible to assure the oncologist that this patient was any different than a patient with negative nodes reported (Figures 22-1 and 22-2). If the pathologist and oncologist wanted to differentiate between patients with negative nodes and 0.2 mm metastases, then the lymph node blocks would need to be prospectively cut at 0.2 mm (200 micron) intervals completely through the block. The thickness of any unexamined residual tissue determines the maximum size of any potential occult metastases. This guiding principle is why it is so critical to control the sectioning and embedding of the sentinel node prior to histologic examination.

The discussion above is easiest to conceptualize when a single metastasis is present in a lymph node. When several metastases are present, the likelihood of detecting at least one metastasis is higher than if only a single metastasis were present. If the identification of one metastasis is associated with additional independent metastases in the lymph node, then prognosis could potentially be worse for these patients due to higher tumor burden. As might be expected, there is little data to support or refute this hypothesis. The problem, of course, is that only what is identified is known; there is always the opportunity to miss metastatic disease unless all nodal tissue is histologically sectioned and examined. Furthermore, the metastatic cascade is more complex than statistical mathematics. Changes in the overall micrometastatic tumor burden in lymph nodes may effect changes in the immunologic microenvironment

that enhance, suppress or have no effect on tumor cell proliferation. Until more is known about tumor cell proliferation and propagation in lymph nodes, it is best to follow the simple statistical strategy of pre-determined sectioning intervals and understand when a metastasis may have been identified by chance. Even more important is the recognition that patients with no metastases identified constitute a heterogeneous group of patients with and without occult metastases. Pathologists can control the sectioning interval; they cannot control the statistical chance associated with identifying metastases smaller than the sectioning interval.

SYSTEMATIC AND PRACTICAL APPROACH TO MICROSCOPIC EXAMINATION

Detection of ITC clusters and small micrometastases in sentinel nodes probably has minimal additive prognostic importance and when minimal nodal disease is present therapeutic decisions should be influenced by primary tumor characteristics and prognostic factors. This approach may change when less toxic, more efficacious regimens are developed but, at present, the more important goal of sentinel node examination is to exclude metastases that are most likely to impact outcome. The existing literature would suggest we exclude metastatic disease in the range of 2 mm in greatest dimension. This can be accomplished by sectioning sentinel nodes as close to 2 mm as possible prior to embedding then histologically examining each resulting tissue section. A single histologic section from the surface of the cut node surfaces will detect virtually all metastases larger than 2 mm although the size of the detected metastasis in the plane of section may not represent its maximum dimension. To exclude smaller metastases, the histologic sectioning plan must include sections from deeper within the paraffin tissue block. For example, a section from the surface and a section 1 mm deeper into the block will detect virtually all metastases larger than 1 mm. A slightly weighted approach was utilized on the experimental component of the NSABP B-32 sentinel node trial. Assuming that most sentinel nodes are ellipsoids that can be bisected on the long axis, the volume of nodal tissue will be more concentrated in the upper portion of the tissue block when cut surfaces are oriented downward during embedding. This would imply some statistical detection advantage to over sampling nearer to the surface.

The B-32 sectioning plan included a surface section, a section approximately 0.5 mm into the block and a final section 1 mm into the block. Only the first section was utilized for clinical management; the two deeper sections were performed at a later time and the findings on these additional sections will be correlated with outcome. The maximum thickness of unexamined node is therefore 1 mm with this strategy but a much higher proportion of the node volume has been sampled. Immunohistochemical stains can be added to increase screening efficiency and detection sensitivity but their

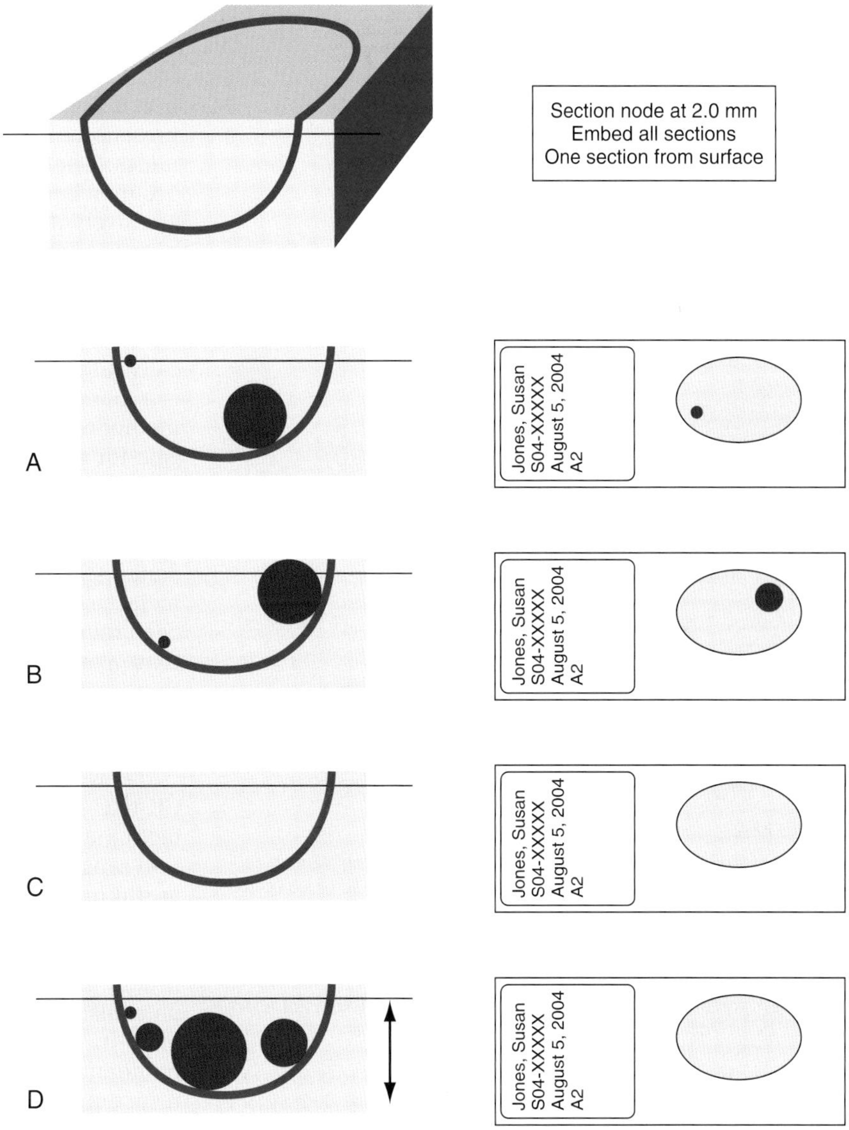

Section node at 2.0 mm
Embed all sections
One section from surface

FIGURE 22-1

Patterns of success and failure in identifying sentinel node metastases. The diagrams are a schematic representation of a single half of a bisected node 2 mm thick embedded in a paraffin block. (a–d) A cross-section through the paraffin block and a single slide prepared from the surface of the block (black line) after facing the tissue. (a) An isolated tumor cell (ITC) cluster has been identified and a 1.2 mm metastasis deeper in the block has been missed. (b) A 1.2 mm metastasis has been identified and an ITC cluster deeper in the block has been missed. Note that the size of the metastasis in the plane of section may not represent the largest dimension. A patient may be arbitrarily placed in the pN0 or pN1mi category depending on the metastasis location and probability of detection. (c) No metastasis has been identified. (d) No metastasis has been identified but metastases of varying size may be missed deeper in the paraffin block. Although C and D produce the same histologic section, a negative section does not guarantee the absence of micrometastases. The size of the largest potential missed metastasis is determined by the thickness of unexamined tissue (double-ended arrow; approximately 1.8 mm). This sectioning strategy, tissue sections no thicker than 2 mm and a single histologic section, would be expected to identify all metastases larger than 2 mm but may miss smaller micrometastases.

prognostic value is still unproven. It must be understood that any node without metastases detected may still contain small tumor cell clusters. Ultimately, the pathologist and clinician must decide the maximum acceptable size for undetected metastases and the pathologist must design a cutting strategy that meets those criteria. At present, exclusion of metastases larger than 2 mm is the most defensible strategy and allows stratification of patients within the AJCC/UICC defined nodal classifications. Future data may or may not require modification of the 2 mm size threshold.

ANCILLARY STUDIES

IMMUNOHISTOCHEMISTRY AND DETECTION SENSITIVITY

The third factor contributing to heterogeneity in node classification is the use of immunohistochemical

(IHC) stains in the evaluation of sentinel nodes. In breast cancer, anti-cytokeratin (CK) immunohistochemistry is generally employed. The use of CK-IHC rarely aids in the detection of larger, clinically significant metastases that are usually readily identified with routine stains. What is most frequently identified with CK-IHC stains are ITCs and small clusters of tumor cells that meet the AJCC/UICC definition for ITCs or are metastases at the lower end of the spectrum of micrometastases. ITCs are metastatic tumor deposits that are no larger than 0.2 mm and are expected to have the least impact on prognosis. The small size of ITC clusters means that there is a high probability that they will be missed with typical lymph node evaluation strategies; ITCs represent approximately 75 % of the occult metastases identified on CK-IHC stained deeper sections of sentinel nodes. From the perspective of staging and predicting outcome for groups of patients, the overlap that exists between patients with and without micrometastases partially obscures the clinical

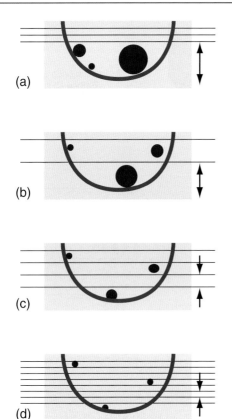

FIGURE 22-2

Patterns of failure in identifying micrometastases utilizing various sectioning strategies. (a–d) A cross-section through a single half of a bisected node 2 mm thick embedded in a paraffin block. Black lines indicate where tissue sections are mounted on glass slides. (a) Three levels separated by 200 microns are represented. This strategy over samples the surface of the block and metastases have been missed deeper in the block. The size of the largest potential missed metastasis is equal to the thickness of unexamined tissue (double ended arrow). (b) Two levels separated by 1000 microns (1 mm). Although only two sections have been examined, the largest potential missed metastasis (double ended arrow) is smaller than the strategy depicted in (a). (c) Four levels separated by 500 microns (0.5 mm). The maximum size of any missed metastasis has been reduced further by systematically controlling the thickness of each step section. (d) Multiple levels each separated by 200 microns (0.2 mm) through the tissue block. This is a comprehensive and time-consuming strategy designed to detect all metastases larger than 0.2 mm (micrometastases). ITCs and clusters may be detected or missed by chance. The maximum size of any potential missed metastasis correlates with the section interval (distance between black arrows). The clinical prognostic significance of identifying micrometastases and ITCs is currently unknown. The pathologist and clinician must determine prospectively the largest acceptable size of any missed metastasis and design a sectioning strategy that will systematically detect metastases larger than the agreed upon threshold.

utility of the separate grouping. In single institution observational studies, patients with metastases identified only by CK-IHC have recurrence and survival similar to patients with no metastases identified. The studies of sentinel nodes do not have long follow-up at this point but do suggest that large differences in outcome are not likely to be identified in randomized prospective trials.

The sensitivity of CK-IHC techniques may also be detecting artifacts associated with the diagnosis and surgical management of breast cancer. When prior biopsy type is correlated with the presence of H&E detected metastases, no statistically significant association is identified. However, a statistically significant association is observed between prior biopsy procedure and the presence of CK-IHC detectable tumor cells in lymph nodes. The lowest rate of CK-IHC detected tumor cells occurs when no prior biopsy is performed and rates progressively increase after fine needle aspirate, core needle biopsy and finally excision biopsy. This suggests that some proportion of patients with tumor cells detected with CK-IHC in lymph nodes do not have true metastatic disease in the traditional sense but have iatrogenically displaced tumor cells. Although size of metastasis is a more objective measure of tumor burden, detection methodology (H&E or CK-IHC) is a reasonable surrogate for tumor burden when size is not available. Cytologically bland and presumably benign epithelial cells have also been described in the subcapsular sinuses of lymph nodes after breast biopsy. It is impossible to demonstrate whether these iatrogenically induced metastases have biologic significance because they have been removed. Presumably, outcome would be no worse than patients with excision biopsy and no axillary surgery. Historical differences in axillary recurrence rates for patients with and without axillary dissection are not unacceptably large.

There are advantages and disadvantages to utilizing CK-IHC stains for sentinel node evaluation. The advantages include more rapid screening and increased detection sensitivity. Increased sensitivity may potentially be useful in determining whether to perform a completion axillary dissection. Additional sections and CK-IHC stains of sentinel nodes can reduce the false negative rate by approximately 18 % but cannot entirely eliminate false negative examinations. This relative improvement in the false negative rate may not be necessary if randomized trials demonstrate no difference in axillary recurrence rates between sentinel node only and axillary dissection. The disadvantages of CK-IHC staining include additional expense and identification of micrometastases that may have marginal prognostic value. Perhaps more worrying is the false sense of security created by using a sensitive technique. The issue of systematic screening of the lymph node is not addressed with CK-IHC stains and the amount of unexamined node still determines the magnitude of any occult metastasis.

INTRA-OPERATIVE ASSESSMENT

Single institution, longitudinal observational data from patients undergoing a sentinel node biopsy alone suggest that this will prove to be a safe alternative to axillary dissection when the sentinel node(s) are negative. What still needs to be determined definitively is whether there will be excess axillary recurrences or decreased survival when no axillary dissection is performed. This will have to wait until results from multi-institution, randomized, prospective trials comparing sentinel node biopsy to axillary dissection are available. In the interim, there is a willingness on the part of patients and physicians to forego axillary dissection, dependent on the results of the sentinel node biopsy. For this reason, an intra-operative assessment of sentinel nodes may be requested by the surgeon to determine whether an immediate completion axillary dissection will be performed. Several related issues must be considered by the pathology laboratory prior to embarking on intraoperative assessment of sentinel nodes. These include: false negative rates, detection of ITCs and economic issues. In addition, issues relating to cytologic or frozen section evaluation must be considered.

The false negative rate for intra-operative assessment of sentinel nodes is approximately 25–30 % on a per case basis and somewhat higher on a per node basis. Demonstrated rates for frozen section are only slightly better than cytologic examination, but this may be subject to interpretation bias as many surgical pathologists are more comfortable interpreting frozen sections than cytologic preparations. The intra-operative false negative rate is largely dependent on sampling and detecting or missing micrometastases, problems inherent to both cytologic and frozen section interpretation. As a clinical decision making tool, the two techniques are essentially equivalent with respect to false negative rate. Frozen section has the advantage of displaying architectural features and location of the metastasis, usually the subcapsular sinus. The disadvantage of frozen section is the possibility of cutting through small metastases during preparation, facing and obtaining satisfactory sections of the frozen tissue block. This may be a particular problem for laboratories with a low volume of frozen sections or in training programs where resident's experience can vary widely. Lymph nodes substantially replaced by adipose tissue can also be problematic. The tendency of these nodes to fold and tear during section preparation and to loosen from the slides during staining will contribute to false negative rates and over-consumption of nodal tissue prior to permanent section analysis.

Intra-operative cytologic evaluation can be accomplished with either cytologic smears or touch imprints. Smears provide more cells for examination and imprints can transfer some architectural orientation to the slide. The disadvantages of cytologic preparations include the loss of metastasis architecture and the difficulty identifying rare events within a background of lymphocytes and histiocytes during the brief time allowed and expected for an intra-operative examination. The fact that no tissue is consumed is the main advantage to cytologic evaluation but this may also contribute to the slightly higher false negative rate, as a small metastasis would still have the opportunity to be detected on permanent sections. When false negative smears were retrospectively reviewed at the University of Vermont in a blinded experiment, together with true positive and true negative smears, trained cytotechnologists were able to detect rare tumor cells on virtually all of the false negative smears, underscoring the difficulty in detecting minimal nodal tumor burden. Rapid intra-operative CK-IHC stains have been developed and proposed as a solution to this problem; however, this raises the larger issue of detection strategies and significance of different size metastases (see below).

The final issue with regard to intra-operative assessment of sentinel nodes involves the complexity of medical economics. Approximately 75 % of candidates for sentinel node biopsy will have pathologically negative axillary lymph nodes. The 25 % of patients with positive sentinel nodes are candidates for completion axillary dissection but 25–30 % of these will be missed on intra-operative examination. Only 17 or 18 patients for each 100 patients evaluated will have the opportunity for immediate completion axillary dissection. For smaller hospitals and laboratories it may not be economically feasible to perform an intra-operative examination when an elective completion axillary dissection can be performed after permanent section analysis. For larger hospitals with larger pathology laboratories, busy operating rooms, difficult schedules and large referral populations, the opportunity to complete the axillary dissection immediately in 17 or 18 of 25 expected cases may outweigh the 75 true negative examinations and the 7 or 8 false negative examinations. A complicating factor may be opportunistic detection of ITC clusters intra-operatively. Some institutions are foregoing completion axillary dissection when only ITC clusters are identified in sentinel nodes. The size of the metastasis would not be known on a cytologic preparation and thus some patients may receive an axillary dissection outside institution guidelines. Alternatively, size may be inaccurately assessed on a frozen section and a decision to forego axillary dissection may need to be reconsidered after evaluation of permanent sections. Another approach to sentinel node evaluation is to examine all sentinel nodes entirely with serial frozen sections. This approach has the advantage of immediate examination of the entire node with no residual tissue for permanent section analysis and no risk for subsequent identification of metastases. When combined with intra-operative IHC, the likelihood of missing significant metastases is low. Although successfully practiced by a few specialized referral centers, this approach is not generally feasible in most hospital settings.

Multiple approaches to intra-operative assessment have been proposed and applied successfully in sentinel node biopsy. There is no universally accepted method; each approach has its advantages and disadvantages; however, a systematic permanent section analysis is the standard by which all intra-operative assessments will be measured. The risk associated with a second anesthetic procedure is relatively low; therefore, individual institutions must evaluate the potential inconvenience of a second procedure for the patient and balance that against the time commitment, technical expertise and accuracy of the pathology assessment available to determine whether an intra-operative assessment will be performed, and if so, what technique will be utilized.

SUGGESTED READINGS

Fitzgibbons PL, Page DL, Weaver D, *et al.* Prognostic Factors in Breast Cancer: College of American Pathologists Consensus Statement 1999. Arch Pathol Lab Med 2000;124:966–978.

Hansen NM, Ye X, Grube BJ, Giuliano AE. Manipulation of the primary breast tumor and the incidence of sentinel node metastases from invasive breast cancer. Arch Surg 2004;139:634–640.

Lyman GH, Givliano AE, Somerfield MR, *et al*. American Society of Clinical Oncology Guideline Recommendations for sentinel lymph node biopsy in early stage breast cancer. J Clin Oncol 2005;23:7703–7720.

Moore KH, Thaler HT, Tan LK, *et al*. Immunohistochemically detected tumor cells in the sentinel lymph nodes of patients with breast carcinoma: Biologic metastases or procedural artifact? Cancer 2003;100:929–934.

Smith PAF, Harlow SP, Krag DN, Weaver DL. Submission of lymph node tissue for ancillary studies decreases accuracy of conventional breast cancer axillary node staging. Mod Pathol 1999;12:781–785.

Weaver DL, Krag DN, Manna EA, *et al*. Comparison of pathologist detected and automated computer-assisted image analysis detected sentinel lymph node micrometastases in breast cancer. Mod Pathol 2003;11:1159–1163.

Weaver DL. Occult "micrometastases" in ductal carcinoma in situ (DCIS): Investigative implications for sentinel lymph node biopsy. Cancer 2003;98:2083–2087.

Weaver DL. Sentinel lymph nodes and breast carcinoma: which micrometastases are clinically significant? Am J Surg Pathol 2003;27:842–845.

23

Sentinal Node Biopsy and Lymph Node Classification in the 6ᵗʰ Edition Staging Manual

Donald L Weaver

The growth and spread of breast cancer is a complex, multi-step process that constitutes an infinite continuum of potential prognostic subsets with opportunities for intervention. Regrettably, the continuum is far more complex than available treatment options, which are directed toward three simplified scenarios:

- Local disease with a low likelihood of metastatic spread and a higher likelihood of local recurrence;
- Local disease with regional spread and a quantifiable likelihood of distant metastases; and
- Distant metastatic disease with or without clinically detected local disease.

Therapeutic intensity is based on probability of recurrence and extent of disease. Toward this end, the American Joint Committee on Cancer (AJCC) and the International Union Against Cancer (UICC) have established objective criteria to quantify disease burden in the primary tumor (T), regional lymph nodes (N) and distant sites (M). Based on available outcome data, the individual criteria are combined to create four major prognostic groups, stage I, II, III and IV, including several clinically relevant subsets. Determining the presence or absence, and extent of regional lymph node metastases is currently the most important prognostic variable in invasive breast cancer. Pathologic evaluation and its inescapable influence on staging were discussed in Chapter 22. In this chapter, communication and documentation of the findings with an emphasis on stratification into the AJCC/UICC categorical node classification is discussed.

INTRODUCTION TO BREAST CANCER STAGING

Over the past four decades, quite remarkable changes have occurred in surgical and medical therapy for breast cancer. The most significant of these changes was the incredible transformation from a paradigm based on radical surgical excision of breast cancer that had progressed to include mastectomy, axillary dissection, removal of the latissimus dorsi, pectoralis major and minor muscles and dissection of the internal mammary lymph nodes to a paradigm that recognized the potential for and importance of subclinical systemic dissemination at the time of clinical diagnosis. This recognition

of subclinical metastatic disease prompted advances in medical chemotherapy, local radiation therapy and less radical surgery. Total mastectomy remains an important surgical option but the days of radical and super radical mastectomy are fading from the collective memory of physicians. In the absence of advanced local disease, treatment generally follows the strategy of removing the primary breast cancer with a varying amount of surrounding normal breast tissue (lumpectomy, tylectomy, excision biopsy, partial mastectomy, or quadrantectomy), treating the remainder of the breast with radiation and the remainder of the body with cytotoxic and/or hormonal chemotherapy. The decision between total mastectomy or partial mastectomy and radiation is not entirely non-biologic but is primarily driven by patient choice and recognition of the importance of maintaining a patient's positive body image. Numerous studies have demonstrated equivalent survival for the two primary surgical approaches to breast cancer and a few recent studies suggest a survival advantage for strategies utilizing radiation therapy, an observation that will need additional confirmation.

Following these tenets of primary breast cancer treatment, options for conservative therapy have now been extended to the surgical management of axillary lymph nodes. A sentinel node biopsy removes only a few nodes and these nodes are 3–4 times more likely than non-sentinel nodes to contain metastases when they are present. The technique is also accurate in predicting the final axillary node status. There is, however, a definable false negative rate, indicating that some patients who are classified as node negative will have undetected metastatic disease in the axilla. This raises an old question and a long-standing debate: is axillary dissection a diagnostic procedure providing prognostic information or is there therapeutic benefit to removal of the axillary nodes? The prevailing opinion favors prognosis but this is a hypothesis that is difficult to prove; removing positive nodes, whether an axillary dissection, low axillary sampling or sentinel node biopsy, may alter the natural history of the disease. Sentinel node trials cannot answer this question but they will determine whether directed removal of a few nodes is equivalent to axillary dissection. Results from large prospective clinical trials in the United States, Europe and Australia comparing sentinel node biopsy alone to axillary dissection are not currently available. Smaller studies and observational data suggest the procedure is a safe alternative to axillary dissection, thus it is being offered to patients as a surgical option. The overall false negative rate for an experienced surgeon will probably approach 5–6 %, which is higher than the 3 % recurrence rate after axillary dissection. However, the recurrence rate after sentinel node biopsy will be influenced by systemic chemotherapy and tangent field radiation to the lower axilla, both of which have the potential to decrease the maximum potential recurrence rate to a rate that may be much closer to or no different from axillary dissection. Those are the ethical arguments on which the trials offering sentinel node biopsy alone as one treatment arm are based. The fact that the expected differences in outcome are quite small is why the studies need to include thousands of patients and why it was important to include an axillary dissection control arm.

A discussion of sentinel lymph node biopsy and staging invariably gravitates toward discussion of the clinical significance of micrometastases warranting a brief discussion of established definitions for staging. A study from Memorial Hospital in New York City, published in 1971, demonstrated that patients with nodal metastases no larger than 2 mm had survival equivalent to patients with negative nodes. The lymph nodes were processed and evaluated by methods routine for that era. A subsequent study from the National Surgical Adjuvant Breast and Bowel Project (NSABP) confirmed the observation but also found that using a slightly smaller stratification threshold (1.3 mm) produced a more statistically significant outcome. Following these observations, the definition for micrometastases was established and incorporated into the AJCC/UICC staging system. Patients with no nodal metastases larger than 2 mm were classified as having micrometastases but were still included in stage IIA. A footnote in the manuals indicated that patients with micrometastases had survival similar to node negative patients.

An adequate axillary dissection should include at least 8–10 lymph nodes and often includes more. The median number of nodes available for evaluation after a sentinel node biopsy is two to three. This drastic reduction in number of nodes available for analysis has facilitated more thorough evaluation of sentinel nodes, including deeper sections and immunohistochemical stains, leading to an increased rate of micrometastasis detection. Many studies have investigated potential differences in outcome between patients with and without occult lymph node metastases. With rare exception, these studies have been retrospective. Utilizing deeper sections and special stains prospectively to identify micrometastases in sentinel nodes is strikingly similar in technique to historical retrospective studies evaluating the significance of occult metastases, the exceptional difference is the potential to influence treatment planning. The earliest retrospective studies utilized deeper sections from paraffin embedded lymph node tissue blocks from node negative patients. In some studies, the original glass slides were also reviewed and occasionally revealed metastases that had been overlooked by the original pathologist. Thus, two categories of occult metastases were created; those identified by additional sections and 'missed' metastases. In either case, the initial report of negative nodes determined treatment.

Occult metastases and micrometastases are not synonymous terms. A micrometastasis is defined by size and must be less than or equal to 2 mm in largest dimension. Metastases larger than 2 mm are often referred to as macrometastases. Occult metastases are not defined by size but are metastases that are initially overlooked then detected after additional evaluation. Most published studies evaluating occult metastases have not distinguished between micrometastases (≤2 mm) and macrometastases (>2 mm) and some have freely acknowledged that metastases larger than 2 mm were identified, therefore an appropriate lower threshold for metastases that are clinically significant cannot be extrapolated from these studies. In addition, sentinel nodes are evaluated more comprehensively than previous practice for axillary nodes. These issues indicate that further research is needed on sentinel nodes to determine the clinical significance of micrometastases and isolated tumor cell clusters within the context of current clinical practice. Two unresolved questions remain:

- Are micrometastases clinically and/or statistically significant; and
- If clinicial significance is demonstrated, what is the appropriate lower threshold for a significant metastasis?

Fortunately, the general approach to gross evaluation of sentinel nodes will limit the magnitude of undetected macrometastases and studies will be truly focused on the significance of micrometastases. A more complex issue is the potential difference in significance between micrometastases in the sentinel nodes of patients who elect no further axillary surgery and those who elect completion axillary dissection and have no further metastases detected. The former group represents a population that may have undetected macrometastases in regional lymph nodes.

PROGNOSIS AND THERAPY

BIOLOGIC AND CLINICAL SIGNIFICANCE OF MICROMETASTASES

From a biologic perspective, the expectation is that a difference in outcome exists between patients with and without micrometastases. It has been repeatedly demonstrated that survival decreases with increasing number of positive lymph nodes. The relationship is nearly linear when more than two lymph nodes are positive for metastatic disease; however, the incremental decrease in survival when only one or two lymph nodes is positive is less pronounced. This is primarily due to other risk factors that are highly correlated with positive nodes, including tumor size and grade. As the nodal tumor burden decreases from macrometastases to micrometastases to isolated tumor cells to negative nodes, the importance of the primary tumor variables takes precedence. The confounding variables make it extremely difficult to prove the hypothesis that micrometastases are biologically significant. Large, prospective randomized trials will have the best chance to demonstrate a statistical difference because the confounding variables should be randomly distributed between groups. However, establishing the risk of recurrence or survival for various combinations of tumor size, grade, and micrometastases will exceed the practical limits of a clinical trial. Answering these questions can only be determined within the context of large population-based registries or by combining data from many clinical trials.

A further complicating factor in exploring the biologic potential of micrometastases in lymph nodes is the bias that detection exerts on clinical behavior. In quantum physics, this is known as the Heisenberg uncertainty principle. In medicine, the lymph nodes must be removed in order to detect micrometastases and this alters the natural history of the disease. Modern oncologic practice is founded on the theory that once a tumor cell colony is vascularized, tumor cells have the potential to be shed into the blood or lymphatics, disseminate systemically, and potentially implant at distant sites. Vascularization occurs when a tumor colony reaches approximately 1 mm in greatest dimension, a size generally accepted to be below the threshold for clinical detection and therefore early in the course of clinical disease. However, this point of vascularization is a late event in the biologic course of any cancer and occurs much closer to the end of the maximum number of tumor doublings. This paradox has driven the modern approach to breast cancer, minimizing local surgical therapy and optimizing systemic therapy. The newest evidence supporting this approach can be found in gene expression profiling of breast cancer. This technique has demonstrated that a metastatic phenotype can be detected early in the clinical life of a breast tumor. In fact, even pre-invasive cancer has accumulated many of the genetic defects identified in metastatic cancers. This suggests that the biologic natural history of a breast tumor is set long before it can be clinically detected.

Thus, a primary tumor proliferates, interacts with the vascular system, and has the potential to colonize other sites systemically. The daughter colonies, whether in lymph nodes, bone marrow, or visceral organs, also have the potential to shed cells into the circulatory system. The standard surgical approach to breast cancer modifies the natural history of the disease by removing the primary tumor and lymph node metastases. Some tumors will be cured by this approach; however, without systemic therapy, most tumors would artificially re-enter a sub-clinical stage only to re-emerge clinically at some later point. Once tumor cells have disseminated from the primary tumor to the systemic circulation, opportunistic, clinically undetectable, distant tumor implants probably influence outcome more than the presence of detected and removed micrometastases in regional lymph nodes. An interest in understanding and exploring this latter hypothesis is driving research into the significance of bone marrow micrometastases and circulating tumor cells in blood. Preliminary studies suggest that bone marrow micrometastases are more predictive of outcome than regional lymph node micrometastases.

If it is accepted that increasing nodal tumor burden represents a continuum of increasingly worse biologic potential, with respect to tumor dissemination, then the more important question of clinical, not biologic, significance can be asked. Clinical significance balances the risk of recurrence and survival with the benefits and complications of therapy. Therapeutic decisions are based on empiric evidence and must be evaluated in the context of available treatment options; small differences in clinical outcome may not necessarily translate into differential treatment plans.

CONSEQUENCES OF COMPREHENSIVE NODAL EXAMINATION

It is highly unlikely that the biology of breast cancer has changed over the past decade or two and yet there has been a relative increase in the proportion of patients with node positive, stage II breast cancer between 1994 and 2000 despite advances in breast cancer screening. This is most likely attributable to the rapid dispersion of sentinel node biopsy and more comprehensive analysis of lymph nodes. These patients have been recruited from a group of patients that historically would have been classified as node negative. Any difference in prognosis would be expected to fall between patients with negative nodes and a single positive node. Relatively old data from the American College of Surgeons demonstrated a 9 % difference in overall survival and an 11 % difference in disease free survival at five years between patients with negative nodes and one positive node, however, these data did not control for tumor size. For patients with tumors less than 1 cm, more recent data from the early 1980s recorded in the United States Surveillance, Epidemiology and End Results (SEER) national database demonstrated a 4–5 % difference in 5 year overall survival between patients with negative nodes and those with 1–3 positive nodes. The difference increased to 9 % for patients with 1–2.9 cm tumors.

These data overstate the risk when only one node is positive and do not distinguish between micro and macrometastases. The relative outcome for the new group of patients with micrometastases detected should fall between historical node negative patients and patients with a single positive node. Thus, data in the literature can only help define the maximum potential differences; actual survival would be predicted to be much closer to the node negative group. Absolute 5-year survival ranges from 98–99 % for tumors under 1.0 cm and from 92–96 % for tumors 1–2.9 cm when nodes are negative. If a 2–3 % decrease in outcome can ultimately be demonstrated for patients with micrometastases, and chemotherapy can reduce the relative recurrence risk by 20 %, then the potential benefit of adding chemotherapy for treatment of patients with micrometastases is only about 0.5 %. Many patients may decide that this small incremental benefit does not outweigh the risk of chemotherapy. Alternatively stated, when only micrometastases are present in lymph nodes, therapeutic decisions should be influenced almost exclusively by primary tumor characteristics.

PREDICTIVE VALUE OF MICROMETASTASES

Two fundamental research questions, alluded to above, are being evaluated with sentinel node biopsy. The first is whether it is safe to omit axillary dissection when sentinel nodes are negative for metastases; the second is whether it is safe to omit axillary dissection when sentinel nodes are positive. The second question is associated with higher risk and is based on the observation that metastases are confined to the sentinel nodes in the majority of node positive patients. The clinical significance of micrometastases in these two situations is fundamentally different as well. The overall prognostic significance of micrometastases in sentinel nodes must first be determined in the context of the entire axilla. For this reason, the sentinel node trials evaluating the safety of sentinel node biopsy are ideal for posing this question because completion axillary dissection is required when sentinel nodes demonstrate any level of metastatic disease. The final axillary status can be used to evaluate the prognosis of micrometastases and small tumor cell clusters. When a sentinel node is positive and no further surgical examination of the axilla is undertaken, the categorical classification of any residual disease is unknown and macrometastases, micrometastases or isolated tumor cell clusters may remain undetected. In other words, the recurrence risk for a patient with micrometastases in sentinel nodes that foregoes axillary dissection may not be equivalent to a patient with micrometastases in sentinel nodes with no further disease detected in a completion axillary dissection. The AJCC/UICC staging manuals group these two patients into different categories by utilizing the '(sn)' suffix modifier when nodal classification is based only on examination of sentinel nodes. Patients and clinicians electing sentinel node biopsy alone when sentinel nodes are positive must understand the risk of residual disease and the options for alternative non-surgical treatment, including directed axillary radiation and/or the effects of adjuvant chemotherapy.

When sentinel nodes are positive for metastatic disease, the risk of involvement of non-sentinel nodes is 13 times higher than in patients with negative sentinel nodes. Approximately 40 % of patients with positive sentinel nodes will have additional axillary disease. If sentinel node metastases are no larger than 1 mm, the rate of non-sentinel node involvement is reduced to about 20 %. When stratified according to AJCC/UICC categories, it has been estimated that patients with micrometastases (>0.2 mm but not more than 2 mm) have a 35 % risk of non-sentinel node macrometastases (>2 mm) and patients with isolated tumor cell clusters (≤0.2 mm) have a 12 % risk of non-sentinel node macrometastases. These risks are somewhat higher than

the 5–6 % false negative rate when sentinel nodes are negative for metastases. The risk of non-sentinel node involvement is not equivalent to the risk of axillary recurrence; recurrence risk is influenced by any systemic or regional treatment. Although it may appear intuitive to assume the risk of axillary recurrence is higher in patients with positive sentinel nodes and no further axillary dissection, this has not yet been demonstrated in clinical trials.

COMMUNICATING AND DOCUMENTING THE LYMPH NODE EXAMINATION

The 6th edition of the AJCC/UICC staging manual is relatively robust in its options for categorizing nodal disease and places much more emphasis on semiquantitative nodal tumor burden than previous editions of the manual. It is not perfect and will undoubtedly need further refinement in the future. In the interim, there are ways in which pathologists can enhance communication of nodal tumor burden to clinicians through accurate documentation of nodal metastases. Throughout Chapter 22, there has been an emphasis on systematic and standardized approaches to the gross and microscopic examination of sentinel and non-sentinel lymph nodes. The same approach can be applied to documenting nodal disease. In general, the total number of involved nodes and the total number of examined nodes should be recorded. The College of American Pathologists also recommends that the size of the largest metastasis be recorded. Accurate nodal classification under the 6th edition staging manual requires this information; documenting metastasis size in the pathology report facilitates appropriate staging by clinicians and tumor registrars. The pathologist can most accurately determine node classification and, ideally, the pathology report should include the appropriate AJCC/UICC notation. In addition, axillary and/or systemic recurrence risks may be different for patients staged exclusively with sentinel node biopsy. When axillary dissection is omitted, the '(sn)' notation should always be appended to the N-classification.

RULES FOR MEASURING METASTASES

Nodal metastases are divided into three size categories that include metastases larger than 2 mm (macrometastases), metastases larger than 0.2 mm but no larger than 2 mm (micrometastases), and metastases less than or equal to 0.2 mm (isolated tumor cells or tumor cell clusters; ITCs). The most significant change in the 6th edition manual is a formal recognition of the prognostic significance of increasing numbers of positive nodes and the direct impact it has on overall stage (Table 23-1). One to three positive nodes are classified pN1, four to nine positive nodes are classified pN2 and 10 or more positive nodes are classified pN3.

TABLE 23-1

Summary of Lymph Node Staging (N-classification) AJCC/UICC Staging Manual, 6th edition

N-classification	#AN pos	IM SLN+	IM Clin+	IC	SC
pN0	No metastases or no metastases >0.2 mm				
pN1mi	Metastases >0.2 mm but none >2 mm				
pN1a	1–3	–	–	–	–
pN1b	0	+	–	–	–
pN1c	1–3	+	–	–	–
pN2a	4–9	–	–	–	–
pN2b	0	–	+	–	–
pN3a	≥10	–	–	–	–
	n.a.	n.a.	n.a.	+	–
pN3b	>3	+	–	–	–
	≥1	n.a.	+	–	–
pN3c	n.a.	n.a.	n.a.	n.a.	+

#AN pos = number of positive axillary lymph nodes; IM SLN+ = internal mammary lymph nodes positive by sentinel lymph node biopsy; IM Clin+ = internal mammary lymph nodes positive by clinical examination or by imaging studies (CT or ultrasound but not lymphoscintigraphy); IC = infraclavicular, level III axillary lymph nodes; SC = supraclavicular lymph nodes; '–' = negative; '+' = positive; n.a. = not applicable to the definition; the highest N-classification takes precedence

Solitary metastases pose no significant problem in measurement; the largest dimension in the plane of section is utilized for determining classification. When multiple metastases are present, the rules for measurement are the same as those for measuring the primary tumor; the size of the largest metastasis is used for classification. The rationale behind this method is that size of the metastasis is a surrogate for volume. Adding metastases over estimates volume more than utilizing the size of the largest metastasis which under estimates volume. When multiple small metastases are clustered, the size of the largest confluent metastatic focus is used. Occasionally, an additional section from the tissue block will demonstrate a larger confluent focus.

ISOLATED TUMOR CELLS AND TUMOR CELL CLUSTERS

Isolated tumor cells and small tumor cell clusters no larger than 0.2 mm (ITCs) represent a new category of metastases in the 6th edition of the staging manual. This category was created specifically to accommodate the increased incidence of minute micrometastases detected in sentinel nodes. For reasons discussed above and primarily due to statistical issues related to detection, ITCs are considered to have a prognosis similar to negative

nodes and are classified as pN0. As might be expected for a new category, ITCs have been problematic with respect to classification and documentation. The pN0 designation has been used synonymously with negative nodes and the conflict between the prognostic and colloquial use of pN0 has created some confusion. Lymph nodes containing ITCs should be reported as positive nodes regardless of the prognostic implication, and appropriate descriptors can alleviate some of the confusion. Positive lymph nodes in this category can be descriptively reported as 'positive for isolated tumor cell clusters' to more clearly communicate the findings. In addition, the size of the largest metastasis should be reported. Microscopic field diameters for each objective can be utilized to estimate metastasis size with sufficient accuracy for nodal classification. For example, a patient with a 0.1 mm metastasis in one of two sentinel nodes without examination of additional axillary nodes would be reported as 'one of two nodes positive for isolated tumor cell clusters (1/2) (pN0(i+)(sn)), largest metastasis measures 0.1 mm'. The '(i+)' designation was originally intended to indicate that metastases were detected by immunohistochemical stains. However, many pathologists recognized that ITCs could be detected with routine stains. The '(i+)' designation was subsequently modified to include all ITCs identified regardless of whether IHC was used. Therefore, 'i+' can be considered synonymous with 'isolated tumor cells or clusters identified'. Although redundant, use of text descriptors, size of metastasis, and the pN0(i+) notation ensure accurate clinical interpretation of the pathology findings.

MICROMETASTASES

In past editions of the staging manuals, micrometastases were distinctively notated and in a footnote to the overall stage table, prognosis was suggested to be similar to patients with negative nodes. Despite the prognostic implication of the footnote, metastases have always had equal influence on overall stage regardless of their size. The increasing incidence of detecting metastases at the extreme lower end of the spectrum of micrometastases necessitated creation of a lower defining threshold. In the 6th edition, the presence of micrometastases still influences overall stage but their prognostic implication has been left open with the omission of the footnote. Micrometastases are currently defined as any tumor deposit larger than 0.2 mm but none larger than 2 mm and are separately notated as pN1mi. Considering the more comprehensive analysis to which sentinel nodes are subject, the categorical distinction between micro and macrometastases should now be more reliable.

Use of text descriptors, metastasis size and AJCC/UICC notation can also enhance reporting of micrometastases. For example, a patient with two of ten axillary nodes positive, one containing a 1.2 mm metastasis and the other containing a few isolated tumor cells in the subcapsular sinus would be reported as 'two of ten nodes positive for micrometastases (2/10)(pN1mi), largest metastasis measures 1.2 mm'. When axillary dissection has been omitted and only sentinel node biopsy performed, the '(sn)' designator should be appended to the notation.

SPECIAL SITUATIONS WITH MICROMETASTASES

There are rare occasions when strict application of the staging rules may not serve patients' best interest and in these situations, the pathologist's judgment and common sense must prevail. The overall objective is to place patients into groups with similar risk of recurrence based on tumor burden. Thus, when tumor burden is not fairly represented by the nodal classification, this should be communicated to the clinician in the pathology report. The most blatant example can be observed in metastatic lobular carcinoma when a large part of a node contains single tumor cells; no focus is larger than 0.2 mm but the total of the tumor cells would exceed the volume of a micrometastasis. Frequently, a deeper section or CK IHC stain can demonstrate a confluent focus larger than 2 mm and the conflict will be resolved; however, this will not always be the case. If the node is of average size and 10–20 % of the lymph node section surface area demonstrates a moderately dense single cell, infiltrating pattern, there is a fair chance that the recurrence risk will be more closely aligned with a higher node classification. In our own practice, we would describe this discrepancy in a comment explaining that although the strict nodal classification would be pN0 we would expect the recurrence risk to be closer to a patient with an axillary macrometastasis (pN1a). If four or more nodes are involved in this fashion, the pN2a classification may be appropriate. When a pathologist chooses to deviate from the strict rules, the best defense is an accurate description of the findings so that another pathologist can easily understand the predicament. In the example above, features that would be useful to describe include the cross sectional size of the node, the size of the area of involvement, the proportional (%) area of involvement, and the density of the tumor cell infiltrate (e.g., moderately dense, or nearly confluent).

Involvement of four nodes with minimal tumor is much more problematic as the pathologist is faced with a conflict between pN0 (ITCs) or pN1mi (micrometastases) and a pN2 classification. Most sentinel node series document a median number of two or three sentinel nodes but four or more sentinel nodes is not so unusual that it is surprising. It is surprising to observe more than three sentinel nodes positive with minimal disease. The pN2 classification group contains patients with at least four and as many as nine positive nodes. It is unlikely that patients with minimal nodal involvement would have a recurrence risk equivalent to macrometastases in four or more nodes and, as in the

example of lobular carcinoma; variation in interpretation of the rules may under or over estimate recurrence risk. The presence of only rare isolated tumor cells or clusters in four nodes should not dissuade a pathologist from utilizing the pN0(i+) classification. Likewise, one or two nodes with micrometastases and additional nodes with only isolated tumor cell clusters should not dissuade use of the pN1mi classification. However, the true dilemma arises when the metastases are at the threshold between ITCs and micrometastases or between micrometastases and macrometastases. Additional sections and CK IHC stains may resolve the issue, particularly when several clusters of tumor cells are adjacent to one another and one or more clusters is at the 0.2 or 2 mm size threshold. When four or more nodes each contain one or more metastases at or near a size threshold, recurrence risk should again be considered and a more thorough description of the extent of nodal involvement should be documented in the pathology report. For example, a patient with four axillary nodes positive, each containing one or more metastases that are close to 2 mm should receive a descriptive comment that suggests node classification and recurrence risk may be closer to a patient with one to three nodes positive for macrometastases (pN1a). In each imagined exception scenario the pathologist should understand that nodal tumor burden is a continuum and consider whether the total nodal tumor burden, and estimated recurrence risk for that patient, justify altering the nodal classification.

Occasionally, clusters of tumor cells can be identified within afferent lymphatics leading to lymph nodes. This raises the issue of in transit metastases; however, these occurrences should be classified according to AJCC/UICC rules for metastases clearly within the boundaries of a lymph node. When disease in afferent lymphatics is an isolated finding, this can be clarified in a comment. When one or more nodes are positive for metastases, afferent lymphatic disease adjacent to an uninvolved node should be considered equivalent to an additional positive node and the size of the largest metastasis should determine the node classification. Disease in afferent lymphatics should not be confused with extranodal extension. Extranodal extension should be separately noted in the pathology report when metastatic tumor cells are observed within the adipose tissue outside the node capsule. This can occur by direct extension from an involved node or by proliferation and extension of disease from within lymphatics independent of an observed node. Extranodal extension has been associated with increased axillary recurrence risk and when observed in sentinel nodes has been associated with a high risk for non-sentinel node involvement.

IMPORTANCE OF 'SN' MODIFIER

The 'sn' modifier is used to indicate that node classification is based exclusively on evaluation of sentinel nodes. This is a critical distinction because of the potentially different recurrence risks in patients undergoing staging without full axillary dissection. When sentinel nodes are negative, the 'sn' modifier communicates the risk associated with the false negative rate for sentinel node biopsy. As discussed above, clinical trials are still evaluating this risk and it may not be substantially different from patients with negative nodes determined from a complete axillary dissection. Differences in recurrence risk when sentinel nodes are positive and no further axillary dissection is elected may be more significant and deserve to be categorized and tracked separate from complete axillary staging. When sentinel nodes are positive, the incidence of residual disease in non-sentinel nodes ranges from approximately 10–50 % depending on the size and quantity of disease in the sentinel nodes and the primary tumor characteristics.

The risk of recurrence for patients with positive sentinel nodes and no further axillary dissection is based on the risk of undetected subclinical axillary and systemic disease whereas the recurrence risk for an equivalently staged patient after axillary dissection is based primarily on subclinical systemic disease. The importance of separating these two groups of patients at present is based on objective incidence data. Whether true differences exist in recurrence and survival will need to be addressed in ongoing and future clinical trials. When completion axillary dissection is performed after sentinel node biopsy, the 'sn' modifer should be omitted from the revised nodal classification and the total number of positive nodes together with the total number of examined nodes should be clearly documented in the pathology report. When the sentinel node biopsy and axillary dissection are performed at different times or in different institutions, this requires review of the previous sentinel node findings and a summative comment or addendum in the pathology report of the axillary dissection.

MACROMETASTASES

Although the term macrometastases is used colloquially and in this chapter, there is no specific definition for macrometastases within the staging manuals. The category is defined by exclusion for metastases that do not fit the defining characteristics for ITCs or micrometastases and thus are metastases larger than 2 mm in greatest dimension. The important change in the 6th edition manual is the incorporation of the prognostic significance of the number of nodes positive for metastatic disease. When any metastasis is > 2 mm and one to three axillary nodes are positive, the classification is pN1a, four to nine positive nodes is pN2a and, 10 or more positive nodes is pN3a. This change aligned the staging classification with the generally applied clinical risk categories used to guide adjuvant treatment for patients with breast cancer.

INTERNAL MAMMARY NODES

During the era of the radical and super-radical mastectomy, dissection of the internal mammary lymph nodes was undertaken. A positive internal mammary lymph node was regarded as a poor prognostic feature. Most studies of internal mammary node status did not evaluate the interaction between internal mammary node status and axillary node status. In most cases with positive internal mammary nodes, axillary nodes are also positive; therefore, the internal mammary node status would not generally impact decisions regarding systemic chemotherapy. Potential benefits to identifying internal mammary nodes are improved prognostic prediction and opportunity for surgical excision. The morbidity associated with internal mammary excision was not trivial since the procedure historically required a sternotomy. In a randomized study with long-term follow-up of patients with internal mammary excision, there was no improvement in survival. The procedure was generally abandoned as more conservative primary breast surgery was adopted. The data at present demonstrate that patients with either axillary nodes or internal mammary nodes positive have similar survival but patients with involvement of both nodal groups have a relative decrease in survival.

With the introduction of sentinel lymph node biopsy, comparisons between overt internal mammary node metastases detected by imaging studies and microscopic disease has become possible. The 6th edition manual recognizes the additive adverse prognostic outcome associated with co-existent internal mammary and axillary disease. In the absence of axillary metastases, internal mammary disease is classified as pN1b if detected by sentinel lymph node biopsy (SLNB) and pN2b if detected by imaging (CT or ultrasound) or clinical examination. If 1–3 axillary nodes are positive and internal mammary nodes are positive, they are classified pN1c if detected by SLNB and pN3b if detected by imaging or clinical examination. If more than 3 axillary nodes are positive and internal mammary nodes are positive, regardless of detection method, they are classified pN3b (see Summary of Node Staging table).

INFRACLAVICULAR NODES

It used to be more common for surgeons to submit axillary lymph nodes to the pathologist either separated or marked into the three traditional axillary levels. More recently, surgeons performing an axillary dissection have omitted dissecting level III infraclavicular nodes in favor of a level I–II dissection with intra-operative palpation of level III nodes and removal only if an abnormality is detected. Only in rare instances are level III nodes involved in the absence of level I or II metastases. The usual scenario with level III nodal disease is a high number of positive axillary nodes. Involvement of infraclavicular level III nodes is classified pN3a and no less than overall stage IIIC. This is a significant change from previous staging practice. Pathologists must be sure that level III nodal specimens are separately submitted and that surgeons specify the axillary level on sentinel node biopsies. Involvement of level III nodes will usually be accompanied by locally advanced disease and is often detectable by ultrasound examination of the infraclavicular region allowing fine needle aspirate of suspicious nodes. In one recent series, approximately one-third of patients with locally advanced disease demonstrated positive infraclavicular nodes. Overall survival was 58 % with positive infraclaviclar nodes compared to 83 % overall survival for patients without infraclavicular disease. Patients with known infraclavicular disease detected by ultrasound and positive fine needle aspirate biopsy can be evaluated for metastatic disease and immediately treated with chemotherapy without any further immediate surgery.

SUPRACLAVICULAR NODES

For nearly 100 years, metastases to supraclavicular nodes have been associated with very poor prognosis and 5-year survival rates have ranged from 5–30 %. Classification of patients with positive supraclavicular nodes has vacillated with each recent revision of the staging manual. The 5th edition recognized the very poor prognosis associated with supraclavicular disease and classified these patients as M1, equivalent to metastases to bone, brain, liver or lung. Patients with stage IV (M1) disease are usually treated with palliative therapy focused on alleviating symptoms rather than curative therapy. When pre- and post-operative chemotherapy are combined with surgery and radiation, patients with supraclavicular metastases have 5 and 10-year survival rates of 41 % and 31 %, respectively. These more recent outcomes are similar to survival rates for patients with locally advanced breast cancer without supraclavicular metastases and are considerably better than patients with distant metastases. In recognition of these improved outcomes, patients with supraclavicular disease are classified as pN3c and, providing no distant metastatic disease is present, as overall stage IIIC. The special stage IIIC classification is new for the 6th edition and will assist in further data accumulation and evaluation of this subset of patients with positive supraclavicular, infraclavicular, or combined axillary and internal mammary lymph nodes.

ANCILLARY MOLECULAR STUDIES

Another unresolved issue in sentinel node analysis is the degree to which special techniques should be applied

to enhance the pathologist's ability to detect microscopic disease. Three general strategies for enhanced detection of metastases have been employed including serial or deeper sections into the paraffin tissue block, immunohistochemistry and molecular techniques employing reverse transcriptase polymerase chain reaction (RT-PCR) to detect tumor derived messenger RNA. RT-PCR appears to be an overly sensitive technique; in some studies virtually any patient can be converted to PCR node positive. When tissue has been removed from sentinel nodes for molecular analysis, this should be clearly documented in the pathology report because of the high incidence of histologic misclassification when less than the entire node has been examined. When results of molecular studies are known, the 'mol' modifier should be used; positive results are indicated by '(mol+)' and negative results by '(mol–).' Tissue sparing techniques, including scraping the cut surfaces of lymph nodes or fine needle aspiration, reduce the incidence of histologic misclassification and allow for more objective evaluation of the utility of molecular evaluation of sentinel nodes. Adjusting the sensitivity of the assay may also provide more useful clinical stratification.

SUGGESTED READINGS
Breast Cancer Staging

Benson JR, Weaver DL, Mittra I, Hayashi M. The TNM staging system and breast cancer. Lancet Oncol 2003;4:56–60.

Greene FL, Page DL, Fleming ID, et al. eds. AJCC Cancer Staging Manual (6th edition). New York: Springer, 2002.

Singletary SE, Allred C, Ashley P, et al. Revision of the American Joint Committee on Cancer Staging System for Breast Cancer. J Clin Oncol 2002;20:3628–3636.

Singletary SE, Greene FL, Sobin LH. Classification of isolated tumor cells: clarification of the 6th Edition of the American Joint Committee on Cancer Staging Manual. Cancer 2003;98:2740–2741.

Sobin LH, Witteking Ch (eds). TNM Classification of Malignant Tumours, 6th Edition. New York: Wiley-Liss, 2002.

Internal Mammary, Infraclavicular and Supraclavicular Metastases

Brito RA, Valero VV, Buzdar AU, et al. Long-term results of combined-modality therapy for locally advanced breast cancer with ipsilateral supraclavicular metastases: The University of Texas M.D. Anderson Cancer Center experience. J Clin Oncol 2001;19:629–633.

Newman LA, Keurer HM, Fornage B, et al. Adverse prognostic significance of infraclavicular lymph nodes detected by ultrasonography in patients with locally advanced breast cancer. Am J Surg 2001;181:313–318.

Veronesi U, Marubini E, Mariani L, et al. The dissection of internal mammary nodes does not improve the survival of breast cancer patients: 30-year results of a randomized trial. Eur J Cancer 1999;35:1320–1325.

24 Molecular Markers in Invasive Breast Cancer

Syed K Mohsin

In the management of patients with invasive breast cancer (IBC), two important questions must be answered about the use of systemic therapy: is the risk-to-benefit ratio high enough to use *any* form of adjuvant therapy, and which type of treatment would be most beneficial in reducing the risk of recurrence and death? In this setting, a prognostic factor is defined as any measurement available at the time of diagnosis or surgery that is associated with disease-free (DFS) or overall survival (OS) in the absence of systemic adjuvant therapy. A predictive factor is defined as any measurement associated with response to a particular therapy. Molecular markers in breast cancer refine the prognostic value of staging and histopathologic variables, such as histologic grade, and predict response to a particular systemic therapeutic agent. This chapter will focus on molecular markers as defined above in clinical management of breast cancer, including those that are well established as well as those which are currently considered potentially important for new targeted therapies on the horizon.

Nearly all the molecular markers discussed here are assessed by immunohistochemistry (IHC) in pathology laboratories. The evaluation of these markers has such an important impact on treatment decision in breast cancer patients that without strict quality control and standardized assays, there exists a marked potential to report meaningless results to the treating physicians. Panels of experts endorsed by the National Institute of Health have published guidelines to conduct studies to establish technically and clinically validated for molecular markers to make them useful in the clinical setting. Unfortunately, these guidelines have not been fully adopted and for most molecular markers, there are several issues about standardization and validation. These will be highlighted for all those markers for which such information exists.

ESTABLISHED MOLECULAR MARKERS

HORMONE RECEPTORS

Estrogen receptor (ER) is a nuclear transcription factor that is involved in breast development, growth,

---

HORMONE RECEPTORS – FACT SHEET

Biology and Indication to Test

▶ ER is the main molecular pathway involved in breast development, growth, differentiation, and tumorigenesis and regulates expression of many genes including PR
▶ It is the most well-established biomarker in breast cancer
▶ ER and PR are assessed in all primary invasive breast cancers today to predict response to endocrine therapy, such as SERMS, aromatase inhibitors, etc.

Methods of Assessment

▶ Both ER and PR can be assessed by biochemical ligand binding assay (LBA) on frozen tissue or immunohistochemistry (IHC) on paraffin sections
▶ Nearly all the clinical data utilized today to make treatment decisions is based on standardized LBA, but no laboratory offers ER or PR measurements by this method
▶ Laboratories worldwide measure ER and PR by IHC but only a handful of standardized methods exist for these two markers
▶ The cut-off to define positive varies from 1–20%, 10% being the most common, but patients with even 1% ER/PR-positive tumors benefit from hormonal therapy

Incidence of 'Positivity'

▶ About 70% of all breast cancers are ER positive
▶ About 60–65% of all breast cancers are PR positive
▶ Reported incidence varies because of technical and interpretive problems

Clinical Use

▶ ER and PR are weak prognostic factors in untreated patients, ~10% survival benefit
▶ ER and PR are strong predictors of response to hormonal therapies, both in adjuvant and metastatic settings, with about 50% proportional reduction in risk of recurrence and/or death
▶ ER and PR negative breast cancers generally do not respond to hormonal therapy

Issues

▶ Concordance between LBA and IHC is 85% or less requiring proper validation studies for IHC
▶ Paucity of published validated methods for ER and PR and lack of awareness of need for proper validation of these assays

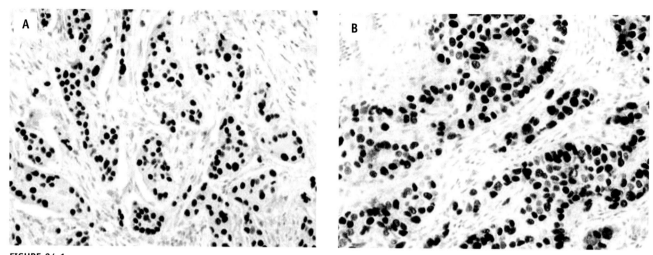

FIGURE 24-1

Estrogen receptor (A) and progesterone receptor (B) are nuclear receptors which often show variable intensity of staining in the tumor cells.

differentiation, and tumorigenesis and it regulates expression of genes, such as pS2, progesterone receptor (PR), and bcl-2. Therefore the presence of PR in a tumor is an indicator of an intact estrogen-response pathway and suggests that ER is present and functional. ER and PR levels are strongly and inversely correlated with histologic grade, proliferation rate, HER-2/neu, and p53. ER and PR determinations are established prognostic and predictive factors in the routine management of patients with breast cancer, and today they are assessed primarily as predictive factors for response to therapeutic and adjuvant hormonal therapy, such as tamoxifen, other selective estrogen receptor modulators (SERM), and aromatase inhibitors.

There are two main methods for assessing hormone receptors in breast cancer, i.e., biochemical ligand binding assay (LBA) and IHC. For nearly two decades, ER and PR used to be measured on frozen tissue using LBA. Using standardized LBA, it was established in numerous randomized clinical trials that about 70 % invasive breast cancers (IBC) express ER and PR. Women with ER-positive tumors derive significant benefit from 5 years of tamoxifen treatment with about a 40–50 % reduction in the odds of recurrence and death, whereas those with ER-negative tumors do not. The benefit is the greatest when the ER level is over 100 fmol/mg protein. The value of PR by itself in predicting benefit from tamoxifen in the adjuvant setting is less established but it is clear that PR adds to the predictive value of ER. Both ER and PR status predict response to therapeutic hormonal therapy in metastatic breast cancer, with about 50–60 % of all patients with ER-positive tumors benefiting from first-line hormone therapy, compared to 5–10 % of patients with ER-negative tumors. Recently, it has been suggested that ER and PR also predict benefit from tamoxifen by reducing recurrence rates in patients with ductal carcinoma *in situ*. As a prognostic factor in the absence of systemic therapy, ER status is a time-dependent variable; as

follow-up time lengthens, the advantage of ER positivity in terms of relapse and death decreases and ultimately disappears. The value of PR status as a prognostic factor is more doubtful.

For the last two decades, IHC has become the method of choice for ER and PR assessment (Figure 24-1). Several comparative studies have compared IHC and LBA and for ER, the reported concordance between the two methods ranges from 70–90 %, while for PR determination it is 70–80 %. This means that the use of IHC for ER and PR requires its own validation studies. Some validation studies for ER and a rare one for PR have been published, but most laboratories have not adopted those assays leading to major problems in the quality of ER and PR testing in breast cancer. This fact is highlighted by data from the UK external quality assurance program showing about 20 % false-negative ER results: there are several reasons for these, including poor fixation, different antigen retrieval methods, antibodies, detection systems, and different cut-offs to define a positive result. For example, the most common cut-off to define ER positively is 10 % but there is convincing data that patients with even 1 % ER positive tumor cells benefit from hormonal therapy. It is therefore, very important to adopt validated methods to measure ER and PR in order to report reliable results to the clinicians.

HER-2/NEU

The proto-oncogene HER-2/*neu* is a member of the human epidermal growth factor receptor family and encodes a transmembrane tyrosine kinase receptor. It is involved in several important regulatory pathways involving proliferation, survival, cell motility, and invasion. The most common methods used to assess HER-2/*neu* are fluorescent *in situ* hybridization (FISH) for

HER-2/*neu* – FACT SHEET

Biology and indication to test

▸ HER-2/*neu* is a proto-oncogene that encodes for a transmembrane tyrosine kinase growth receptor
▸ It is involved in several regulatory pathways in breast involving proliferation, survival, cell motility and invasion
▸ It is assessed for both prognosis and prediction of response to trastuzumab, chemotherapy, and endocrine therapy

Methods of Assessment

▸ HER-2/*neu* has been mostly measured by IHC, but also by FISH
▸ There are more than 20 IHC antibodies available for this marker, but none have become the standard, however, HercepTest is an FDA approved test and is the most commonly employed in several countries
▸ For treatment decisions, equivocal IHC results should be verified by FISH
▸ The cut-off to define HER-2/*neu* positivity by IHC is moderate to strong complete membrane reactivity in at least 10 % of tumor cells and a HER-2-to-chromosome 17 ratio of ≥2 by FISH
▸ The best method to assess this marker to predict response to trastuzumab remains to be established

Incidence of 'Positivity'

▸ Overexpression/amplification is reported in 10–34 % IBC
▸ Protein overexpression and gene amplification are concordant in over 90 % cases
▸ Reported incidence varies because of technical and interpretation problems

Clinical Use

▸ HER-2/*neu* is associated strongly with shorter DFS and OS in all IBC
▸ HER-2/*neu* predicts response to trastuzumab, which targets this receptor
▸ There is growing data, although still controversial, that HER-2/*neu* overexpression predicts for a relative sensitivity to adriamycin-based therapy

Issues

▸ No standardized IHC tests have been validated in appropriate clinical settings
▸ There is some data suggesting FISH may be more reliable test for HER-2/*neu* assessment, but it is technically difficult and 5–10 times more expensive than IHC
▸ Reliability for testing HER-2/*neu* by both IHC and FISH may be related to laboratory experience

gene amplification and IHC for protein overexpression. In over 90 % of cases, gene amplification is associated with protein overexpression. Using FISH or IHC, HER-2/*neu* is found in 10–34 % of breast cancers. High HER-2/*neu* in breast cancer is associated with high histologic grade and tumor aggressiveness.

Studies that measured HER-2/*neu* gene amplification found that it was predictive of shorter DFS and OS in node-positive and node-negative patients. More recent studies assessed HER-2/*neu* protein expression by IHC (Figure 24-2) with conflicting results, particularly in

the node-negative subgroups. Deficiencies in the design of the studies, different definitions for scoring positivity and lack of a widely accepted standard methodology for detection are largely responsible for these unclear results, but it appears that there are specific clinical settings where HER-2/*neu* status is potentially useful. In the absence of systemic therapy, HER-2/*neu* is a marker of shorter DFS and OS. For patients receiving adriamycin-based therapy HER-2/*neu* may be a marker of relative sensitivity. Finally, HER-2/*neu* is a marker of response to its targeted therapy, i.e., trastuzumab.

Most studies that have assessed the value of HER-2/*neu* in these clinical settings have used IHC with different antibodies, detection systems, and cut-offs to define positivity; no standardized validated method exists for HER-2/*neu* testing. In studies looking at the predictive value of HER-2/*neu* for trastuzumab, initially a cocktail of two antibodies was used, but later retrospective concordance studies generated data that led to FDA approval of HercepTest for IHC and PathVysion for FISH. Today, these are the two most commonly used methods for HER-2/*neu* assessment. Both have some problems. For example, IHC testing leads to about 15–30 % indeterminate cases, which need to be resolved by FISH. On the other hand, FISH is technically difficult and costs nearly 8–10 times more than IHC. Overall, assessment of HER-2/*neu* is problematic and requires experience as well as the establishement of rigorous quality control procedures. Laboratories performing HER-2/*neu* testing should also be involved in an external quality assurance program. It is hoped that results of currently ongoing large clinical trials will help establish the best approach to measure this marker in breast cancer.

Ki-67 PROLIFERATION INDEX

Assessment of proliferative activity is one of many promising prognostic factors. Several IHC methods have been utilized, including thymidine-labeling index, BrdU index, Ki-67, MIB-1, Ki-S5, Ki-S11, proliferating cell nuclear antigen (PCNA), topoisomerase II alpha (Ki-S1), mitosin and Ki-S2. Among these markers, Ki-67, which is expressed in all phases of the cell cycle except G0, is considered to be the best. MIB-1 antibody detects the Ki-67 protein in paraffin sections (Figure 24-3). Ki-67 proliferation is ideally measured by point counting or image analysis of 500 to 1000 cells and reported as percent positive. A high Ki-67 proliferation index is associated with higher histologic grade, absence of hormone receptors, larger tumors and nodepositivity.

Several studies have shown a significant correlation between a high Ki-67 proliferation index and shorter DFS or OS by univariate analysis, but only a half of these confirmed its significance in multivariate analysis. In the absence of adjuvant therapy in node-negative breast cancer, a high Ki-67 proliferation index is associated with significantly shorter DFS and OS. Since cytotoxic chemotherapeutic agents target the dividing cells,

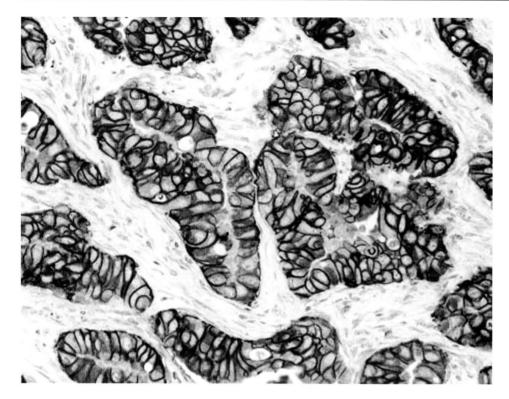

FIGURE 24-2

HER-2/*neu* is a transmembrane receptor. IHC signal is membranous but tends to show a cytoplasmic blush next to the cell membrane. This should not be mistaken for cytoplasmic staining because it simply reflects a sectioning artifact.

Ki-67 PROLIFERATION INDEX – FACT SHEET

Biology and Indication to Test

▸ Proliferative activity is one measure of tumor aggressiveness
▸ It is a potential target of certain therapies used in breast cancer
▸ High proliferation rates in breast cancer are associated with poor outcome

Methods of Assessment

▸ Ki-67 protein is expressed in all phases of the cell cycle, except G0
▸ MIB-1 antibody measures Ki-67 in paraffin-embedded tissue sections
▸ Other antibodies include PCNA, Ki-S5, Ki-S11, Ki-S2 and Ki-S1, which also measure proliferation-related proteins, but MIB-1 is the most commonly used antibody
▸ MIB-1 proliferation index ideally requires point-counting of 500–1000 cells or image analysis and is reported as percent positive

Incidence of 'Positivity'

▸ Difficult to ascertain the true incidence of 'high' proliferation rate due to lack to standard definition

Clinical Use

▸ High proliferation rate is used in a subset of patients with equivocal prognosis to identify those who may be at risk of recurrence or death and may benefit from adjuvant therapy

Issues

▸ Lack of standardized methods to assess Ki-67 proliferation index
▸ The cut-off to define 'high' proliferation index is not established
▸ Validation studies using standardized methods have not been performed

it is hypothesized that patients with rapidly proliferating tumors may derive more benefit from such therapies. However, the data on the predictive value of Ki-67 proliferation index, as well as other markers of proliferation is conflicting, showing either no difference in benefit in tumors with low versus high Ki-67 index or increased responsiveness in tumors with high Ki-67 index in the neoadjuvant setting.

Although the assessment of Ki-67 index is technically not difficult, its interpretation/scoring is somewhat tedious and the major issue is lack of a well-defined cut-off to identify slowly versus rapidly proliferating tumors. It is also not uncommon to see an extremely high Ki-67 index, i.e., > 75 % positive cells, which may be related to the fact that cells in all phases of the cell cycle express Ki-67. Therefore, S-phase fraction or phosphorylated histones may be better markers of tumor proliferation. S-phase fraction assessed on frozen tissue by flow cytometry is a validated method for determining tumor proliferation but this is not true for flow cytometry on paraffin sections. Studies on other IHC markers have not been performed. It is recommended that a measure of tumor proliferation is routinely reported on all IBC but the pathologists need to validate their method.

p53

The p53 tumor suppressor gene encodes a 53 kD nuclear phosphoprotein, which is involved in cell cycle regula-

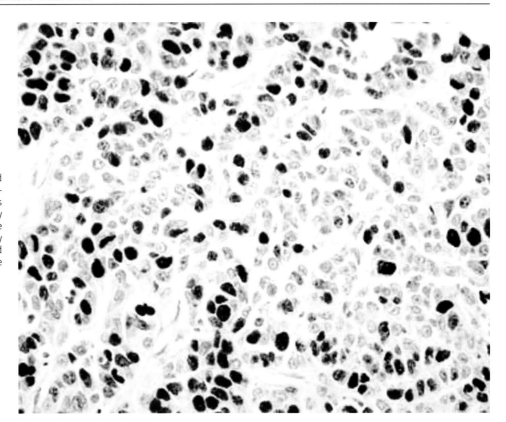

FIGURE 24-3

Ki-67 proliferation index as assessed by MIB-1 antibody. The amount of Ki-67 antigen varies in different phases of the cell cycle and it is reflected by variable intensity of staining in the nuclei. The index is calculated by point counting 500–1000 cells and reportig the percentage of positive cells.

---

p53 – FACT SHEET

Biology and Indication to Test

▶ p53 is a classic tumor suppressor gene that encodes for a nuclear phoshoprotein
▶ It is involved in regulation of cell cycle, DNA repair, and apoptosis
▶ Loss of p53 function is associated with poor outcome and it is one of the most established poor prognostic factors in breast cancer

Methods of Assessment

▶ IHC detects mutated (non-functional) p53 protein due to its prolonged half-life
▶ Other methods include SSCP and sequencing
▶ IHC is the most common method and a number of antibodies are available against p53
▶ Arbitrary cut-off for p53-positivity is 10%

Incidence of 'Positivity'

▶ About a third or more breast cancers have mutated p53

Clinical Use

▶ p53 inactivation is associated with worse clinical outcome, i.e., ~50% increased risk of recurrence or death
▶ p53 overexpression may predict response to certain types of chemotherapies in breast cancer but the data is controversial

Issues

▶ The sensitivity of different antibodies to p53 is variable and nearly 13 antibodies are available to choose from
▶ Some antibodies may detect wild-type p53 and results from such assays require caution
▶ p53 is not very useful in the clinical setting

---

tion, DNA repair, and apoptosis. Alterations in this gene are the most frequent genetic changes reported in many malignancies, including breast cancer. Overexpression of p53 seems to be relatively independent of axillary node status and menopausal status, weakly related to tumor size, and strongly associated with DNA ploidy, other measures of proliferation, steroid receptors and nuclear grade. It is considered to be a modest, but not very useful, prognostic factor in breast cancer.

Techniques to measure p53 overexpression/mutation include IHC, based on the prolonged half-life of mutated p53, or PCR-based amplification with screening using single-strand conformation polymorphism assays (SSCP) and sequencing. Most p53 abnormalities occur as spontaneous somatic events. IHC is the most commonly employed method (Figure 24-4), and several antibodies exist that detect mutated p53. Nearly one-third of breast cancers have mutated p53 gene. In node-

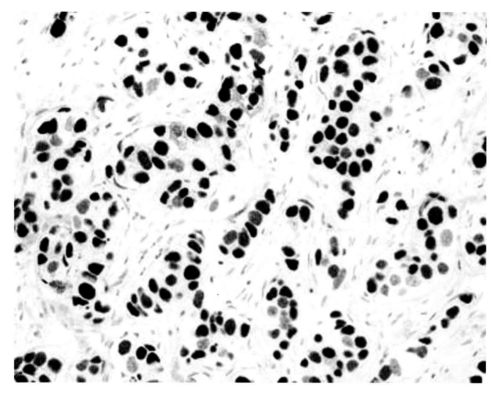

FIGURE 24-4

p53 tumor suppressor protein is detected in the tumor nuclei by IHC because of its prolonged half-life.

negative patients who received no systemic adjuvant therapy, p53 combined with other prognostic factors appeared to be a modestly effective marker to identify patients at high risk for early disease recurrence and/or death, for whom the use of adjuvant chemotherapy may be justified. There is some data suggesting that patients with p53-positive tumors may benefit from radiation therapy, CMF and adriamycin-based therapy, however, the findings have not been consistent.

Besides not being very useful in the clinical settings, there are several issues in measuring p53 by IHC. At least 13 antibodies have been used in different studies and some compared IHC to SSCP analysis, showing different sensitivities of these antibodies with staining rates for the different antibodies ranging from 18–36 %. Lack of unanimity of results in the studies mentioned above may be due to differences in technique, study design and variety of treatments, or the population. At this time, p53 is not routinely measured in IBC.

POTENTIALLY USEFUL MARKERS WITH TARGETED THERAPIES

ANGIOGENESIS

Angiogenesis is a process by which new vessels generate from existing ones. It is a critical step in tumor

---

ANGIOGENESIS – FACT SHEET

Biology
▶ Angioinvasion is an essential process of malignant behavior and angiogenesis is one component of this process
▶ The process is regulated by stimulators, such as VEGF, VEGFRs, TP, Tie-2, and inhibitors, such as HIF, TSP-1, TIMPs, etc.

Methods of Assessment
▶ IHC using antibodies to Factor VIII-related antigen, CD-31 and CD-34 and imaging modalities such as Doppler ultrasound, and thermography
▶ IHC is the most commonly used and number of IHC-positive endothelial cells per unit area or in 10 HPF are reported as 'microvessel density'
▶ Experts in the field have established guidelines for MVD assessment but these are not usually followed

Data in Clinical Breast Cancer
▶ High MVD is associated with poor clinical outcome in both node-negative and node-positive breast cancer
▶ Reduction in MVD with endocrine and chemotherapy may be a predictor of response

Future Clinical Use
▶ Direct targeting of endothelial cells or regulators of angiogenesis has been in clinical trials but results are not encouraging
▶ If standardized methods become available to assess angiogenesis, it may potentially be added to the list of useful prognostic factors
▶ Possible role in breast cancer prevention using targeted therapy since angiogenesis is a key element in all stages of tumorigenesis

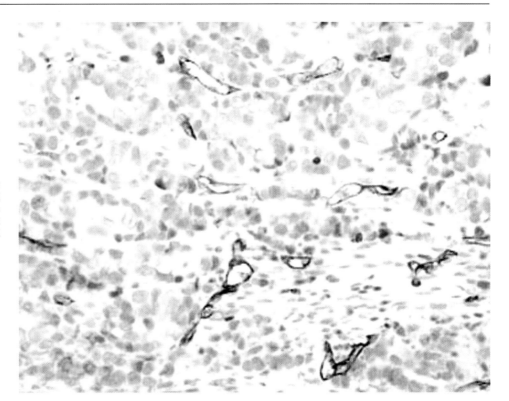

FIGURE 24-5

Microvessel density as assessed by IHC using CD-31 antibody. All immunostained endothelial cells are counted over a unit area, such as 1 mm² and reported as microvessel count.

growth, invasion, and metastasis. This is a dynamic process regulated by several inducers, such as vascular endothelial growth factor (VEGF), VEGF receptors, thymidine phosphorylases, and Tie-2 and inhibited by factors such as hypoxia induced factor (HIF), thrombospondin, and tissue inhibitor of metalloproteinases (TIMP). Besides neovascularization, other mechanisms of establishing tumor blood supply include intussusception (insertion of columns of tumor cells into existing vessels), and vascular mimicry (creation of new vascular network composed of tumor cells acting as endothelial cells). Angiogenesis has been shown to be an independent prognostic factor in breast cancer.

A variety of methods are available to assess angiogenesis, including dynamic radiologic techniques such as Doppler ultrasound, thermography and MRI, and static methods such as IHC in tissue sections. A number of antibodies have been used for IHC and include but are not limited to type IV collagen, laminin, factor VIII-related antigen, CD-34, and CD-31. The number of IHC stained endothelial cells are counted per 10 high power fields or unit area and the count is reported as 'microvessel density' (MVD). This is the most commonly employed method to assess angiogenesis in breast cancer (Figure 24-5).

Some investigators have shown a strong association between high vascular density and poor clinical outcome. MVD is an independent predictor of DFS and OS in node negative and positive patients in some series, but most have included only small numbers of patients of mixed stage and treatment and relatively short follow-up and therefore do not meet the criteria for validation.

Well-designed studies following recommended methodology from an international consensus conference are needed before this marker will become useful in the clinical setting. An attractive feature of angiogenesis is that it may offer a target for novel therapeutic interventions. Several antiangiogenic agents, including enzymes that control the vascularization process, steroids and steroid-related substances, antibiotics and synthetic antibiotic derivatives and specific immunotherapies, have been tested in both animal models and human trials, however, at least in late stages of breast cancer, the results have not been promising. Since angiogenesis is critical in all steps of tumorigenesis, therapeutic targeting still remains an attractive option for early breast cancer.

EPIDERMAL GROWTH FACTOR RECEPTOR

Epidermal growth factor receptor (EGFR) is the first member of the HER family and is a 170 kD transmembrane tyrosine kinase activated by both EGF and TGFα. Its main role in breast cancer may be its ability to heterodimerize with HER-2/*neu*, which plays a very significant role in breast cancer progression. Although the data on EGFR overexpression in breast cancer is confusing, there is evidence that even normal levels of EGFR may be important in cross-talk between EGFR family members and ER and has implications in response to targeted therapies to ER, such as tamoxifen.

EPIDERMAL GROWTH FACTOR RECEPTOR – FACT SHEET

Biology

▶ First member of the family with a transmembrane receptor with tyrosine kinase activated by EGF and TGF-alpha
▶ Its role in breast tumorigenesis alone is controversial but may be important because it heterodimerizes with HER-2/*neu*

Methodologies for Measuring

▶ Radioligand binding assay, autoradiography, immunoenzymatic methods, RT-PCR, and IHC
▶ No established assay or cut-off exist to define 'overexpression'

Data in Clinical Breast Cancer

▶ Reported incidence of 'expression' is 10–50 % using various techniques
▶ Associated with aggressive phenotype, i.e., ER negative, high grade, high proliferation index, p53 alterations, etc
▶ Associated with poor clinical outcome
▶ EGFR expression may be associated with resistance to hormonal therapy

Future Clinical Use

▶ In the metastatic setting, EGFR tyrosine kinase inhibitors may be useful as second or third line therapy
▶ May delay resistance to hormonal therapy and clinical trials are ongoing addressing these issues

---

COX-2 – FACT SHEET

Biology

▶ Cox–2 catalyzes a rate-limiting step in prostaglandin and thromboxane biosynthesis
▶ Cox-2 can be induced by growth factors, oncogenes and cytokines
▶ In vitro and in vivo models show that overexpression of Cox-2 is associated with mammary tumor development, and Cox-2 knock out animals do not develop tumors

Methods for Measuring

▶ IHC, RT-PCR, Northern blot

Data in Clinical Breast Cancer

▶ Cox-2 expression is associated with HER-2/*neu* overexpression, angiogenesis, lymph node metastasis, large tumor size, high grade, and a high proliferation rate
▶ Cox-2 overexpression is associated with poor clinical outcome
▶ In case–control studies of NSAID use, which non-selectively inhibit Cox-1 and -2, there was a 40 % decreased incidence of breast cancer in users of NSAIDs

Future Clinical Use

▶ Selective Cox-2 inhibitors are being considered for breast cancer treatment

---

EGFR has been measured by several methods, including radioligand-binding assays, autoradiography, immunoenzymatic assays, measurement of EGFR transcripts and IHC; no clear difference is seen among the different assay techniques. EGFR has been reported to be 'overexpressed' in 40–50 % of breast carcinomas, particularly those with a poor prognostic phenotype. Studies have generally reported a correlation between EGFR and absence of steroid receptor status, high tumor grade and high proliferation indices. Recent studies suggest that EGFR positivity may be correlated with overexpression of abnormal p53 and angiogenesis. These studies, however, have provided mixed results regarding the prognostic significance of EGFR overexpression, with only some showing correlation with a poor DFS. Several groups have demonstrated that tumors expressing EGFR are more likely to be resistant to endocrine therapy. Conversely, EGFR-negative tumors, especially if they are also ER positive, tend to have higher response rates.

There are a limited number of antibodies available for EGFR. Standardized methods of assessing EGFR do not exist and our understanding of the biology of EGFR and its role in breast cancer is still evolving. The most exciting reason to measure EGFR in breast cancer today is its potential use as a target for new therapies. Several monoclonal antibodies directed against EGFR (known as EGFR tyrosine kinase inhibitors) are under evaluation in breast cancer patients and clinical trials testing tyrosine kinase inhibitors in metastatic breast cancer patients are either ongoing or being planned. There is also some preliminary evidence that these agents alone or in combination with established chemopreventive agents such as tamoxifen may be useful in breast cancer prevention.

COX-2

Cyclooxygenase (Cox) catalyzes the conversion of arachidonic acid to prostaglandin H2, which is the rate-limiting step in PG and thromboxane synthesis. Cox-2 is present at low levels in breast tissue but can be rapidly induced by several stimuli including hormones, cytokines, growth factors, mitogens, and oncogenes. Tyrosine kinase, protein kinase C and A mediate its effects. Cox-2 derived prostanoids can induce angiogenesis, invasion, and metastasis. Cox-2 overexpression has been demonstrated in many human malignancies including breast cancer.

Cox-2 can be measured by IHC in tissues where it is detectable in the cytoplasm, often in a granular pattern. A few monoclonal and polyclonal antibodies are now available for IHC, however, in the past Cox-2 specific antibodies have been a problem. There are a relatively few good studies that have evaluated Cox-2 expression in the breast. Its expression has been reported to be weak and heterogeneous in 81 % of normal breast epithelium, and in DCIS the expression varies from

50 % in low intermediate grade to 13 % in high grade lesions. In invasive breast cancer, its expression varies from 20–50 % in the reported series. In survival analyses, Cox-2 overexpression has been found to be associated with poor outcome

The interest in Cox-2 has come from *in vitro* and *in vivo* data showing elevation of Cox-2 mRNA in breast cancer cell lines, induction of mammary tumors in transgenic mice with Cox-2 overexpression and delay in tumor development either by Cox-2 inhibitors or knocking out the gene. In a case–control study of human subjects, use of NSAIDs, which are non-selective inhibitors of Cox, resulted in 40 % reduction in the incidence of IBC. Based on these data, Cox-2 inhibitors are being tested in breast cancer trials.

SUGGESTING READING

Adjuvant therapy for breast cancer. NIH consensus statement 2000;17:6–7.

McGuire WL. Breast cancer prognostic factors: evaluation guidelines. J Natl Cancer Inst 1991;83:154–155.

Hormone Receptors

Harvey JM, Clark GM, Osborne CK, Allred DC. Estrogen receptor status by immunohistochemistry is superior to the ligand-binding assay for predicting response to adjuvant endocrine therapy in breast cancer. J Clin Oncol 1999;17:1474–1481.

Mohsin SK, Weiss H, Havighurst TC, *et al.* Progesterone receptor by immunohistochemistry and clinical outcome in breast cancer; a validation study. Mod Pathol 2004;17;1545–1554.

Rhodes A, Jasani B, Balaton AJ, Miller KD. Immunohistochemical demonstration of oestrogen and progesterone receptors: correlation of standards achieved on in house tumours with that achieved on external quality assessment material in over 150 laboratories from 26 countries. J Clin Pathol 2000;53:292–301.

HER-2/neu

Slamon DJ, Clark GM, Wong SG, *et al.* Human breast cancer: correlation of relapse and survival with amplification of the HER-2/neu oncogene. Science 1987;235(4785):177–182.

Ross JS, Fletcher JA, Linette GP, *et al.* The Her-2/neu gene and protein in breast cancer 2003: biomarker and target of therapy. Oncologist. 2003;8:307–325.

Ki-67 proliferation index, p53, angiogenesis, EGFR, and Cox-2

Allred DC, Clark GM, Elledge R, *et al.* Association of p53 protein expression with tumor cell proliferation rate and clinical outcome in node-negative breast cancer. J Natl Cancer Inst 1993;85:200–206.

Jansen RL, Hupperets PS, Arends JW, *et al.* MIB-1 labelling index is an independent prognostic marker in primary breast cancer. Br J Cancer 1998;78:460–465.

Ristimaki A, Sivula A, Lundin J, *et al.* Prognostic significance of elevated cyclooxygenase-2 expression in breast cancer. Cancer Res 2002;62:632.

Sainsbury JR, Farndon JR, Needham GK, *et al.* Epidermal-growth-factor receptor status as predictor of early recurrence of and death from breast cancer. Lancet 1987;1(8547):1398–402.

Vermeulen PB, Gasparini G, Fox SB, *et al.* Quantification of angiogenesis in solid human tumors: an international consesus on the methodology and criteria of evaluation. Eur J Cancer 1996;32A:2474–2484.

25 Overview of Immunohistochemistry in Breast Lesions

Syed K Mohsin · Frances P O'Malley · Sarah E Pinder

The use of immunohistochemical stains as an adjunct to diagnosis in breast pathology has become routine in many laboratories. While breast pathologic diagnoses should be based primarily on the morphologic changes recognized on hematoxylin and eosin (H&E) stained sections, there are certain diagnostically challenging cases where immunohistochemistry can be useful in confirming the H&E diagnosis. This can certainly be the case in distinguishing an invasive lesion from a benign mimic, such as radial scar versus tubular carcinoma. Other areas where immunohistochemistry is used with varying degrees of success is in differentiation of *in situ* lobular from ductal proliferations. This is covered in Chapter 15 so it will only be briefly discussed here. The use of immunohistochemistry in the evaluation of sentinel lymph nodes remains a controversial topic and has been thoroughly addressed in Chapter 22. Recently, the utility of immunohistochemistry to differentiate usual ductal hyperplasia from atypical ductal hyperplasia has been assessed, although in our experience, this is relatively rarely of assistance in diagnostically difficult cases.

This chapter highlights the immunohistochemical stains that may be helpful in clinical practice. Topics include differentiating benign lesions that can mimic an invasive process from invasive carcinoma, distinguishing *in situ* ductal from lobular proliferations and the confirmation of systemic metastases from a breast primary. We also cover some recent data elucidating possible distinct paths of differentiation of tumors based on cytokeratin immunohistochemical profiles.

IN SITU DUCTAL VERSUS LOBULAR DIFFERENTIATION

The distinction between *in situ* ductal and lobular lesions is usually readily made using well-established cytologic and morphologic criteria. There are cases, however, that have ambiguous histologic features leading to difficulty in categorization. The importance of this differentiation is critical when these lesions are diagnosed in core needle biopsies or lumpectomies, as the management varies. Most patients diagnosed with incidental lobular carcinoma *in situ* (LCIS) on a core needle biopsy have not traditionally been subjected to

---

IN SITU DUCTAL VERSUS LOBULAR DIFFERENTIATION – FACT SHEET

Indication
▸ Distinction between DCIS and LCIS is critical in both core needle biopsies and surgical excisions, because of different treatment options

Markers
▸ E-cadherin – usually negative in LCIS
▸ Beta-catenin – usually negative in LCIS
▸ CK8 – DCIS shows peripheral cytoplasmic staining while LCIS has perinuclear, granular staining
▸ 34βE12 – negative in DCIS, positive in LCIS

Problems
▸ E-cadherin is positive in 10% of LCIS cases
▸ Beta-catenin is focally positive in 25–30% of LCIS cases
▸ Differences in staining patterns of CK8 may be difficult to interpret
▸ Data are limited on 34βE12

Recommendation
▸ E-cadherin with or without beta-catenin are the most useful markers

---

surgical excision (provided that there is a pathologic–mammographic correlation; see Chapter 15) because of the belief that LCIS is a risk factor and not a direct precursor of invasive breast cancer. Patients who have a diagnosis of LCIS in a lumpectomy will not require any further therapy. In contrast, patients with ductal carcinoma *in situ* (DCIS) diagnosed in a lumpectomy will often require adjuvant radiation therapy.

Several studies have shown that E-cadherin, a cell adhesion molecule, is almost uniformly retained in ductal lesions, but nearly always lost in lobular lesions. Antibodies to E-cadherin have proved very useful in distinguishing DCIS from LCIS. This has been addressed in detail in Chapter 15. Caution must be exercised, however, not to interpret staining in entrapped myoepithelial and benign epithelial cells as evidence of presence of E-cadherin. This is important in ALH/LCIS involving large ducts, where there may be a complex mixture of residual benign epithelium with lobular neoplastic cells. Goldstein et al have also reported that distinct and unequivocal membrane staining for E-cadherin can be seen in about 10 % of cases of LCIS, which could lead to interpretative problems, particularly in a CNB.

In addition to E-cadherin, expression of beta-catenin has also been used to differentiate ductal from lobular lesions; however, this marker is less reliable for this purpose. Another useful immunohistochemical marker is cytokeratin 8 (CK8), which can be detected by the antibody CAM 5.2. Ductal lesions show CK8 staining in peripheral cytoplasm, while lobular lesions tend to have a perinuclear pattern and the staining is more granular. Also, high-molecular weight keratin antibody 34βE12, which contains antibodies to cytokeratins 1, 5, 10, and 14, may be helpful in some equivocal lesions. With this antibody, ductal lesions are negative, and lobular lesions show a perinuclear staining similar to that seen with CK8.

Although the typing of invasive breast cancer into ductal, no special type and lobular subtypes is important, it usually does not impact on the clinical management. Also, this distinction can generally be easily made based on morphologic criteria. Thus, E-cadherin staining in invasive carcinomas is usually not necessary.

NEUROENDOCRINE DIFFERENTIATION

It has been suggested that invasive breast cancers (IBC) showing neuroendocrine differentiation (NED) may have prognostic implications (see also Chapter 18). However, the literature on this topic is relatively limited and controversial. Miremadi *et al* studied 99 cases of IBC with three standard IHC markers for NED, i.e, neuron-specific enolase (NSE), chromogranin A, and synaptophysin and reported an incidence of NED in 10–18 %

of IBCs. They did not find any significant prognostic value of NED in IBC. A few other studies have suggested that NED in breast cancer is associated with better survival. In our opinion, it is best to state that the diagnostic and clinical utility of NED in IBC is questionable and not important for routine diagnostic work up.

MYOEPITHELIAL MARKERS IN THE ASSESSMENT OF STROMAL INVASION

One of the most used applications of immunohistochemistry in breast pathology is in the differential diagnosis of benign lesions or *in situ* malignant proliferations mimicking invasive breast cancer. Some of the common scenarios include carcinoma *in situ* involving areas of sclerosing adenosis mimicking invasive breast carcinoma (Figure 25-1), entrapped benign ducts in a radial scar/complex sclerosing lesion mistaken for a tubular carcinoma, or distortion of ducts involved by DCIS overinterpreted as stromal invasion. In all these instances, the approach has been to identify an intact myoepithelial layer as evidence of an *in situ* process rather than invasion. Loss of myoepithelial cell staining can also help confirm the presence of microinvasion (Figure 25-2). A search for a specific marker of myoepithelial cells in breast has been ongoing for many years. There are four markers that are commonly used in current clinical practice, so our discussion will be limited to these markers.

NEUROENDOCRINE DIFFERENTIATION – FACT SHEET

Indication
▶ NED in breast cancer may potentially be a useful prognostic factor

Markers
▶ Chromogranin A
▶ Synaptophysin
▶ Neuron specific enolase (NSE)

Problems
▶ 30–50 % of breast cancers show at least some staining with these markers
▶ Definition of NED in breast cancer is not standardized
▶ Definite prognostic values of NED in breast cancer is not established

Recommendation
▶ Establishing NED in breast cancer has no clinical utility at this time

---

MYOEPITHELIAL MARKERS – FACT SHEET

Indications
▶ Distinction between carcinoma *in situ* involving sclerosing adenosis versus invasive breast cancer
▶ Identification of tubular carcinoma versus entrapped benign tubules in radial scar

Markers
▶ Smooth muscle actin – cytoplasmic staining in myoepithelial cells
▶ Calponin – cytoplasmic staining in myoepithelial cells
▶ p63 – nuclear staining in myoepithelial cells
▶ Smooth muscle myosin heavy chain – cytoplasmic staining in myoepithelial cells

Problems
▶ SMA and calponin tend to stain myofibroblasts and blood vessels
▶ p63 staining can be incomplete and about 10% invasive breast cancers express this marker

Recommendation
▶ SMM-HC with or without p63 are currently the most useful markers

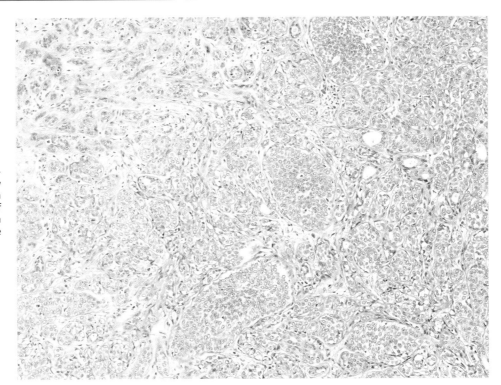

FIGURE 25-1

Lobular carcinoma in situ in sclerosing adenosis. Acini are expanded by cells of lobular neoplasia. This, in combination with the irregularity of the acini and stromal fibrosis, can lead to a misdiagnosis of invasive carcinoma.

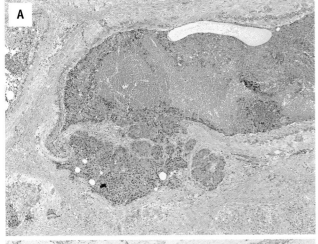

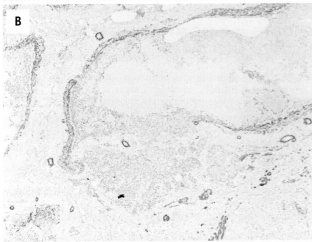

FIGURE 25-2

Microinvasive carcinoma. (A) Ductal carcinoma in situ with a focus of microinvasion. (B) Absence of a myoepithelial cell layer is confirmed on immunohistochemical staining with SMM-HC.

SMOOTH MUSCLE ACTIN
(Figures 25-3A and 25-4A)

The smooth muscle actin (SMA) marker has a relatively long track record of use in this situation. The two most commonly employed antibodies are anti-SMA and muscle-specific actin (clone HHF-35). SMA is a sensitive marker of myoepithelial differentiation, but it is not specific, because any cell with substantial expression of actin is positive for SMA. In the breast, myofibroblasts and blood vessels are generally positive for SMA. This becomes problematic in lesions such as sclerosing adenosis, radial scars, papillary lesions, or DCIS where there are either myofibroblasts or blood vessels in close proximity to the epithelial lesion in question. Nevertheless, SMA still remains a fairly useful marker because of its high sensitivity and helps resolve the differential diagnoses in a significant number of cases.

CALPONIN (Figures 25-3B and 25-4B)

This protein is associated with contractile apparatus in smooth muscle cells. Calponin has been shown to be a useful marker of myoepithelial cells and is considered nearly as sensitive as SMA. But like SMA, staining of myofibroblasts and smooth muscle in blood vessels is seen. Compared to other markers, such as p63 and smooth muscle myosin-heavy chain, it tends to show more complete staining of the myoepithelial layer.

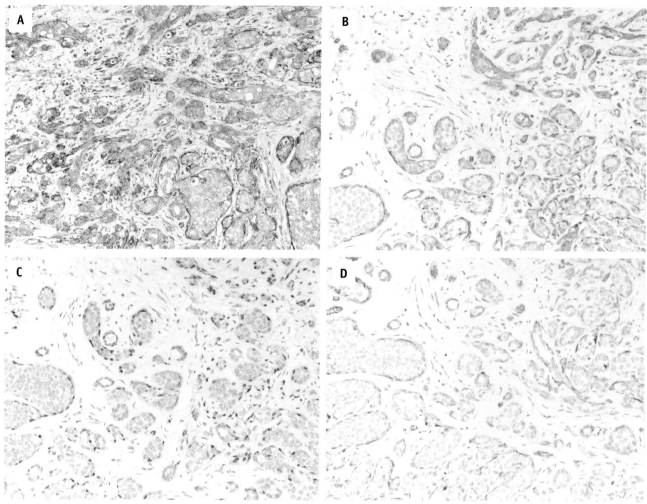

FIGURE 25-3

Myoepithelial cell markers in the assessment of stromal invasion. Lobular carcinoma in situ in sclerosing adenosis mimicking invasive carcinoma. The myoepithelial cell layer is preserved, confirming the in situ nature of the lesion. (A) SMA is a sensitive marker of myoepithelial differentiation, but it lacks specificity and also marks myofibroblasts and blood vessels. (B) Calponin is almost as sensitive a myoepithelial cell marker as SMA; however, it, too, marks fibroblasts and blood vessels. (C) p63 is a nuclear stain and is absent in myofibroblasts and blood vessels. (D) SMM-HC stains myoepithelial cells and blood vessels but shows less cross-reactivity to myofibroblasts than SMA.

P63 (Figures 25-3C and 25-4C)

p63 is a homolog of p53, and has been shown to be expressed exclusively in myoepithelial cells in normal breast. The advantage of using p63 is its nuclear localization and absence of staining in smooth muscle cells, such as myofibroblasts and blood vessels. Thus, it provides almost 100 % specificity, but its sensitivity has been reported to be about 90 %. This is demonstrated by 'focal gaps' in staining in the myoepithelial layer. Also, it has now been shown that about 10–15 % of invasive tumors, particularly high grade carcinomas, express p63, although the staining is usually weaker than that seen in the myoepithelial cells. Despite these shortcomings, p63 can be very useful in differential diagnoses involving sclerosing adenosis, radial scars and papillary lesions (Figure 25-5).

SMOOTH MUSCLE MYOSIN-HEAVY CHAIN
(Figures 25-3D and 25-4D)

Like other smooth muscle markers, smooth muscle myosin-heavy chain (SMM-HC) is associated with contractile elements and is present in all cells with such capabilities. In the breast, it is expressed primarily in myoepithelial cells but also stains blood vessels. An advantage of SMM-HC is that it demonstrates less cross reactivity to myofibroblasts than calponin and SMA.

Overall, the studies so far suggest that among smooth muscle markers, SMM-HC provides the best results, both in terms of sensitivity and specificity. In most laboratories, however, the choice between SMA, calponin and SMM-HC depends on individual experience and preference. It is possible to use a combination of a nuclear myoepithelial marker such as p63 with a cyto-

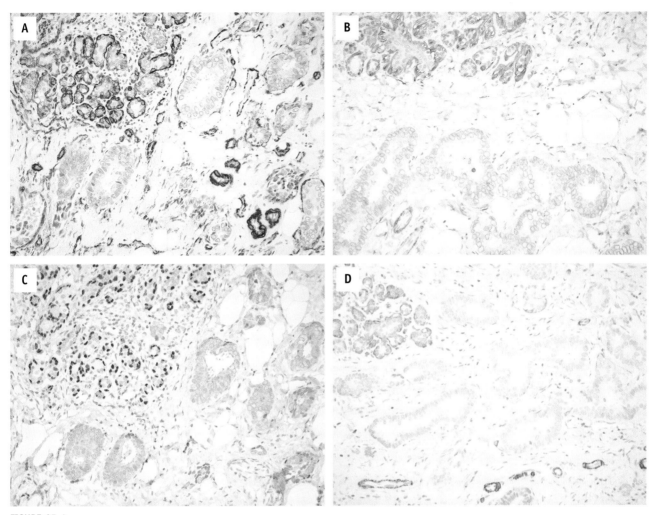

FIGURE 25-4
Myoepithelial cell markers in the assessment of stromal invasion. Invasive ductal carcinoma with tubular features. The absence of a myoepithelial cell layer is confimed immunohistochemically with (A) SMA, (B) calponin, (C) p63 and (D) SMM-HC. Adjacent benign ducts act as an internal positive control.

plasmic protein, such as SMA, calponin, or smooth muscle myosin heavy chain to increase the diagnostic utility of these markers.

DIFFERENTIATING USUAL DUCTAL HYPERPLASIA FROM DCIS

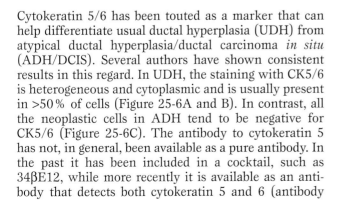

Cytokeratin 5/6 has been touted as a marker that can help differentiate usual ductal hyperplasia (UDH) from atypical ductal hyperplasia/ductal carcinoma *in situ* (ADH/DCIS). Several authors have shown consistent results in this regard. In UDH, the staining with CK5/6 is heterogeneous and cytoplasmic and is usually present in >50% of cells (Figure 25-6A and B). In contrast, all the neoplastic cells in ADH tend to be negative for CK5/6 (Figure 25-6C). The antibody to cytokeratin 5 has not, in general, been available as a pure antibody. In the past it has been included in a cocktail, such as 34βE12, while more recently it is available as an antibody that detects both cytokeratin 5 and 6 (antibody

UDH VERSUS ADH/DCIS – FACT SHEET

Indication
▸ Distinction between UDH and ADH/DCIS is critical because of breast cancer risk implications and therapeutic options

Markers
▸ Antibodies containing keratin 5
  ▸ 34βE12 – UDH is heterogeneously/diffusely positive while ADH/low grade DCIS is negative
  ▸ D5/16B4 – UDH is diffusely positive, while ADH/DCIS is focally positive
▸ ER/PR usually show heterogeneous positivity in UDH, while ADH/low grade DCIS are usually diffusely positive

Problems
▸ Both markers contain keratins other than CK5
▸ Data are limited on the utility of these markers

Recommendation
▸ The distinction between UDH and ADH/DCIS is currently based on morphology alone; use of these markers should be limited to select cases and interpreted with some caution

BASAL VERSUS LUMINAL PHENOTYPE – FACT SHEET

Indication

▸ Basal phenotype in breast cancer may be associated with poor prognosis

Markers

▸ CK5/6 and 14 – markers of basal phenotype (seen in about 13–17 % cancers)
▸ CK7/8, 18, and 19 – markers of luminal phenotype

Problems

▸ Staining patterns of some keratins, such as CK5/6 and CK7/8 may be difficult to interpret
▸ Data are limited on this subject
▸ Clinical utility of this distinction is not established at this time

Recommendation

▸ Routine use of these markers to classify breast cancer is not recommended

D5/16B4). Otterbach *et al*, using the antibody 34βE12, found that in their series 87 % of UDH lesions were diffusely positive while none of the DCIS or LCIS were positive. ADH either completely lacked staining or showed only focal staining. Another study compared 34βE12 and D5/16B4 and reported that D5/16B4 was

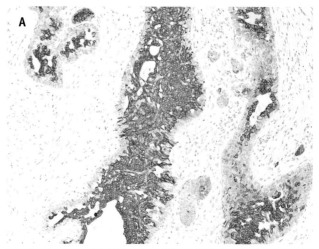

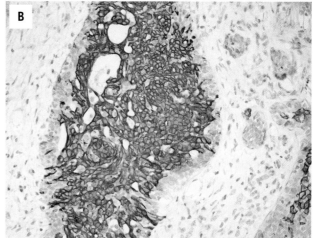

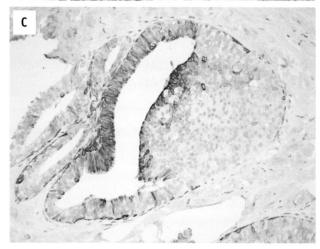

FIGURE 25-6

High-molecular weight cytokeratin in epithelial hyperplasia of usual type. (A, B) Staining with HMW-CK is diffuse and cytoplasmic in >50% of cells. (C) In contrast, the neoplastic cells in atypical ductal hyperplasia tend to be negative.

FIGURE 25-5

Intraductal papillary carcinoma. (A) H&E showing a well-circumscribed lesion composed of fibrovascular cores, lined by malignant epithelium. (B) The preservation of the myoepithelial cell layer around the periphery of the duct is confirmed with p63.

more helpful (Lacroix-Triki *et al.*). However, in their hands D5/16B4 did not provide a clear cut distinction between UDH and ADH/DCIS. It is suggested that CK5/6 IHC may be used in difficult lesions, but it is possible that it may not resolve the diagnostic dilemma in these cases.

DISTINCTION OF BASAL FROM LUMINAL BREAST CANCER PHENOTYPES

Another indication for the use of CK5/6 is in the classification of invasive breast cancer as basal versus luminal subtypes. This is based on studies following up on the data from gene expression profiling of invasive breast cancer showing that sub-categorizing these lesions into basal and luminal types was associated with both different molecular profiles and different prognoses. One such study (Abd El-Rehim *et al*), using a panel of keratins to define basal (CK 5/6 and 14-positive) and luminal (CK 7/8, 18, and 19-positive) invasive breast cancer by IHC, showed that about 13–17 % of cancers can be classified as having a basal phenotype. The CK5/6-positive basal-type breast cancers are associated with other known poor prognostic factors and have a somewhat aggressive biologic behavior. As more data become available, this marker has the potential to be a useful prognostic factor in invasive breast cancer.

CONFIRMATION OF SYSTEMIC METASTASES FROM A BREAST PRIMARY

This is an important distinction and pathologists are routinely asked to confirm the source of metastatic car-

---

SYSTEMIC METASTASES FROM A BREAST PRIMARY – FACT SHEET

Indication

▶ Confirm or rule out metastatic cancer from a breast primary for therapeutic considerations

Markers

▶ ER and PR – about 70–75 % of metastatic breast cancers are positive
▶ GCDFP-15 – about 50–75 % of metastatic breast cancers are positive
▶ BCA225 – about 60 % of metastatic breast cancers are positive

Problems

▶ Negative staining for these markers does not necessarily rule out metastatic breast cancer
▶ None of these markers are specific for breast cancer

Recommendation

▶ A panel of ER, PR, and GCDFP-15 is the most useful in this setting

---

cinoma, sometimes with an unknown primary and at other times with a past history of breast cancer but an unusual clinical presentation. Often, the sample from the metastatic disease is limited and typically a cytologic preparation. Fortunately, it is rare today to diagnose metastatic breast cancer (MBC) without a history of breast cancer or a concurrent suspicious lesion in the breast. IHC can be very helpful in this setting; however, no single marker is sensitive or specific enough. Depending on the case, markers of breast cancer need to be combined with some specific markers of a possible other primary to workup such cases. It is also important to remember that a negative IHC result is not usually helpful in most clinical settings.

The markers used in establishing metastatic breast carcinoma include gross cystic disease fluid protein (GCDFP)-15 (Figure 25-7), estrogen receptor (ER), progesterone receptor (PR), CEA and BCA225. The pattern of cytokeratin 20 (CK20) and cytokeratin 7 (CK7) expression may also be extremely valuable in cases where no known primary site is recognized

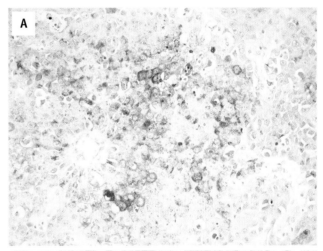

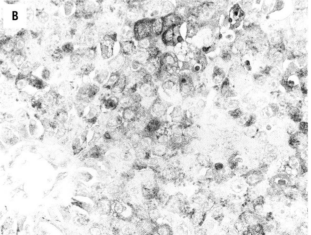

FIGURE 25-7

Evaluation of systemic metastases from a breast primary. (A) Medium and (B) high-power view of a poorly differentiated metastatic carcinoma staining positive with GCDFP-15. This marker, while specific, lacks sensitivity, and must be used as part of a wider immunohistochemical panel.

clinically. However, although CK7 is usually present in carcinomas in, and from, the breast, it is also present in a range of other carcinomas including serous ovarian and endometrial carcinoma as well as lung adenocarcinomas; these are all typically CK20 negative. Conversely, tumors from the colon usually express CK20 but not CK7. Other lesions such as renal and hepatocellular carcinoma tend to express neither CK20, nor CK7.

GCDFP-15 is the most specific marker for MBC, and carries a high positive predictive value of 95 % but its sensitivity is about 50–75 %. ER, though considered fairly specific for breast and gynecologic malignancies in the past, has been shown to be positive in other primaries, such as gastric and lung tumors. However, the results of these studies have not been consistent and depend on the antibody used, i.e., 6F11 or 1D5. Although with a history of ER-positive breast cancer in the past, ER positivity strongly favors a metastasis from a breast primary. PR has been shown to be more specific than ER for a workup of metastatic cancer, but it is much less sensitive. CEA is a sensitive but non-specific marker for adenocarcinoma. Polyclonal CEA antibodies stain a majority of breast carcinomas, but it has been suggested that a new clone, CEAD-14, stains only a subset of high-grade breast cancers (~13 %) and this can be helpful in certain settings in a panel of antibodies. BCA225 has been shown to have a sensitivity of about 60 % in detecting MBC; however, this marker can be positive in metastatic lung adenocarcinoma. TTF1 expression is seen in 75 % of lung adenocarcinomas but is not seen in breast carcinomas and this may also be valuable in distinguishing tumors arising from the two sites. Thus, a combination of ER, PR and GCDFP-15 is 83 % sensitive and 93 % specific for metastatic carcinoma of breast origin and, at present, this is the most useful panel for confirming MBC.

SUGGESTED READINGS

Abd El-Rehim DM, Pinder SE, Paish CE, et al. Expression of luminal and basal cytokeratins in human breast carcinoma. J Pathol 2004;203:661–671.

Dabbs DJ. Diagnostic immunohistochemistry of the breast. In: Dabbs DJ, editor. Diagnostic immunohistochemistry. Philadelphia: Churchill Livingstone; 2002. p. 536–558.

Goldstein NS, Kestin LL, Vivini FA. Clinicopathologic implications of E-cadherin reactivity in patients with lobular carcinoma in situ of the breast. Cancer 2001;92:738–477.

Kaufmann O, Deidesheimer T, Muehlenberg M, et al. Immunohistochemical differentiation of metastatic breast carcinomas from metastatic adeno-carcinomas of other common primary sites. Histopathology 1996;29:233–240.

Lacroix-Triki M, Mery E, Voigt JJ, et al. Value of cytokeratin 5/6 immuno-staining using D5/16 B4 antibody in the spectrum of proliferative intraepithelial lesions of the breast. A comparative study with 34betaE12 antibody. Virchows Arch 2003;442:548–554.

Miremadi A, Pinder SE, Lee AH, et al. Neuroendocrine differentiation and prognosis in breast adenocarcinoma. Histopathology 2002;40:215–222.

Otterbach F, Bankfalvi A, Bergner S, et al. Cytokeratin 5/6 immunohisto-chemistry assists the differential diagnosis of atypical proliferations of the breast. Histopathology 2000;37:232–240.

Ribeiro-Silva A, Zamzelli Ramalho LN, Garcia SB, Zucoloto S. Is p63 reliable in detecting microinvasion in ductal carcinoma in situ of the breast? Pathol Oncol Res 2003;9:20–23.

Werling RW, Hwang H, Yaziji H, Gown AM. Immunohistochemical distinction of invasive from noninvasive breast lesions: a comparative study of p63 versus calponin and smooth muscle myosin heavy chain. Am J Surg Pathol 2003;27:82–90.

Wick MR, Lillemoe TJ, Copland GT, et al. Gross cystic disease fluid protein-15 as a marker of breast cancer: immunohistochemical analysis of 690 human neoplasms and comparison with alpha-lactalbumin. Hum Pathol 1989;20:281–287.

Other Malignant Lesions of the Breast

Sunil Badve

LYMPHOID AND HEMATOPOIETIC LESIONS

Involvement of the breast in hematopoietic malignancies is relatively uncommon. In most cases, clinical history and physical examination will show the breast lesions to be part of a disseminated process. Secondary involvement of the breast can be seen in nearly all types of hematopoietic lesions including leukemias, lymphomas, myeloma and even myeloid metaplasia. The criteria adopted by the World Health Organization (WHO) for the diagnosis of a primary breast lymphoma are tissue documentation of a lymphomatous infiltrate within the breast tissue with no concurrent nodal disease (apart from axillary nodes) and no prior history of involvement of other organs or tissues.

LYMPHOMAS AND LEUKEMIAS

CLINICAL FEATURES

Primary breast lymphoma has been described in a broad age group of patients, mostly women, with an age range of 13–90 years. Similar to lymphomas at other sites, a bimodal age distribution can be seen. The presentation is usually in the form of a unilateral mass lesion; however, bilateral masses and multi-nodular lesions have been described. An inflammatory carcinoma-like presentation has also been documented. The lesion shows a slight predilection for the right side and, as with breast carcinoma, often involves the upper outer quadrant. Enlarged axillary lymph nodes are present in a significant number of cases. Primary mammary lymphomas have been described during pregnancy, in women with silicone implants and in men in association with gynecomastia.

RADIOLOGIC FEATURES

Mammographically, the tumor is often well circumscribed but can have an infiltrating, irregular outline, mimicking carcinoma (Figure 26-1). Microcalcifications

---

LYMPHOMAS AND LEUKEMIAS – FACT SHEET

Definition
- Primary breast lymphoma is diagnosed when the lesion is confined to the breast with or without involvement of the axillary lymph nodes (in the absence of systemic disease)
- Leukemic deposits are usually synchronously or metachronously associated with systemic disease

Incidence and Location
- Primary involvement of breast by hematopoietic malignancies is relatively uncommon
- Predilection for the right breast

Morbidity and Mortality
- Depending on the type and extent of disease

Gender, Race and Age Distribution
- Bimodal distribution
- Wide age range

Clinical Features
- Unilateral or bilateral mass lesions
- Enlarged axillary lymph nodes are present in a significant number of cases

Radiologic Features
- Well circumscribed mass(es)
- Rarely infiltrative lesions

Prognosis and Treatment
- Primary breast lymphoma can be treated with conservative surgery
- Chemotherapy required for systemic disease

---

are rare but may be seen secondary to necrosis or incidental benign breast disease. The presence of multiple ill-defined lesions of varying sizes associated with increased stromal density but with only rare microcalcifications could provide a hint to the pre-operative diagnosis of lymphoma. Ultrasonography reveals an ill-defined, round hypoechoic mass (or masses) with skin thickening. Pre-contrast T1-weighted MRI images demonstrate single or multiple well-defined, hypointense mass(es), which show rapid rim enhancement in dynamic post-contrast sequence. The enhancement rate indicates malignant pathology.

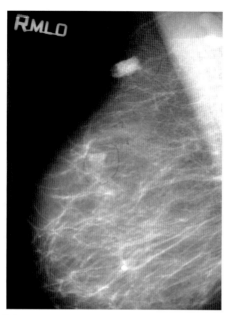

FIGURE 26-1

Mammograhic image of breast lymphoma. The tumor has irregular margins, mimicking carcinoma.

LYMPHOMAS AND LEUKEMIAS – PATHOLOGIC FEATURES
Gross Findings
▶ Gray-white to pink nodular masses
▶ Hemorrhage and necrosis may be seen
Microscopic Findings
▶ Diffuse infiltration without any specific pattern
▶ Interstitial infiltration of fat
▶ Low grade lesions may mimic lobular carcinoma
Ultrastructural Features
▶ N/A
Fine Needle Aspiration Biopsy Findings
▶ Diffusely scattered single cells
▶ Cellular monotony
Immunohistochemical Features
▶ Most lesions are B-cell lymphomas
Differential Diagnosis
▶ Inflammatory infiltrate
▶ Lobular carcinoma

PATHOLOGIC FEATURES

On macroscopic examination, the lesions tend to be gray-white to pink with a nodular configuration, with or without focal areas of necrosis and hemorrhage. Additional smaller lesions may be present. Tumors as large as 12 cm have been described. In recent years, it is extremely unusual to see resection of large lesions due to the routine use of needle core biopsies prior to excision of breast lesions.

Microscopic examination varies to some extent, depending on the type of disease; however, the predominant picture is that of a diffuse cellular infiltrate composed of relatively small cells (Figure 26-2). The tumor cells may show a periductal targetoid growth pattern (Figure 26-3) and may be mistaken for invasive lobular carcinoma. The presence of lymphoid cells with clear cell or signet ring cell features may compound this problem (Figure 26-4A). However, lymphoid cells, unlike cells of lobular carcinoma, do not have intracytoplasmic mucin or true lumina. The patterns of nondestructive invasion and infiltration into fat also help to distinguish these lesions from lobular carcinoma. Infiltration of co-existing benign structures can complicate the morphology and lead to a false impression of *in situ* lobular carcinoma (Figure 26-4B).

Most primary breast lymphomas are of the non-Hodgkin type with a diffuse growth pattern composed of mixed small and large cells. A follicular growth pattern is distinctly uncommon. Most cases of primary breast lymphomas are now classified as diffuse large B cell lymphomas, according to the recent WHO classification. A few cases of lymphoplasmacytic lymphomas have been reported. Other types of lymphomas reported in the breast include Burkitt lymphoma, extra-nodal marginal zone lymphoma of mucosa associated lymphoid tissue (MALT), follicular lymphomas and lymphoblastic lymphomas. T-cell lymphomas are extremely uncommon; angiotrophic lymphoma may present as a vasculitic process (Figure 26-5). Involvement of the breast with Hodgkin lymphoma is almost always secondary to nodal involvement.

Leukemic involvement of the breast can be seen in association with both acute and chronic leukemias but is distinctly less common in lymphoid (Figure 26-6) than in myeloid lesions (Figure 26-7A). The resulting mass lesions have been called chloromas or myeloblastomas. These lesions can be synchronous or metachronous with hematogenous evidence of myeloid leukemia. Histochemical stains, such as chloracetate esterase (CAE), are useful in identifying the more differentiated cells (Figure 26-7B).

ANCILLARY STUDIES

FINE NEEDLE ASPIRATION CYTOLOGY

Fine needle aspiration (FNA) cytology has been successfully used to diagnose breast lymphomas. In a recent series that included cases of both primary and secondary breast lymphomas, a diagnosis of lymphoma could

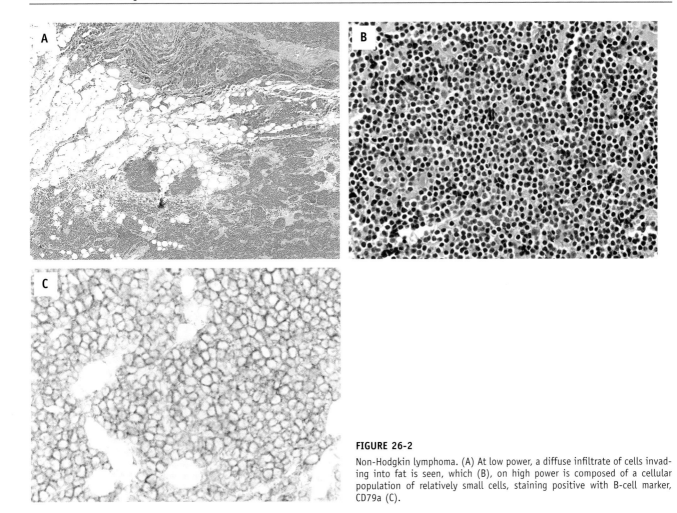

FIGURE 26-2

Non-Hodgkin lymphoma. (A) At low power, a diffuse infiltrate of cells invading into fat is seen, which (B), on high power is composed of a cellular population of relatively small cells, staining positive with B-cell marker, CD79a (C).

FIGURE 26-3

Non-Hodgkin lymphoma. Follicle center cell, low-grade. Note the targetoid infiltration of small lymphoid cells around lymphovascular spaces.

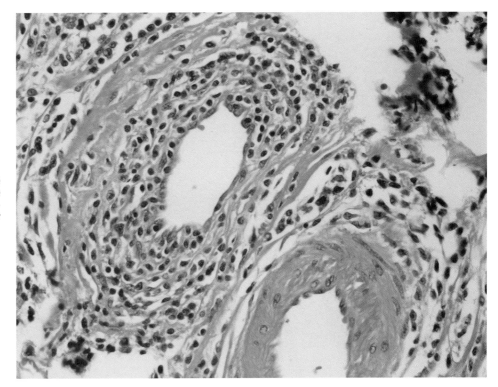

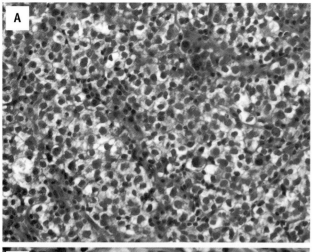

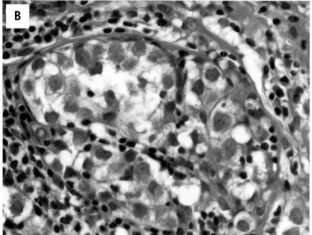

FIGURE 26-4

Non-Hodgkin lymphoma. Follicle centre cell, high-grade. Note the infiltration of breast tissue by large cells, which have pale to clear cytoplasm, mimicking both (A) invasive and (B) *in situ* lobular carcinoma.

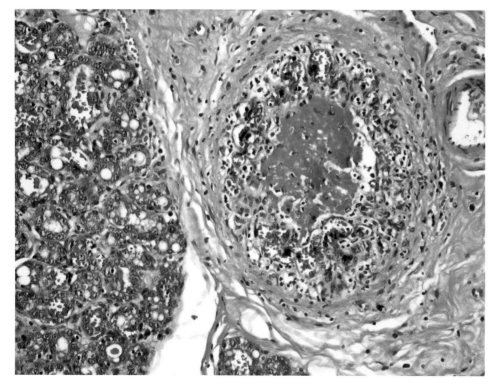

FIGURE 26-5

Section from a breast mass of a 35-year-old woman showing vasculitis. Additional investigations (including lung biopsy) led to the diagnosis of non-Hodgkin lymphoma, angiotrophic T-cell.

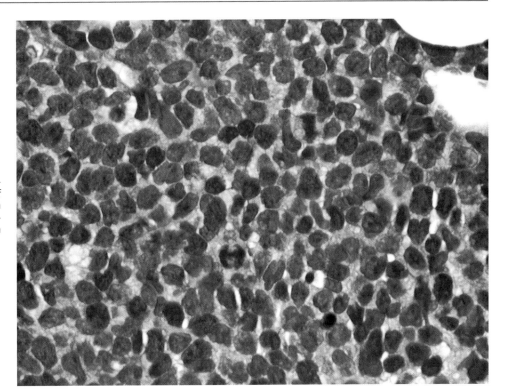

FIGURE 26-6

Diffuse infiltration by acute lymphoblastic leukemia. Involvement of the breast can be seen with both acute and chronic leukemias, lymphoid lesions far less frequently than myeloid.

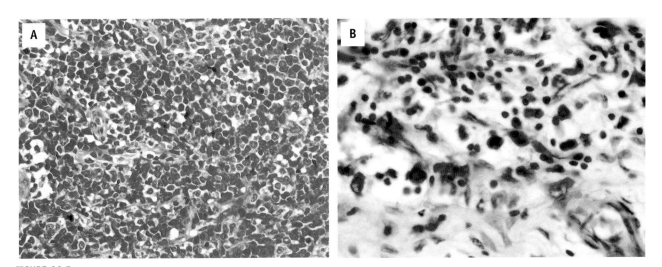

FIGURE 26-7

(A) Diffuse infiltration by acute myeloid leukemia. (B) Histochemical stains, such as chloracetate esterase (CAE), are often positive.

be made by FNA cytology in all cases; however, subtyping of lymphomas was possible in only a small number of cases. Nevertheless, the suspicion of lymphoma on FNA cytology can enable organization of a full hematologic work-up of the patient and the collection of material for flow cytometry which may be extremely helpful in the diagnosis and sub-typing of lymphomas.

IMMUNOHISTOCHEMISTRY

Immunohistochemistry plays a vital role in differentiating lymphomas and leukemia deposits from benign lymphoid infiltrates and from carcinoma, particularly of invasive lobular type. The lack of estrogen receptor (ER) and progesterone receptor (PR) expression in a lesion that superficially looks like an invasive lobular carcinoma may provide a clue to the correct diagnosis in some cases; this can be further confirmed by the lack of cytokeratin expression. Most lymphomas in the breast are of B-cell origin. A panel composed of CD45RO, CD3, CD20 and CD45 with the addition of CD23 for MALT lymphomas and CD56 for the diagnosis of leukemia infiltrates is usually adequate in investigating a suspicious lesion. If possible, material should be sent for flow cytometric analysis.

DIFFERENTIAL DIAGNOSIS

The differential diagnosis of leukemia and lymphoma in the breast includes intramammary lymph nodes and lymph nodes low in the axilla, inflammatory conditions including lymphocytic mastitis and invasive lobular carcinoma. Intramammary lymph nodes are not uncommon; these can be recognized by mammography and will often not be biopsied. The commonest cause of biopsy of intramammary lymph nodes is the lack of a fatty center, which is typically seen in lymph nodes, on ultrasound examination. Histology, in most cases, shows a typical lymph node architecture, however, on occasion, special stains are needed. A reticulin stain, for example, can be performed to highlight the follicular architecture. In troublesome cases, a panel of immunohistochemical stains, as detailed above, may be necessary. Intramammary lymph nodes can show additional pathologies, as may be seen in axillary lymph nodes, such as granulomatous inflammation, silicone reactions and metastatic deposits. Lymphocytic mastitis (Figure 26-8) and diabetic mastopathy are uncommon fibro-inflammatory breast diseases in which the associated lymphoid infiltrates are composed predominantly of B-cells. Histologic examination shows variable amounts of fibrosis in association with lymphoid and plasma cell infiltrates (plasma cell mastitis). The inflammatory infiltrate tends to be most prominent around vascular structures and lobules and may be associated with granulomatous and/or xanthomatous features. Lymphoepithelial lesions, similar to those seen in MALT lymphomas, can be present. However, these lesions are not clonal and do not appear to be associated with an increased risk of lymphoma. Rare cases of sinus histiocytosis with massive lymphadenopathy (Rosai-Dorfman disease) have been described.

Malignant lymphoid infiltrates may show many of the features considered classical of invasive lobular carcinoma. Lack of nuclear pleomorphism, periductal 'targetoid' infiltration and non-destructive invasion of the stroma are features common to both lesions. Lymphomas may also show cytoplasmic clearing that can mimic cells of lobular carcinoma. However, true cytoplasmic lumina or the presence of intra-cytoplasmic mucin are seen only in lobular carcinoma. In rare cases, cytokeratin immunohistochemical stains may be required to distinguish between the two lesions. An additional point to remember is that lobular carcinomas are seldom negative for hormone receptors; any lesion that is called lobular carcinoma but is negative for ER and PR requires a critical second look.

PROGNOSIS AND TREATMENT

The prognosis of primary breast lymphoma is dependent on the stage of disease. Disease confined to the breast can be treated with conservative surgery and radiation. Chemotherapy may be needed in cases with disseminated disease. Leukemic deposits are associated with synchronous or metachronous appearance of systemic disease; it is the latter that determines long term prognosis.

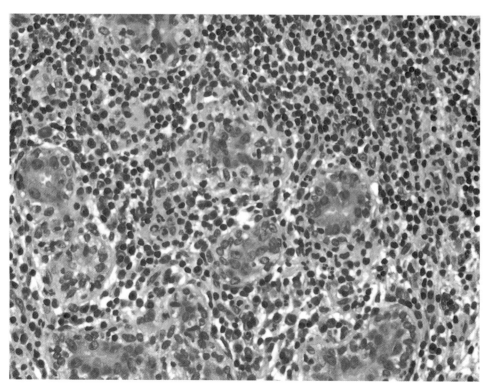

FIGURE 26-8

A dense chronic inflammatory infiltrate surrounds breast lobules, indicative of lobular mastitis.

SARCOMAS

The term stromal sarcoma has been applied by some authors as a collective noun to identify sarcomas that arise in the breast. In recent years, this term has fallen out of favor and sarcomas of the breast are classified in a manner similar to those that arise elsewhere in the body. In general, these lesions are rare; angiosarcomas appear to be the most common type of sarcoma reported at this site.

ANGIOSARCOMA

CLINICAL FEATURES

Angiosarcomas of the breast are seen in two distinct settings. In older women, it is usually related to breast cancer, where it is secondary to chronic lymphedema following surgery (Stewart-Treves syndrome) or secondary to radiotherapy for breast cancer. In the latter setting, it is typically seen 3–12 years after radiotherapy and primarily affects the skin with or without involve-ment of the underlying breast parenchyma. The risk of developing angiosarcoma does not correlate with the amount of radiation received or the use of a 'boost' dose. In younger women, it presents as a painless mass often without any skin changes. It may occur in pregnant women, in whom the tumors tend to be of higher grade and concomitantly more aggressive in behavior. Unlike breast cancers, angiosarcomas are as common in the right as in the left breast.

RADIOLOGIC FEATURES

Mammography in primary angiosarcomas usually shows architectural distortion without micro-calcifications. On ultrasound examination, the lesion is usually seen as an ill-defined lobulated tumor with areas of hyper- and hypoechogenicity. MRI has been used successfully to characterize these lesions and is particularly useful in post-radiation angiosarcomas to define the extent of the lesion.

PATHOLOGIC FEATURES

Although most malignant lesions tend to be larger than 2 cm, the gross features of low grade angiosarcomas are non-specific. High grade tumors, on the other hand, tend

---

ANGIOSARCOMA – FACT SHEET

Definition
▶ Malignant vascular tumor

Incidence and Location
▶ Rare tumor
▶ Equally affects right and left breasts
▶ Associated with radiotherapy or surgery for breast carcinoma

Morbidity and Mortality
▶ 5-year survival: 15–75 %, depending on tumor grade

Gender, Race and Age Distribution
▶ Wide age range
▶ In older women it is associated with lymphedema post surgery for breast cancer or radiotherapy

Clinical Features
▶ In young women, painless mass
▶ In older women, skin erythema with or without mass lesions

Radiologic Features
▶ Architectural distortion
▶ MRI is useful in defining the extent of the lesion

Prognosis and Treatment
▶ Surgery with clean margins
▶ Role of chemotherapy is not clear

ANGIOSARCOMA – PATHOLOGIC FEATURES

Gross Findings
▶ Non-specific
▶ Larger lesions may have areas of hemorrhage and necrosis

Microscopic Findings
▶ Vasoformative, sieve-like or solid patterns
▶ Endothelial tufting, cytologic atypia prominent in high grade lesions

Ultrastructural Features
▶ Weibel-Palade bodies
▶ Intra-cytoplasmic lumina

Fine Needle Aspiration Biopsy Findings
▶ Difficult lesion to diagnose on FNA

Immunohistochemical Features
▶ CD31, CD34, B72.3 positive
▶ Ki-67 expression useful in low grade lesions

Differential Diagnosis
▶ Benign vascular lesions
▶ Pseudoangiomatous stromal hyperplasia
▶ Carcinoma with pseudovascular growth pattern

to be large and are often friable; some lesions appear spongy and resemble placental tissue.

Histologically, angiosarcomas show vasoformative (Figure 26-9), sieve-like (Figure 26-10) and solid growth patterns. Low grade angiosarcomas can exhibit a capillary hemangioma-like growth pattern, an anastomosing branching pattern (Figure 26-11) or, rarely, a diffuse, infiltrating growth pattern. The endothelial cells lining the vascular spaces are cytologically bland and do not show endothelial tufting or significant mitotic activity. Distinction from benign lesions can be difficult; a high index of suspicion is required. As normal vascular

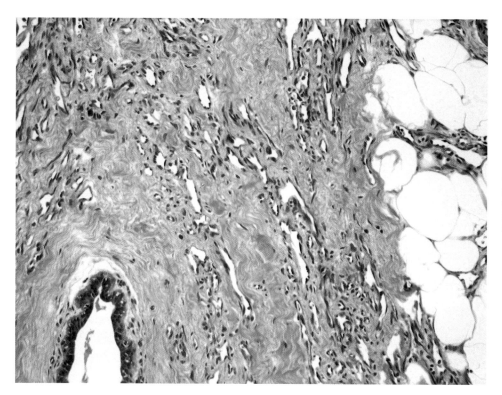

FIGURE 26-9

Angiosarcoma. Vasoformative pattern showing neoplastic well-formed vascular channels, lined by a single layer of endothelial cells.

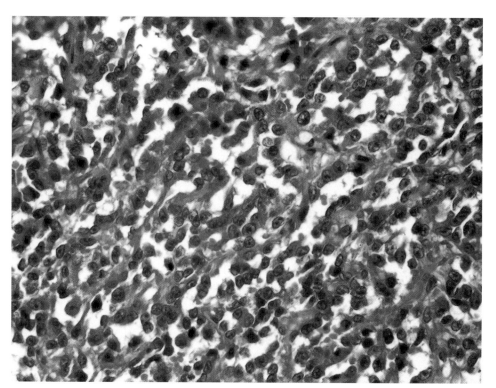

FIGURE 26-10

Angiosarcoma. Sieve-like pattern. The vascular channels are lined by a, predominantly, single layer of plump, hyperchromatic endothelial cells.

endothelial cells have a very low proliferation rate (less than 0.1%), analysis of proliferation markers, such as Ki-67, can be of value in difficult cases.

Intermediate grade angiosarcomas are relatively rare in most series. These show areas of cellular proliferation with endothelial tufting (Figure 26-12). Although a spindle cell growth pattern can be seen, it is usually not prominent in intermediate grade tumors.

High grade lesions are characterized by prominent endothelial tufts, solid papillae and large vascular cisterns (blood lakes) (Figure 26-13). The endothelial cells show marked cytologic atypia and frequent mitoses

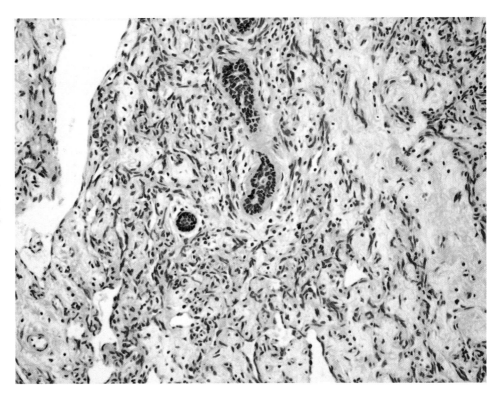

FIGURE 26-11

Angiosarcoma, low-grade. An anastomosing branching pattern is present, exhibiting a capillary hemangioma-like appearance. Infiltration of the breast parenchyma is seen.

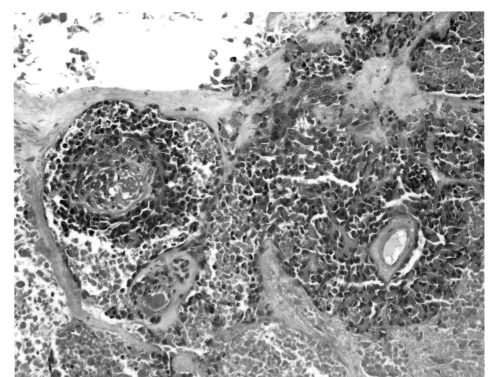

FIGURE 26-12

Angiosarcoma, intermediate grade. Endothelial cell proliferation is greater than that seen in low-grade lesions. Perivascular growth and endothelial tufting are present.

(Figure 26-14). Focal areas of necrosis, interstitial hemorrhages and solid growth mimicking carcinoma are common and helpful in both diagnosis and grading.

Post-radiation angiosarcomas are superficial and an ill-defined purple discoloration of the skin is all that is seen in early lesions. The tumor is located in the skin with or without involvement of the breast parenchyma.

Although these tumors can be low-grade, most lesions show mixed morphologic patterns and are associated with cytologically malignant endothelial cells showing nuclear anaplasia and frequent mitotic activity.

On electron microscopy, the tumor cells show the expected characteristics of endothelial cells such as Weibel-Palade bodies and intra-cytoplasmic lumina. In

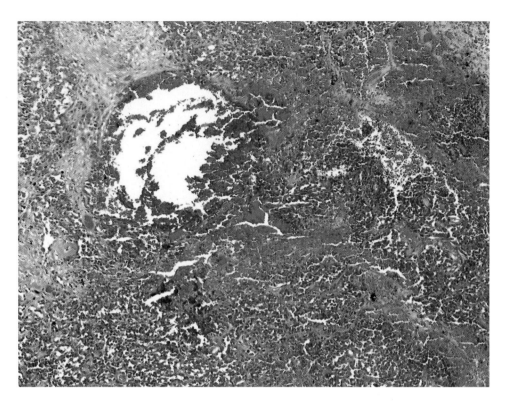

FIGURE 26-13

Angiosarcoma, high grade. A more solid pattern of growth is seen with areas of necrosis and large vascular cisterns (blood lakes).

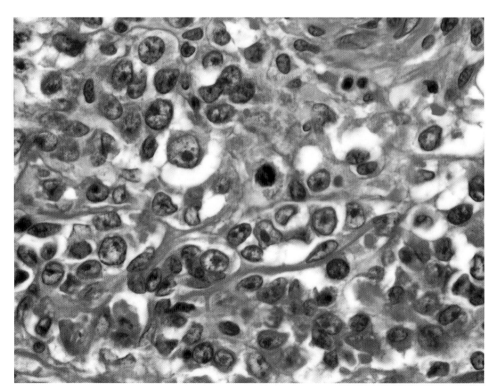

FIGURE 26-14

Angiosarcoma, high grade. On higher magnification, marked cytologic atypia is seen with a mitotic figure (center). The growth is more solid; however, red blood cells can still be identified in a paranuclear location and in small vascular channels.

addition, features such as endothelial cell overlap and spider web-like spaces are seen on scanning electron microscopy.

ANCILLARY STUDIES

Fine needle aspiration diagnosis of angiosarcoma is difficult; this is particularly so for low-grade lesions. In the irradiated breast, angiosarcoma needs to be distinguished from recurrent carcinoma. Features such as marked cell discohesiveness, elongated cytoplasmic processes (pseudopodia), heterogeneous cell size, large nucleoli or macronucleoli, and cytoplasmic lumina have been suggested to be of help in the differential diagnosis. Morphologic and immunohistochemical characteristics of tumor cells in cell blocks can help in making the correct diagnosis.

Immunohistochemistry is extremely valuable in the diagnosis of angiosarcoma. The tumor cells show expression of vascular markers, such as factor VIII-related antigen (FVIIIAg), Ulex europaeus agglutinin-I, CD31 and CD34. Expression of B72.3 directed against tumor associated glycoprotein-72 has been reported in epithelioid angiosarcomas. Although focal expression of cytokeratin may be seen in epithelioid lesions, it tends to be weak and unlike the diffuse positivity seen in carcinomas. Analysis of expression of proliferation markers in endothelial cells is useful in the diagnosis of low grade angiosarcomas, as noted above.

DIFFERENTIAL DIAGNOSIS

The differential diagnosis of low grade angiosarcoma includes hemangioma, lymphangioma, angiolipomas, papillary endothelial hyperplasia (Masson's tumor) and pseudoangiomatous stromal hyperplasia (PASH). Perilobular hemangiomas are a relatively common incidental finding in breast specimens. They lack endothelial atypia and do not show evidence of proliferation. Angiolipomas can show small vessel proliferation and the growth pattern may appear infiltrative, particularly in small biopsies. The presence of hyaline thrombi in the vessels is a good clue to the correct diagnosis. Pseudoangiomatous stromal hyperplasia is characterized by the presence of prominent slit-like spaces lined by spindle cells, which can mimic the anastomosing pattern seen in angiosarcomas. In the commoner benign lesions, the presence of keloidal collagen is a helpful finding. However, in some lesions the cellularity is prominent enough to raise the differential diagnosis of a sarcoma. These cells do not react with vascular markers except for CD34 and show expression of actin and/or desmin. In the irradiated breast, the skin can show small vascular lesions designated as atypical vascular lesions. These lesions tend to be circumscribed, located in the superficial dermis and lack endothelial multi-layering. Breast carcinomas can show a pseudovascular growth pattern (Figure 26-15), and need to be distinguished from high grade sarcomas. Unlike angiosarcomas, carcinomas show diffuse, strong expression of cytokeratins and do not show expression of vascular markers.

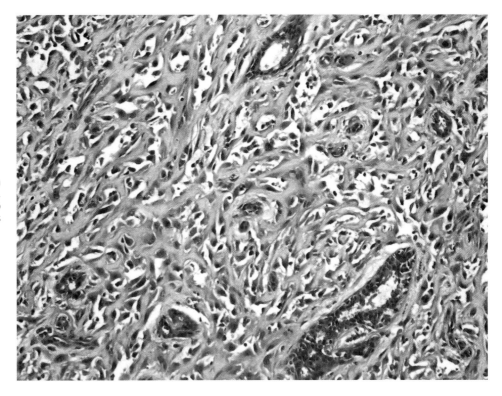

FIGURE 26-15
Pseudo-angiosarcomatous pattern in an infiltrating ductal carcinoma. Immunohistochemistry is needed to confirm the epithelial nature of this infiltrate.

PROGNOSIS AND TREATMENT

The prognosis in angiosarcomas is largely determined by tumor grade. The 5-year survival of patients with low, intermediate and high grade angiosarcomas is reported to be 76 %, 70 % and 15 %, respectively. High grade lesions tend to metastasize to the lungs, contralateral breast and skeleton. Nodal involvement is rare. The treatment consists of local surgery to obtain clear margins, and in some cases, may involve a mastectomy. Chemotherapy does not seem to be very helpful in the control of disease.

OTHER TYPES OF SARCOMAS

CLINICAL FEATURES

Sarcomas of the breast, apart from angiosarcomas, have been described in rare case reports and small series. The majority of sarcomas of the breast arise in association with a phyllodes tumor and the clinical features and presentation of these will therefore be as for the underlying fibroepithelial lesion. Primary sarcomas, except for rhabdomyosarcomas, tend to be tumors of adults with a wide age range. Rhadomyosarcomas in the breast tend to be seen in children, can be primary or metastatic in origin and tend to be of embryonal or alveolar sub-type. Most tend to be rapidly growing masses but, on occasion, the growth might be deceptively insidious.

RADIOLOGIC FEATURES

Mammographic findings are non-specific and in some cases can be negative. Abnormalities, when present, tend to be soft tissue masses with architectural distortion. Ultrasound examination is generally better at delineating the size of the lesion.

PATHOLOGIC FEATURES

In general, primary sarcomas of the breast are seen as poorly circumscribed, infiltrative lesions with areas of necrosis and hemorrhage (Figure 26-16). The size can vary depending on the duration of the lesion and is significantly affected by the location in the breast; superficial lesions tend to be smaller than those located deep in the breast due to ease of diagnosis. The lesions tend to be aggressive and are often associated with a history of rapid growth. One of the main features to be noted on gross examination is the presence or lack of associ-

---

OTHER SARCOMAS – FACT SHEET

Definition
▶ Sarcomas similar in morphology to other soft tissue tumors

Incidence and Location
▶ Extremely rare

Morbidity and Mortality
▶ Depends on the type and extent of disease

Gender, Race and Age Distribution
▶ Wide age range
▶ Rhabdomyosarcoma in young individuals

Clinical Features
▶ Poorly circumscribed, infiltrative lesions
▶ Hemorrhage and necrosis common

Radiologic Features
▶ Depending upon the type
▶ Marked calcifications and ossifications may be seen in osteosarcomas

Prognosis and Treatment
▶ Depends on the type and extent of disease

OTHER SARCOMAS – PATHOLOGIC FEATURES

Gross Findings
▶ Poorly circumscribed, infiltrative lesions
▶ Hemorrhage and necrosis common

Microscopic Findings
▶ Depends on the type

Ultrastructural Features
▶ Depends on the type

Fine Needle Aspiration Biopsy Findings
▶ Malignant appearing spindle to polygonal cells
▶ Sub-typing of sarcoma is difficult

Immunohistochemical Features
▶ Depends on the type

Differential Diagnosis
▶ Benign soft tissue tumors such as nodular fasciitis, granular cell tumor
▶ Phyllodes tumor
▶ Metaplastic carcinoma
▶ Metastatic melanoma

ated carcinoma or phyllodes tumor. Examination of the periphery of these lesions is often very informative in making the correct diagnosis.

Primary sarcomas of the breast are rare; every effort should be made to exclude a metaplastic carcinoma and/or phyllodes tumor with stromal overgrowth. Sarcomatous areas in these tumors can show features of leiomyosarcoma, liposarcoma, osteosarcoma and/or malignant fibrous histocytoma (pleomorphic sarcoma, not otherwise specified).

Of the primary sarcomas of the breast, leiomyosarcomas are said to be the most common. These may arise from the smooth muscle of the nipple or from vascular smooth muscle. The morphology of these tumors is similar to those arising elsewhere. In terms of behavior, they are related to their counterparts in the extremities rather than those arising in the uterus. Any degree of mitotic activity or pleomorphism is worrisome and tumors with 1–2 mitoses per high power field can metastasize. It is not known whether these tumors express estrogen and/or progesterone receptors.

Liposarcomatous differentiation (Figure 26-17) in metaplastic carcinomas or phyllodes tumors is not uncommon. These tumors also need to be differentiated from those arising in the skin and soft tissue of the chest. The diagnosis of liposarcoma of the breast is thus one of exclusion. All grades of liposarcomas have been described with the myxoid variant being more frequent.

Primary osteosarcoma of the breast is also rare (Figure 26-18); focal osteosarcomatous differentiation in metaplastic carcinomas or phyllodes tumors is, however, much more common. The entire spectrum of morphologic types including osteoblastic, spindle cell,

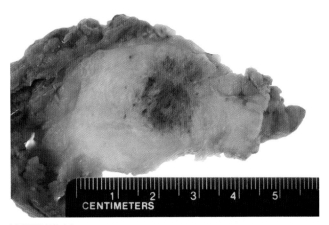

FIGURE 26-16

Sarcoma in the breast. The tumor is seen as a poorly circumscribed, infiltrative lesion, with areas of necrosis and hemorrhage.

chondroid, osteoclastic, telangiectatic and small cell have been described.

Sarcomas can also be undifferentiated; these have, in some cases, been designated as fibrosarcoma, malignant fibrous histiocytomas or pleomorphic sarcomas, not otherwise specified. A significant number of these lesions arise in the irradiated breast (Figure 26-19), but, lesions of similar morphology can arise in the absence of radiation. These tend to be high grade lesions with frequent mitotic activity and areas of necrosis.

Electron microscopy can be of use in classifying stromal lesions of the breast and this technique was

FIGURE 26-17

Liposarcoma of the breast. Variably-sized fat cells with lipoblasts in a myxoid background. Liposarcomatous differentiation can be seen in metaplastic carcinomas and phyllodes tumours.

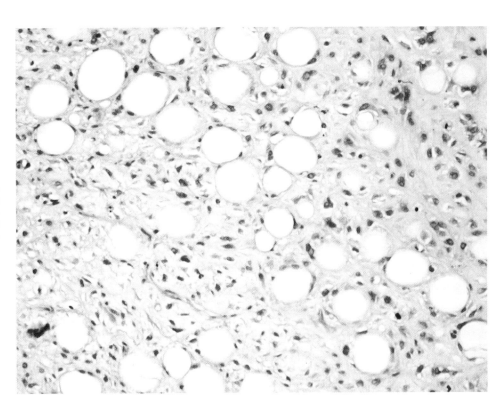

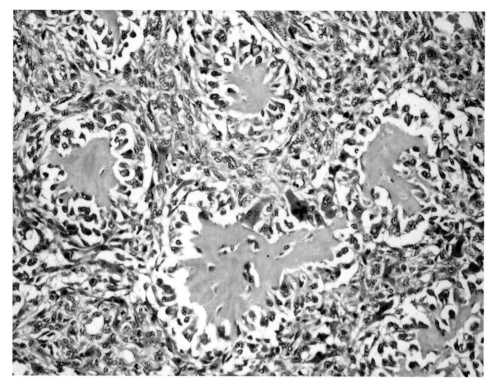

FIGURE 26-18

Osteogenic sarcoma of the breast. A malignant spindle-cell population producing osteoid is identified. Primary osteosarcomas of the breast are rare. Osteosarcomatous differentiation is more often seen in metaplastic carcinomas or phyllodes tumors.

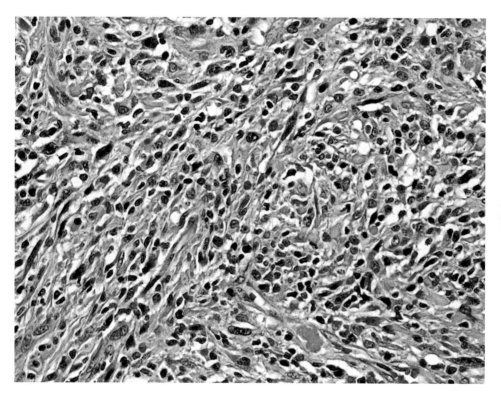

FIGURE 26-19

Post-radiation sarcoma of the breast. A diffuse infiltrate of malignant spindle cells is seen, lacking any differentiating features.

commonly used prior to the immunohistochemistry era. The finding of epithelial features, such as tight junctions, would enable recognition of a carcinoma masquerading as a sarcoma. Similarly, the presence of melanosomes could confirm the diagnosis of melanoma. Apart from excluding carcinoma and melanoma, ultrastructural features could also identify specific differentiating features associated with different sarcomas such as myofilaments in leiomyosarcoma.

ANCILLARY STUDIES

Fine needle aspiration cytology usually shows the presence of discohesive clusters of pleomorphic malignant cells. The cells tend to be spindled to polygonal with a high nuclear to cytoplasmic ratio. Although sampling issues make a definite diagnosis of primary sarcoma difficult, a preliminary diagnosis of these lesions can on occasions be made.

IMMUNOHISTOCHEMISTRY

Sarcomas of the breast exhibit an immunophenotype that is similar to their counterparts elsewhere in the body and, in general, are negative for cytokeratins. Although focal expression may be seen in the epithelioid variants, the distribution and intensity is never similar to that seen in carcinomas. Leiomyosarcomas tend to stain positively for smooth muscle actin and desmin while liposarcomas are positive for S100 protein. Osteosarcomas and undifferentiated sarcomas are only positive for vimentin.

DIFFERENTIAL DIAGNOSIS

A malignant spindled cell lesion of the breast is likely to represent a metaplastic carcinoma rather than a primary sarcoma. Thus, the diagnosis of primary sarcomas of the breast is one of exclusion, and metaplastic carcinoma, phyllodes tumor and metastatic lesions such as malignant melanoma need to be excluded. Metaplastic carcinomas very often show strong positivity with only one or two of a range of cytokeratins and a panel of anti-cytokeratin antibodies should be applied. Similarly, a phyllodes tumor may demonstrate significant stromal overgrowth and thorough blocking should be undertaken to search for the cleft-like spaces of the epithelial component of such a lesion. In addition, S100 protein and HMB-45 are useful in the differential diagnosis if malignant melanoma is to be excluded. Tumors of the skin and subcutaneous tissue, such as dermatofibrosarcoma protuberans, also need to be considered. These tumors are composed of fibroblastic cells that show a characteristic storiform pattern and lack significant pleomorphism.

The differential diagnosis of low grade spindled cell/fibrous tumors includes inflammatory myofibro-

blastic tumor and fibromatosis of the breast. The morphology of fibromatosis is similar to that at other sites and consists of fascicles of infiltrating fibroblastic cells in a collagenous matrix. Rare mitotic figures may be present. In addition, benign stromal lesions, such as granular cell tumors, nodular fasciitis and myofibroblastomas may require exclusion in some cases. The latter is composed of small spindle cells that have a characteristic growth pattern. They can exhibit mild to moderate nuclear pleomorphism and can show mitotic activity although this is unusual.

Leiomyomas and leiomyomatous hamartomas need to be considered in the differential diagnosis of leiomyosarcoma. The latter is a rare condition in which mature smooth muscle bundles are seen as part of a benign hamartomatous proliferation. The differential diagnosis of lipomatous tumors includes angiolipoma and atypical and pleomorphic lipomas.

PROGNOSIS AND TREATMENT

The behavior of primary sarcomas of the breast is similar to their soft tissue counterparts. These tumors are treated with local surgery which, at times, consists of a mastectomy. Smaller lesions can be treated with breast conserving therapy.

METASTATIC TUMORS

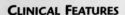

CLINICAL FEATURES

Metastatic tumors in the breast are rare in any age group. In childhood, rhabdomyosarcoma, particularly embryonal type, is the commonest metastatic tumor. In adults, apart from metastatic malignant melanoma, most metastatic lesions to the breast tend to be carcinomas. The primary sites include the usual suspects such as lung, stomach and gastrointestinal tract. Additional primary sites include the ovary in females and prostate in males. Metastatic tumors in the breast can be unilateral or bilateral and although the presence of multiple masses in the breast in a patient with a known history of carcinoma is classical, these lesions are seldom biopsied. Most lesions that undergo biopsy tend to be solitary and the biopsy tends to be performed to rule out primary carcinoma.

RADIOLOGIC FEATURES

Mammographic examination is indicated in the work-up of any breast mass. No typical appearance has been described for metastatic carcinoma and the features can be similar to primary breast carcinoma (Figure 26-20). However, the identification of smaller, non-palpable lesions in a patient with a history of cancer is strongly suggestive of metastatic disease. Similarly, ultrasound examination may be of great value in detecting smaller lesions not associated with calcifications.

PATHOLOGIC FEATURES

Most cases of metastatic carcinoma are diagnosed on needle biopsies. As surgical resection is most commonly performed on cases that lack characteristic features, the classical appearance of multiple masses of varying sizes throughout the breast tissue is seldom seen. Resected metastatic lesions in the breast are typically seen as solitary lesions mimicking breast cancer. In rare instances, metastases from a malignant melanoma may contain enough pigment to be grossly visible.

The wide range of morphologic features seen in primary breast cancer can make diagnosis of metastatic disease difficult; in most cases the diagnosis requires good clinico-pathologic correlation. The recognition of metastatic tumor requires a high index of suspicion and the diagnosis should be considered in any tumor that lacks an *in situ* component. However, the presence of an associated (atypical) intra-ductal proliferation does not always indicate a breast origin (Figure 26-21).

The diagnosis of metastatic tumor is easier when the tumor has an unusual appearance for a breast primary lesion or a typical morphology of its primary site of origin such as extensive squamous differentiation; primary squamous cell carcinoma of the breast is relatively rare and usually is part of a metaplastic carcinoma. A tumor with a signet ring cell morphology in the breast most likely represents a primary lobular carcinoma, however, a metastasis, in particular from a gastric tumor, can have a prominent signet ring appearance (Figure 26-22). The presence of melanin pigment enables the recognition of malignant melanoma. The presence of psammoma bodies might aid the recognition of a papillary serous carcinoma of the ovary. The diagnosis is more difficult to make when the tumor has neuroendocrine features as tumors with similar morphology can be seen in the breast, particularly in older women. In some cases, the diagnosis is made retrospectively following the recognition of a primary elsewhere.

Electron microscopy might aid in the identification of specific cell lineage such as the presence of melanosomes in malignant melanoma. The presence of neuroendocrine granules can be seen in a large number of primary tumors and does not help in the differential diagnosis of primary tumor versus a metastatic deposit.

ANCILLARY STUDIES

Fine needle aspiration biopsy is useful in making the diagnosis of malignancy. In some cases this is enough to confirm the suspected diagnosis of metastatic

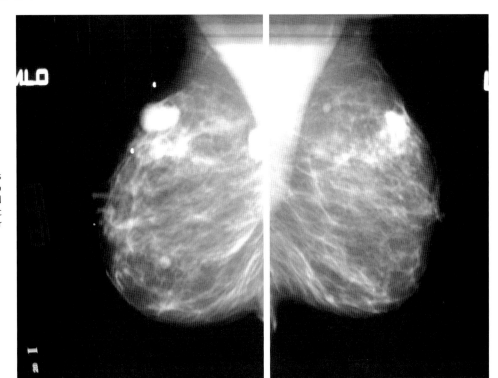

FIGURE 26-20

Mammogram showing metastases from a malignant melanoma. No typical features have been described for metastatic lesions to the breast and the appearances can be similar to primary breast carcinoma.

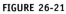

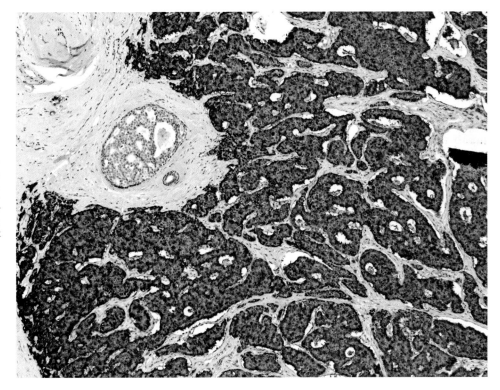

FIGURE 26-21

Chromogranin expression in metastatic carcinoid tumor but not in the associated intraductal proliferation. This image illustrates that the presence of an associated *in situ* or atypical intra-ductal proliferation does not always indicate a breast origin.

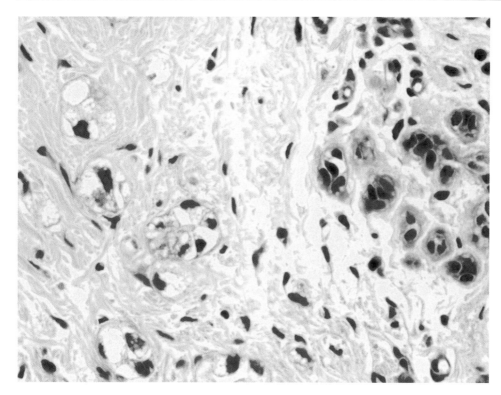

FIGURE 26-22

Metastatic signet ring cell carcinoma from the stomach. Malignant cells with a signet ring cell morphology, mimicking primary lobular carcinoma of the breast.

disease. The diagnosis of melanoma can be suggested on the basis of cytologic features and the presence of melanin pigment. Similarly, the presence of numerous signet ring cells might lead one to suspect metastatic disease.

Immunohistochemistry can play a major role in the diagnosis of metastatic tumors (see Chapter 25). The analysis of differential cytokeratin expression, particularly CK7 and CK20, is useful in suspected cases. Gastrointestinal tumors tend to be CK20 positive and CK7 negative; however, this profile can also be seen in some primary mucinous tumors of the breast. Lung and ovarian tumors have a similar cytokeratin profile as breast cancer; the latter can also show expression of hormone receptors. In males, the expression of PSA and PSAP might help in the recognition of metastatic prostatic carcinoma.

DIFFERENTIAL DIAGNOSIS

The diagnosis of metastatic breast tumors is difficult and requires a high index of suspicion and good clinicopathologic correlation. The recognition of unusual morphologic features and the lack of an *in situ* component are useful features. However, these features are not absolute as illustrated in Figure 26-21, where foci of DCIS or ADH may be seen adjacent to metastatic tumors. The cytokeratin profile may be useful in making the diagnosis. Urothelial tumors tend to express high molecular weight keratins and the CK7/CK20 expres-

sion profile may be of value in recognizing a gastrointestinal primary. However, as noted above, mucin-secreting breast carcinomas may rarely show CK20 expression. Although adenocarcinomas of the lung have the same cytokeratin profile as breast carcinoma, the expression of TTF-1 has not been reported in breast cancers. Additionally, the expression of hormone receptors would be extremely unusual in tumors arising from the lung, gastrointestinal tract or urothelium, although gastric carcinomas may do so. Prostate specific antigen (PSA) can be secreted by normal and malignant breast tissues. The presence of PSA in serum and in tumor cells has been reported. However, the expression of both PSA and PSAP (prostate specific acid phosphatase) is extremely unlikely in breast cancer. Distinction of metastatic neuroendocrine tumors from primary breast tumors on the basis of morphology is extremely difficult. But, unlike metastatic carcinoid tumors, primary breast tumors, at least those of low grade, almost invariably express hormone receptors. The analysis of expression of other breast 'specific' markers such GCDFP-15 is of limited value.

PROGNOSIS AND TREATMENT

The prognosis of patients with metastatic tumors depends on the extent of disease. In most cases, the presence of disease at multiple sites precludes an aggressive approach. However, patients with isolated breast metastases may be treated with conservative surgery.

SUGGESTED READINGS

Leukemia and Lymphomas

Abbondanzo SL, Seidman JD, Lefkowitz M, *et al*. Primary diffuse large B-cell lymphoma of the breast. A clinicopathologic study of 31 cases. Pathol Res Pract 1996;192:37–43.

Aguilera NS, Tavassoli FA, Chu WS, Abbondanzo SL. T-cell lymphoma presenting in the breast: a histologic, immunophenotypic and molecular genetic study of four cases. Mod Pathol 2000;13:599–605.

Brustein S, Filippa DA, Kimmel M, *et al*. Malignant lymphoma of the breast. A study of 53 patients. Ann Surg 1987;205:144–50.

Angiosarcoma

Billings SD, McKenney JK, Folpe AL, *et al*. Cutaneous angiosarcoma following breast-conserving surgery and radiation: an analysis of 27 cases. Am J Surg Pathol 2004;28:781–788.

Branton PA, Lininger R, Tavassoli FA. Papillary endothelial hyperplasia of the breast: the great impostor for angiosarcoma: a clinicopathologic review of 17 cases. Int J Surg Pathol 2003;11:83–87.

Fineberg S, Rosen PP. Cutaneous angiosarcoma and atypical vascular lesions of the skin and breast after radiation therapy for breast carcinoma. Am J Clin Pathol 1994;102:757–763.

Kahn HC, Chin NW, Opitz LM, *et al*. Cellular angiolipoma of the breast: immunohistochemical study and review of the literature. Breast J 2002;8:47–49.

Ritter JH, Mills SE, Nappi O, Wick MR. Angiosarcoma-like neoplasms of epithelial organs: true endothelial tumors or variants of carcinoma? Semin Diagn Pathol 1995;12:270–282.

Other Sarcomas

Adem C, Reynolds C, Ingle JN, Nascimento AG. Primary breast sarcoma: clinicopathologic series from the Mayo Clinic and review of the literature. Br J Cancer 2004;91:237–241.

Callery CD, Rosen PP, Kinne DW. Sarcoma of the breast. A study of 32 patients with reappraisal of classification and therapy. Ann Surg 1985;201:527–532.

Devouassoux-Shisheboran M, Schammel MD, Man YG, Tavassoli FA. Fibromatosis of the breast: age-correlated morphofunctional features of 33 cases. Arch Pathol Lab Med 2000;124:276–280.

Silver SA, Tavassoli FA. Primary osteogenic sarcoma of the breast: a clinicopathologic analysis of 50 cases. Am J Surg Pathol 1998;22:925–933.

Metastatic Carcinoma

Alvarado Cabrero I, Carrera Alvarez M, Perez Montiel D, Tavassoli FA. Metastases to the breast. Eur J Surg Oncol 2003;29:854–855.

Georgiannos SN, Chin J, Goode AW, Sheaff M. Secondary neoplasms of the breast: a survey of the 20th Century. Cancer 2001;92:2259–2266.

27 Diseases of the Male Breast
Sunil Badve

GYNECOMASTIA

The male breast is composed of a small nipple areolar complex with underlying ducts admixed with fatty tissue. The general architecture of the ductal system is similar to the female breast apart from the fact that it is relatively poorly developed. The ductal system ends blindly and the presence of terminal duct lobular units is extremely rare. Enlargement of the male breast due to any cause is termed gynecomastia.

GYNECOMASTIA – FACT SHEET

Definition
▸ Enlargement of the male breast

Incidence and Location
▸ Unilateral or bilateral

Morbidity and Mortality
▸ No increased risk of malignancy

Gender, Race and Age Distribution
▸ Peri-pubertal children
▸ Males older than 50 years

Clinical Features
▸ Soft nodule in the breast
▸ Pendulous breast
▸ Occasionally tender

Radiologic Features
▸ Increased fibro-glandular densities
▸ Increased fat

Prognosis and Treatment
▸ Benign self-limited disorder
▸ Surgery is curative

CLINICAL FEATURES

Gynecomastia can be seen at any age but is typically seen in boys around puberty and in men over the age of 50 years. Mild enlargement of the breast is not uncommon in boys; this tends to be bilateral, often asymmetrical and rarely persists into adulthood. Gynecomastia of a degree which requires surgery is more common in older adults and can be unilateral or bilateral. A broad range of drugs and medical conditions can lead to enlargement of the breast (Table 27-1). Although morphologic changes of gynecomastia can be found in tissues excised for breast cancer, available evidence seems to suggest that gynecomastia does not predispose to malignancy.

Clinically, gynecomastia is seen as a soft, sometimes tender nodular area located behind and slightly above the nipple; this is in contrast to carcinomas which may be peripherally located. The lesions can vary in size from 2–5 cm and can be unilateral or bilateral. Symptoms such as nipple discharge, ulceration, bleeding and skin inversion are distinctly uncommon and may be indicative of underlying malignancy.

RADIOLOGIC FEATURES

Mammography can be used as effectively in males as in females to diagnose breast lesions. The typical findings are a diffuse increase in fibro-glandular densities. Microcalcifications can be identified on occasion. Ultrasound examination can also be used to rule out malignancy. Benign masses and cysts tend to follow the breast parenchyma and are seen on sonogram, typically as lesions that are 'wider than tall'.

PATHOLOGIC FEATURES

The gross features of gynecomastia are non-specific. The tissue is seen as an ill-defined mass of grayish white tissue admixed with fat; no definite mass lesion can be identified. However, in some cases, a circumscribed mass with a pseudo-capsule has been described.

TABLE 27-1

Causes of gynecomastia and their relative frequency

Cause	Frequency (%)
Idiopathic	25
Puberty	25
Drugs	10 ± 20
Cirrhosis or malnutrition	8
Primary hypogonadism	8
Testicular tumor	3
Secondary hypogonadism	2
Hyperthyroidism	2
Renal disease	1
Others	6

Data from Braunstein GD. Gynaecomastia. N Eng J Med 1993;328:490–495.

GYNECOMASTIA – PATHOLOGIC FEATURES

Gross Findings
▸ Non-specific
▸ Ill-defined grayish mass

Microscopic Findings
▸ Florid and fibrous types
▸ Florid type associated with epithelial hyperplasia, stromal edema and increased cellularity. PASH-like changes may be present
▸ Fibrous type characterized by dense fibrous tissue with atrophic glands

Ultrastructural Features
▸ Non-specific

Fine Needle Aspiration Biopsy Findings
▸ Pauci-cellular aspirate with epithelial and myoepithelial cells along with fatty stroma

Immunohistochemical Features
▸ Epithelial cells express 34βE12, CK5 and ER

Differential Diagnosis
▸ Male breast cancer
▸ Fat necrosis, epidermal inclusion cyst
▸ Myofibroblastoma

Gynecomastia can be classified into two types based on morphologic features: the florid type (also referred to as early type) and fibrous type (or late type). The terms early and late may not necessarily indicate duration of disease and are therefore not favored. Additionally, it is not uncommon to see an admixture of these two morphologies. The florid type (Figure 27-1) tends to exhibit epithelial hyperplasia. Epithelial hyperplasia is usually of mild to moderate degree. The proliferation is composed of two or more layers of cells often with finger-like projections extending in to the lumen (Figure 27-2). This, in some cases, might be severe enough to mimic micropapillary type of ductal carcinoma *in situ* (DCIS). The papillary projections, however, tend to lack the bulbous ('drumstick') architecture so characteristically seen in DCIS. In addition, the cells lack cytologic atypia. This 'gynecomastoid' hyperplasia, can also be seen in the female breast where it can be confused with atypical ductal hyperplasia.

Although atypical ductal hyperplasia has been described in gynecomastia, it is extremely rare and the diagnosis should be made with caution. The stroma in the florid type of gynecomastia stage is cellular and edematous (Figure 27-3), and depending on the type of hematoxylin and eosin (H&E) stain used, may show a bluish tinge due to the presence of mucopolysaccharides. Edema is most prominent around the ducts; the stroma gets progressively more fibrotic away from the ducts. The fibrous proliferative process terminates abruptly with a sharp interface at the mammary fat leading in some cases to an exaggerated nodular outline. Keloidal fibrosis may be noted and may, indeed, be prominent. The combination of keloidal fibrosis and stromal cellularity can in several areas give rise to the morphologic changes referred to as pseudoangiomatous stromal hyperplasia (PASH) (Figure 27-4). In the fibrotic type of gynecomastia the epithelial elements are seen in the form of scattered ducts with a minimal

degree of proliferative activity; the stroma is also fibrotic and acellular (Figure 27-5).

Gynecomastia does not have a well-defined capsule; however, on occasion a pseudo-capsule can be present. Some lesions may contain well-developed lobules with an architecture not unlike that seen in fibroadenomas. Cases of mammary hamartomas and phyllodes tumor, both benign and malignant, have also been described. Multi-nucleated stromal giant cells have been reported. These can occur in the absence of a history of radiation and are biologically similar to those described in fibroadenomas of the female breast.

ANCILLARY STUDIES

The morphologic characteristics are typical and ancillary studies, such as immunohistochemistry, are rarely required to confirm the diagnosis. In difficult cases, where there is coincidental co-existing invasive carcinoma, stains for myoepithelial cells are helpful in delineating the areas of invasion. Epithelial hyperplasia is associated with diffuse strong expression of high molecular weight keratins (34βE12) and/or CK5. This pattern is similar to that described in women and may be used as an adjunct in differentiating between intraductal proli-ferations in some cases. Fine needle aspiration (FNA) biopsy of male breast lesions has been

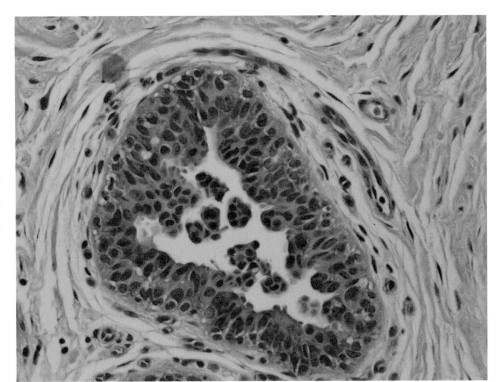

FIGURE 27-1

Gynecomastia, florid type. Note the moderate epithelial hyperplasia with budding, which is characteristically seen in gynecomastia. This 'gynecomatoid' hyperplasia is often seen in female breasts too.

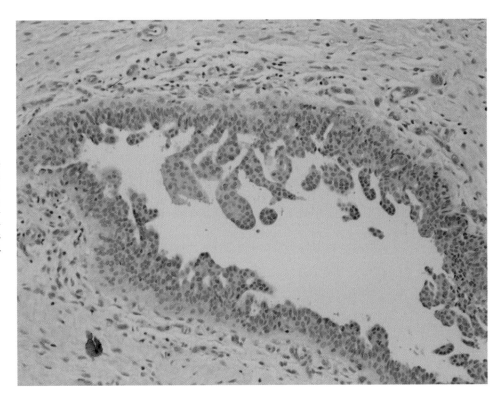

FIGURE 27-2

Gynecomastia, florid type. The epithelial proliferation is composed of two or more layers of cells, often with finger-like, tapered projections, extending into the lumen. This contrasts with the rigid bulbous projections characteristic of some forms of atypical ductal hyperplasia/ductal carcinoma *in situ*.

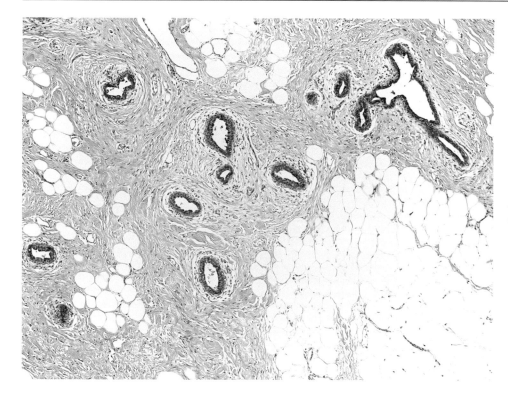

FIGURE 27-3

Gynecomastia, florid type. A cellular fibroblastic stroma and periductal edema is seen.

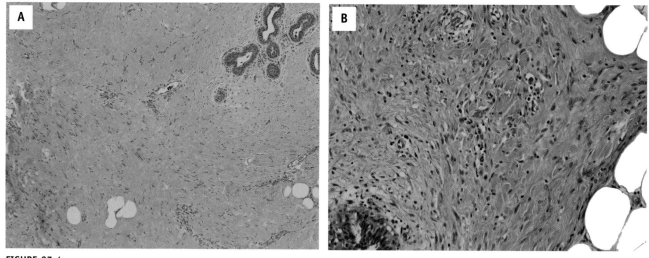

FIGURE 27-4

Gynecomastia with pseudoangiomatous stromal hyperplasia; (A) low power, (B) high power.

performed and, as in the female breast, is extremely valuable in excluding malignancy.

DIFFERENTIAL DIAGNOSIS

The clinical differential diagnosis of gynecomastia includes carcinoma, myofibroblastoma, fibroadenoma (and phyllodes tumor), epidermal inclusion cyst, fat necrosis and other soft tissue lesions such as lipomas and leiomyomas. These lesions are clinically and morphologically similar to those occurring in women and are discussed in detail in other sections of this book.

Mammography and ultrasound are of great value in making the correct pre-operative diagnosis. FNA cytology can be used to differentiate between these lesions. The accuracy is perhaps higher than that in the female breast because of the rarity of fibroadenomas and well-differentiated tubular or lobular carcinomas. Aspirates from malignant lesions are cellular, form three dimensional clusters and show cytologic atypia.

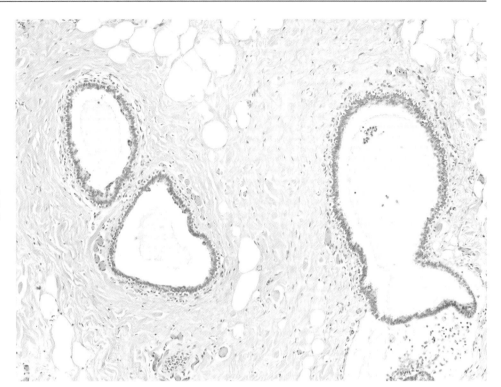

FIGURE 27-5
Gynecomastia, fibrous type. Scattered ducts with a minimal degree of proliferative activity are seen. The stroma is fibrotic and acellular.

PROGNOSIS

Gynecomastia is often a self-limiting disease and, in younger individuals, may not need any form of therapy. In those cases where a specific etiologic agent, such as a drug, can be identified, withdrawal of the causative agent may lead to regression. Although hormonal therapy with androgens can be used, surgical excision is curative. Currently there is very little evidence to suggest that gynecomastia predisposes a patient to malignancy.

MALE BREAST CANCER

CLINICAL FEATURES

Carcinoma of the male breast is rare. In the United States, it is estimated that approximately 1450 new cases of male breast cancer will be diagnosed in the year 2004 and 470 deaths will occur; this represents 0.2 % of all cancers and less than 0.1 % of all cancer deaths in men annually. By contrast, in Tanzania and areas of central Africa, breast cancer accounts for up to 6 % of cancers in men. In the US, the ratio of female to male breast cancer is approximately 100 : 1 in Caucasians, but lower (70 : 1) in African Americans. The data from the

---

MALE BREAST CANCER – FACT SHEET

Definition
▸ Carcinoma of the male breast

Incidence and Location
▸ 0.2% of all cancers
▸ Less than 0.1 % of all cancer related deaths

Morbidity and Mortality
▸ Depends on the histologic grade and stage

Gender, Race and Age Distribution
▸ Males, greater than 50 years of age

Clinical Features
▸ Self-detected painless mass lesion
▸ Occasionally bleeding, ulceration and pain

Radiologic Features
▸ Architectural distortion, spiculated calcifications
▸ Irregular contour on ultrasound with posterior shadowing

Prognosis and Treatment
▸ Stage tends to be higher than female breast cancer
▸ Prognosis similar to female breast cancer (stage by stage)

Surveillance, Epidemiology and End Results (SEER) database seems to suggest that the incidence of male breast cancer, unlike female breast cancer, has remained stable.

High levels of androgens in young men are thought to exert a protective effect against the development of malignancy. This theory is supported by the association of male breast cancer with prolactinomas, a condition often associated with low levels of plasma testosterone. In addition, carcinoma is distinctly uncommon in young men. Carcinoma in these younger individuals tends to be associated with conditions in which low levels of androgens are common. These include hypogonadism from a variety of causes including orchitis, cryptorchidism and testicular injury. Other predisposing causes include prior chest wall radiation and liver disease. Chromosomal disorders such as Klinefelter's syndrome (XXY) may also be associated with male breast cancer. Other predisposing causes include prior chest wall radiation and liver disease. Some reports suggest an increased risk for development of male breast carcinoma after occupational exposure to gasoline and airline fuels.

Familial male breast cancer is an inherited disorder and can be seen in families with *BRCA1/BRCA2* mutations. Men who inherit germline BRCA2 mutations have an estimated 6% lifetime risk of male breast cancer; this represents a 100-fold higher risk than in the general male population. Similarly, male breast cancer has been associated with mutations in p53 and PTEN tumor suppressor genes.

The patients are typically older individuals, median age 65–67 years, who present with a self-detected painless mass lesion. Nipple discharge, ulceration, bleeding, skin inversion, swelling and breast pain can also be the cause for presentation. In rare instances, presentation may be in the form of Paget's disease with excoriation of the nipple. Extremely rare cases of inflammatory carcinoma have been reported. The lesions, unlike those in the female breast, are typically located in the sub-areolar region and can often involve the nipple.

RADIOLOGIC FEATURES

As in the female breast, radiologic evaluation can contribute significantly to the diagnosis of a mass lesion in the male breast. Some reports seem to suggest that mammography is as effective in detecting and diagnosing carcinoma in the male breast as it is in the female breast. The BI-RADS™ system has been shown to be useful for reporting lesions of the male breast. Abnormalities similar to those seen in female breast cancer can be seen in 80–90% of the cases. These include architectural distortion, a mass that is 'taller than it is wide', irregular margins and spiculated, often, coarse calcifications. Unlike gynecomastia, the lesion tends to be located eccentrically in relation to the nipple. Ultrasound examination can also be used to aid in the differential diagnosis of benign cysts and, to a limited extent, fat necrosis.

PATHOLOGIC FEATURES

The gross examination of the specimen usually shows a hard, irregular, stellate mass often associated with yellow streaks. Lesions tend to be around 2 cm in size (1–5 cm). Fixation to the skin or pectoral muscles is not uncommon. Skin involvement may be in the form of edema, an ulcer or, rarely, take the form of Paget's disease.

Microscopically, the tumors look like their counterparts in women and grading of male breast carcinoma should be carried out in a similar manner using the Elston and Ellis (Nottingham) modification of the Scarff-Bloom-Richardson system. Most series describe a preponderance of high and intermediate grade tumors with relatively few well-differentiated tumors. Invasive carcinoma of ductal/no special type, accounts for the majority of the cases (Figure 27-6 and 27-7). However, all subtypes of invasive carcinoma, including cases of secretory type and mucinous type, have been described. Lobular carcinoma is rare (Figure 27-8); this has been (mistakenly) ascribed to the lack of lobules in the male breast.

As in women, invasive carcinoma in men is frequently associated with DCIS. Pure DCIS of the male breast is rare and in some studies accounts for 5% of male breast lesions. All architectural patterns, including papillary (intra-cystic) carcinoma, have been described.

MALE BREAST CANCER – PATHOLOGIC FEATURES

Gross Findings
▸ Hard irregular stellate mass

Microscopic Findings
▸ Similar to female breast cancer
▸ Lobular histology is rare

Ultrastructural Features
▸ Similar to female breast cancer

Fine Needle Aspiration Biopsy Findings
▸ Similar to female breast cancer

Immunohistochemical Features
▸ Similar to female breast cancer

Differential Diagnosis
▸ Gynecomastia
▸ Fat necrosis, epidermal inclusion cyst
▸ Myofibroblastoma

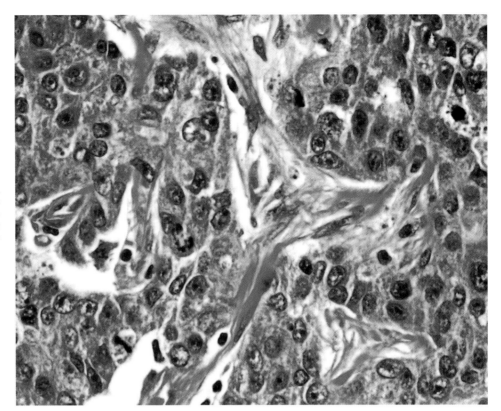

FIGURE 27-6

Invasive ductal carcinoma, no special type. This high power view shows solid nests of malignant cells, with prominent mitoses, similar to an analogous tumor in the female breast.

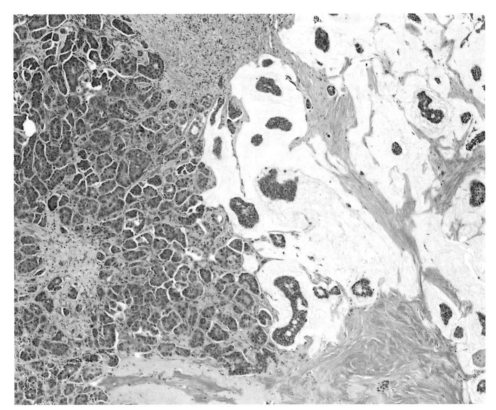

FIGURE 27-7

Invasive ductal carcinoma, with mucinous features. Again the histologic changes are similar to those found in breast cancer in women.

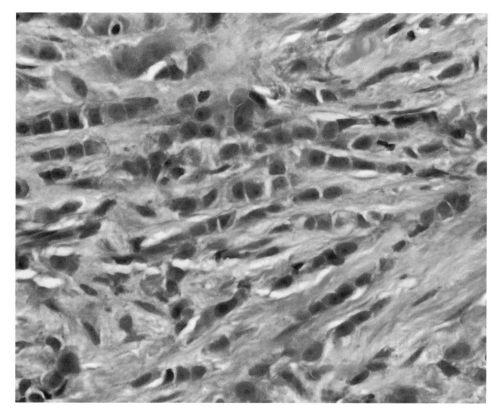

FIGURE 27-8

Invasive lobular carcinoma. The neoplastic cells are arranged in the characteristic single file fashion. This subtype of breast cancer is rare in men.

Comedo type necrosis is relatively uncommon. Whether or not lobular carcinoma in situ occurs in the male breast is controversial.

ANCILLARY STUDIES

RADIOLOGIC IMAGING

Identifying the tumor in the male usually does not require ancillary studies. Imaging studies can be used to define the extent of the lesion, particularly when breast conservation or preservation of the nipple–areolar complex is planned. In the rare situation where axillary metastasis is the presentation, imaging studies may be used to localize the primary tumor in the breast.

FINE NEEDLE ASPIRATION CYTOLOGY

Fine needle aspiration (FNA) cytology can play a significant role in the diagnostic process of male breast carcinoma, since most lesions are palpable. The accuracy is also improved by the fact that fibroadenomas and lobular carcinoma, which can often give rise to misdiagnosis, are relatively rare. The morphologic features seen on FNA cytology are similar to those seen in women and are described in Chapter 3.

IMMUNOHISTOCHEMISTRY

Immunohistochemically, male breast carcinomas are more likely to show expression of estrogen and/or progesterone receptors (ER and PR, respectively) than female breast carcinomas (Figure 27-9). Expression of these receptors has been reported in up to 80 % of cases and does not appear to show the strong association with grade that is seen in female breast cancers; in several studies, this association fails to reach statistical significance. The expression of androgen receptors is extremely common and has been described in up to 90 % of cases. The analysis of *HER2*/neu (c-*erb*B2) has been performed in male breast cancer; over-expression and amplifications are seen. Although experience is limited, it appears that the significance of *HER2*/neu (c-*erb*B2) expression is similar to that in female breast cancer both in terms of an aggressive course and, more importantly, response to Herceptin (trastuzumab). Mutations leading to abnormal expression of p53 are seen in around 30 % of cases. Expression analysis of several markers related to cell proliferation and apoptosis have been performed; in some studies these appear to have a prognostic and/or predictive role. Neuro-endocrine differentiation, as analyzed by histochemistry (silver stains) or immuohistochemistry (chromogranin, synaptophysin, NSE), is not uncommon and does not appear to have prognostic significance.

DIFFERENTIAL DIAGNOSIS

Gynecomastia, myofibroblastoma, fat necrosis, epidermal inclusion cyst, intra-ductal papilloma and stromal lesions can clinically mimic breast cancer; in most cases

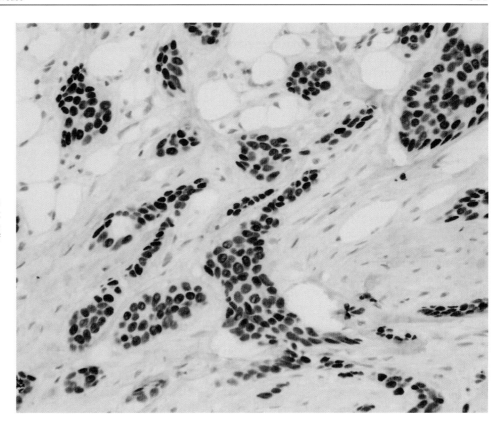

FIGURE 27-9
Estrogen receptor expression in male breast cancer. Most male breast carcinomas are strongly positive for estrogen receptors regardless of grade.

a pre-operative diagnosis can be made by the judicious use of imaging techniques. FNA cytology and/or core biopsy is particularly useful in cases where the imaging results are equivocal. The histology, usually, is sufficient to confirm the diagnosis of breast carcinoma. However, in some cases of gynecomastia and intra-ductal papillomas, intra-ductal epithelial proliferation can be prominent enough to raise the differential diagnosis of intra-ductal carcinoma. Hyperplastic lesions tend to show strong expression of high molecular weight cytokeratins (34βE12). Expression of this marker is either absent or weak and focal in DCIS. Expression analysis of myoepithelial markers such as smooth muscle actin or myosin, CD10 and/or p63 can be helpful in distinguishing intra-ductal from invasive lesions.

Paget's disease can present as a pigmented lesion and needs to be differentiated from melanoma. In addition, cancer cells may also contain prominent pigment. Stains for *HER*-2/neu, EMA, S100 protein and mucin are a useful adjunct in determining the correct diagnosis.

Metastases to the breast can occur from cancers arising at a variety of primary sites including lung, prostate, bladder carcinoma as well as malignant melanomas. Anecdotal evidence suggests that expression of keratins (CK7/CK20), ER/PR, TTF-1 and 'breast markers' such as GCDFP-15 can be used (see Chapter 25). Metastases from prostatic carcinoma are not an uncommon problem, particularly since a large number of patients with this cancer get hormonal therapy which can lead to gynecomastia. It has been suggested that expression of prostate specific antigen (PSA) can be used to differentiate primary breast cancer from metastases. However, a recent study found the expression of PSA in a small number of primary breast tumors; none of the tumors in this study expressed prostate specific acid phosphatase (PSAP).

PROGNOSIS AND STAGING

Although less frequent, male breast cancer has been thought to be more aggressive than its female counterpart. One of the reasons for this is the relatively small size of the male breast, which may permit earlier and/or easier access for the tumor cells to the chest wall. However, recent studies show that, although patients with male breast cancer tend to have a lower overall survival than breast cancer in women, this does not hold true when matched for stage and grade.

Tumor size and axillary lymph node status are important prognostic predictors and the same staging system that is used in female breast carcinoma is applied to male breast cancer. The overall 10-year disease-specific survival for node negative disease is around 80 % while that for node positive disease is around 50 %. However, it falls to around 20 % in patients with four or more positive nodes. Similarly, the 5-year disease-free survival rates are around 90 % for stage 1 disease and under 20 % for stage IV disease.

There is limited experience for the role of sentinel node biopsy in male breast cancer. The few studies that have been performed so far seem to suggest that this procedure is as effective in men as it is in women.

It is presumed that male breast cancer is biologically similar to female breast cancer and hormone receptor status has also been used in predicting prognosis. However, there are differences between the two; the frequency of expression of estrogen receptor (80 %) and progesterone receptor (70 %) is higher in male breast cancer. The association between ER status and grade in male breast cancer is not as strong as in female breast cancer and correlations between ER status and survival are relatively poor. Expression of (mutated) p53 and *HER*-2/neu over-expression are associated with an inferior outcome. Androgen receptor expression correlates with survival in some but not all studies. Expression of proliferation markers (MIB-1), cell cycle markers (p27), growth factors (epidermal growth factor), stromal matrix metalloproteinases and microvessel density, have been correlated with survival.

Due to the rarity of the disease, randomized clinical trials have not been carried out and the treatment of male breast cancer has not been standardized. Male breast cancers are treated, like female breast carcinomas, with surgery followed by adjuvant chemotherapy and radiation, as appropriate. The surgery tends to take the form of mastectomy due to general lack of interest in breast conservation and due to the central location of the tumors.

Tamoxifen has been used in ER positive cases with some success and surgical methods of hormonal therapy such as orchidectomy, adrenalectomy and hypophysectomy have also been used utilized with some success. The role of aromatase inhibitors in the treatment of male breast cancer is unclear; and anecdotal evidence seems to suggest that they may not be as useful as in female breast cancer. The optimal chemotherapy regimen for male breast cancer has not been defined due to the relative rarity of the disease. However, most patients are treated with combination chemotherapy based on their efficacy in women. Herceptin (trastuzumab) appears to be effective in *HER*2/neu positive cases.

SUGGESTED READINGS

Gynecomastia

Badve S, Sloane JP. Pseudoangiomatous hyperplasia of male breast. Histopathology 1995;26:463–466.

Braunstein GD. Gynaecomastia. N Engl J Med 1993; 328: 490–495

Ismail AA, Barth JH. Endocrinology of gynaecomastia. Ann Clin Biochem 2001;38:596–607.

Raju U, Crissman JD, Zarbo RJ, Gottlieb C. Epitheliosis of the breast. An immunohistochemical characterization and comparison to malignant intraductal proliferations of the breast. Am J Surg Pathol 1990;14:939–947.

Male Breast Cancer

Gennari R, Curigliano G, Jereczek-Fossa BA, *et al*. Male breast cancer: a special therapeutic problem. Anything new? Int J Oncol 2004;24:663–670.

Giordano SH, Cohen DS, Buzdar AU, *et al*. Breast carcinoma in men: a population-based study. Cancer. 2004;101:51–57.

Goss PE, Reid C, Pintilie M, *et al*. Male breast carcinoma: a review of 229 patients who presented to the Princess Margaret Hospital during 40 years: 1955–1996. Cancer 1999;85:629–639.

Goyal A, Horgan K, Kissin M, *et al*. ALMANAC Trialists Group. Sentinel lymph node biopsy in male breast cancer patients. Eur J Surg Oncol 2004;30:480–483.

Joshi MG, Lee AK, Loda M, *et al*. Male breast carcinoma: an evaluation of prognostic factors contributing to a poorer outcome. Cancer 1996;77:490–498.

Kidwai N, Gong Y, Sun X, *et al*. Expression of androgen receptor and prostate-specific antigen in male breast carcinoma. Breast Cancer Res 2004;6:R18–23.

Ribeiro G. Male breast carcinoma – a review of 301 cases from the Christie Hospital & Holt Radium Institute, Manchester. Br J Cancer 1985;51:115–119.

SEER website: www.seer.cancer.gov

Siddiqui MT, Zakowski MF, Ashfaq R, Ali SZ. Breast masses in males: multi-institutional experience on fine-needle aspiration. Diagn Cytopathol 2002;26:87–91.

Sun X, Gong Y, Rao MS, Badve S. Loss of BRCA1 expression in sporadic male breast carcinoma. Breast Cancer Res Treat 2002;71:1–7.

Index

Notes: Entries followed by the letters 'f' and 't' refer to figures and tables respectively
Abbreviations: Common abbreviations used in subentries include: DCIS, ductal carcinoma *in situ;* FNA, fine needle aspiration; LCIS, lobular carcinoma *in situ:* SLNB, sentinel lymph node biopsy.

A

Abscess(es), 30, 69–70, 69f, 70f
  differential diagnosis, 146
Acinic cell carcinoma, 221–222
Acute lymphoblastic leukemia (ALL), 287f
Acute myeloid leukemia (AML), 287f
Adenocarcinoma(s)
  mucinous cystadenocarcinoma, 223
  nipple adenoma *vs.,* 146
  with spindle cell metaplasia, 216
Adenoid cystic carcinoma, 209, 220–221
Adenoma(s)
  fibroadenoma *See* Fibroadenoma
  nipple *See* Nipple adenoma
  tubular, 116, 116f
Adenosis tumor, 86
  epithelial hyperplasia of usual type, 159
Adenosquamous carcinoma, 215
  low grade, 214–215
    syringomatous adenoma *vs.,* 147
Adjuvant! program, 239
Adjuvant therapy
  ductal carcinoma *in situ* (DCIS), 200
  NPI score and, 239
AJCC/UICC staging manual 6th edition, 257–264, 261t *See also*
      Lymph node staging (LN)
  micrometastases and, 260
Alcian blue, adenoid cystic carcinoma, 220
Alveolar soft part sarcoma, benign granular cell tumor *vs.,* 137
American Joint Committee on cancer/International Union Against
      Cancer classification system *See* AJCC/UICC staging manual
      6th edition
Amyloid lesions, 127
Androgens, male breast cancer and, 308, 310, 312
Aneuploidy, ductal carcinoma *in situ,* 185
Angiogenesis
  antiangiogenic agents, 271
  assessment, 270, 271, 271f
  clinical use, 270, 271
  as molecular marker with targeted therapy, 270–271
  process, 270–271
Angiolipoma, angiosarcoma *vs.,* 293
Angiomatosis, 134
Angiosarcoma, 289–294
  clinical features, 289
  definition, 289
  differential diagnosis, 289, 293, 293f
    benign lesions *vs.,* 290
    hemangioma, 134
  epidemiology, 289
  incidence/location, 289
  mortality/morbidity, 289
  pathologic features, 289–293
    electron microscopy, 289, 292–293
    FNA biopsy, 289, 293
    growth patterns, 290–292, 290f, 291f, 292f
    high grade lesions, 291–292, 292f
    immunohistochemistry, 289, 293
    intermediate-grade lesions, 291, 291f
    low grade lesions, 290–291, 290f, 291f
    macroscopic, 289
    microscopic, 289
    proliferative rate, 291
  radiologic features, 289

  radiotherapy-induced, 289, 292
  treatment/prognosis, 289, 294
Antiangiogenic agents, 271
APC gene/protein, familial breast cancer, 247
Apocrine carcinoma, 217
  ancillary studies, 217
  clinical features, 217
  differential diagnosis, 217
    benign granular cell tumor *vs.,* 137
  pathologic features, 217
Apocrine cells
  fine needle aspiration, 19–20
  papillomas, 100, 101
Apocrine metaplasia
  differential diagnosis, 156
  fibrocystic change, 150
  nipple adenoma, 143
  sclerosing adenosis, 88f
Apocrine proliferations, differential diagnosis, 26, 156
Archetypical lesions, diagnostic problems, 19
Aromatase inhibitors, male breast cancer, 312
Asynchronous thelarche, 60
Ataxia telangiectasia, familial breast cancer, 246–247
ATM gene, 246–247
Atrophy, sclerosing lymphocytic lobulitis, 75
Atypical ductal hyperplasia (ADH), 30, 164–168, 165f, 166f, 168t
  ancillary studies, 167
    FNA, 20
  BRCA1 associated breast cancer, 244
  clinical features, 165
  columnar cell lesions, 155, 155f
  core biopsy, 21
  differential diagnosis, 167
    ductal carcinoma *in situ* (DCIS) *vs.,* 167f, 197
    epithelial hyperplasia *vs.,* 162
    usual ductal hyperplasia *vs.,* 279–281, 280f
  fibroadenoma and, 113f
  gynecomastia and, 304, 305f
  metastatic tumors and, 299f
  molecular genetics, 187
  papillomas, 100, 103, 103f
  pathologic features, 165–166
    signet ring features, 174f
  radiologic features, 165
  treatment/prognosis, 167–168
Atypical lobular hyperplasia (ALH), 30, 169–184
  ancillary studies, 175–176
    FNA, 20
  clinical features, 169–170
  columnar cell hyperplasia and, 154f
  differential diagnosis, 176–178, 180–181
    lobular carcinoma *in situ vs.,* 172f
    myoepithelial cells *vs.,* 178f
    TDLU *vs.* infiltrating lobular carcinoma, 177f
  extralobular ducts, 172
  molecular genetics, 187–188
  pathologic features, 170, 172–173
  pseudo-acini, 178
  radiologic features, 170
  terminal duct unit, 173f
Autoimmune mastitis, 29–30
Axillary lymph nodes *See also* Lymph node staging (LN)
  dissection
    as diagnostic *vs.* therapeutic procedure, 257

313

differential diagnosis, 297
immunohistochemistry, 297
Leukemia(s), 283–288
  breast deposits, definition, 283
  differential diagnosis, 288
  pathologic features, 284, 287f
    FNA cytology, 284, 287
    immunohistochemistry, 284, 287
  treatment/prognosis, 284, 288
Li Fraumeni syndrome, familial breast cancer, 246
Ligand binding assay (LBA), hormone receptors, 265, 266
Lipid rich carcinoma (LRC), 222–223
Lipomas, gynecomastia *vs.*, 306
Liposarcoma, 295, 295f
  differential diagnosis, 297
  immunohistochemistry, 297
Liposarcomatous differentiation, 295, 295f
Lobar architecture, 55–56, 58f
  changes, 61f
  development, 61
Lobular carcinoma *in situ* (LCIS), 179f
  ancillary studies, 175–176
  BRCA1 associated breast cancer and, 244
  clinical features, 169–170
  collagenous spherulosis, 173f
  comedo type, 175f, 181
  differential diagnosis, 176–178, 180–181
    atypical lobular hyperplasia *vs.,* 172f
    ductal carcinoma *in situ* (DCIS) *vs.,* 180f, 198, 275–276
    immunohistochemistry, 275–276
    importance of, 275
    invasive carcinoma *vs.,* 276, 277, 277f, 278f
    metastatic tumors *vs.,* 300f
    radial scars *vs.,* 96
  ductal carcinoma *in situ* and, 180f
  extralobular ducts, 172
  fibroadenoma in, 112f
  infiltrating lobular carcinoma and, 170
  molecular genetics, 187–188
  non-Hodgkin's lymphoma *vs.,* 286f
  pathologic features, 170, 171f, 172–173
  pleomorphic (PLCIS), 173, 174f
    ancillary studies, 175–176
    clinical features, 169–170
    comedo type, 175f
    diagnostic dilemmas, 180–181
    dyshesive growth pattern, 172–173
    radiologic features, 170
    therapeutic considerations, 183
  pseudo-acini, 178
  radial scars and, 94f, 96
  radiologic features, 169–170
  as risk factor for invasive cancer, 275
  in sclerosing adenosis, 88f, 276, 277, 277f, 278f
  therapeutic considerations, 181, 183–184
Lobular intraepithelial neoplasia (LIN), 169 *See also* Atypical
    lobular hyperplasia (ALH); Lobular carcinoma *in situ*
    (LCIS)
Lobular neoplasia *See also* Atypical lobular hyperplasia (ALH);
    Lobular carcinoma *in situ* (LCIS)
  core biopsy, 21, 184
  definitions/terminology, 169
  ductal *vs.,* 159–160
Lobulocentric pattern, sclerosing adenosis, 85–86, 87
Loss of heterozygosity (LOH)
  atypical ductal hyperplasia, 187
  BRCA1 associated breast cancer, 244
  ductal carcinoma *in situ*, 185
  lobular carcinoma *in situ*, 175
  pleomorphic lobular carcinoma *in situ*, 175
  secretory carcinoma, 219
Luminal cells, syringomatous adenoma, 146
Luminal epithelium, papillomas, 100
Lumps, assessment, 29
Lymphangioma, angiosarcoma *vs.,* 293

Lymphatic drainage, 59
Lymph node(s)
  axillary *See* Axillary lymph nodes
  consequences of comprehensive examination, 259–260
  internal mammary, 288
  mammography, 35
  metastases
    glycogen-rich clear cell carcinoma (GRCC), 222
    infraclavicular nodes, 263–264
    internal mammary nodes, 263
    invasive papillary carcinoma, 219
    lipid rich carcinoma (LRC), 222–223
    male breast cancer, 311–312
    micropapillary carcinoma, 212
    prognostic importance, 257, 259–260, 311–312
    staging *See* Lymph node staging (LN)
    supraclavicular nodes, 264
    tubular carcinoma, 207
    tumor size relationship, 235
    vascular invasion and, 236
  pathological examination, 15–16
    See also Lymph node staging (LN)
  reaction to silicone, 82
  sentinel *See* Sentinel lymph nodes
  ultrasound, 43
Lymph node staging (LN), 257–264
  AJCC/UICC classification, 257, 261t
  axillary in breast carcinoma, 32–33
  communication/documentation, 260, 261
    'i+' notation, 261
    'mi' notation, 261
    'mol' notation, 264
    'sn' suffix, 260, 262–263
  comprehensive examination and, 259–260
  importance, 250
  infraclavicular nodes, 263–264
  internal mammary, 263
  isolated tumor cells/tumor cell clusters, 261
    multiple ITCs/multiple nodes, 262
  macrometastases, 263
  male breast cancer, 311–312
  metastases measurement, 260–261
  micrometastases, 258–259, 260, 261–262
    'special' situations, 262
  molecular studies (RT-PCR), 264
  multiple nodes–minimal tumor, 262
  prognosis/clinical significance, 231, 238, 258–264
  sentinel nodes, 249, 250, 258, 260, 262–263
    See also Sentinel lymph node biopsy (SLNB)
  supraclavicular nodes, 264
  survival *vs.* node positivity, 258, 263
  transit metastases/afferent lymphatics, 262
Lymphoblastic lymphomas, 284
Lymphocytic response
  BRCA1 associated breast cancer, 242, 243f
  mastitis, lymphoma *vs.,* 288, 288f
  non-Hodgkin's lymphoma, 285f
Lymphoid infiltrates
  lymphoma/leukemia differential diagnosis, 288
  normal breast, 64
Lymphoma(s), 283–288
  clinical presentation, 283
  differential diagnosis, 26, 288, 288f
  incidence/location, 283
  morbidity/mortality, 283
  pathologic features, 284
    FNA biopsy, 20, 284, 287
    immunohistochemistry, 284, 287
  primary, definition, 283
  radiologic features, 283, 284f
  treatment/prognosis, 283, 288
  types, 284
Lymphoplasmacytic lymphomas, 284
Lymphovascular invasion, micropapillary carcinoma,
    212

differential diagnosis, 197–198
immunohistochemistry, 276, 277f
Micrometastases
bone marrow, 259
definition, 258, 260, 261
'mi' notation, 261
prognostic/clinical significance, 250, 254f, 258–259, 261–262
confounding variables, 259
predictive value, 260
sentinel nodes, 249, 250, 251–252, 253f
failure to identify, 254f
increased detection of, 258, 261
'special' situations, 262
Micropapillary carcinoma, 213f
ancillary studies, 213
clinical features, 212
differential diagnosis, 213
pathologic features, 212
prognosis treatment, 213
Microscopes, mitotic counts, 227–228
Microvessel density (MVD), 271, 271f
Milk lines, 59
Minimally invasive carcinoma (MIC), tumor size assessment, 235
Mitotic frequency
angiosarcomas, 291–292, 292f
apoptotic figures and, 229f, 230
BRCA1 associated breast cancer, 242, 244f
heterogeneity, 228
histologic grading, 225, 227–228, 229f
fulfilling morphological criteria, 230
scores, 230t
hyperchromatic nuclei and, 230
male breast cancer, 309f
tissue preservation/preparation and, 225, 227, 229f, 230
Molecular biology See also Molecular markers
adenoid cystic carcinoma, 221
apocrine carcinoma, 217
atypical ductal hyperplasia (ADH), 187
atypical lobular hyperplasia (ALH), 187–188
BRCA1/BRCA-2-associated breast cancer, 241, 244, 246
ductal carcinoma in situ (DCIS), 185–187
invasive ductal carcinoma/no specific type (NST), 203
invasive lobular carcinoma, 205
male breast cancer, 308, 310, 311
micropapillary carcinoma, 213
mucinous carcinoma, 210
secretory carcinoma, 219
Molecular markers, 265–274 See also Molecular biology; specific markers
differentiation pathways, 62, 64f
established markers, 265–270
HER2/neu See HER2/neu gene/protein
hormone receptors, 265–266, 266f
p53 See p53 gene/protein
proliferation markers, 267–268
fine needle aspiration, 2
immunohistochemical See Immunohistochemistry (IHC)
male breast cancer, 311
potential markers and targeted therapy, 270–273
angiogenesis, 270–271
Cox-2, 272–273
EGFR, 271–272
quality assurance issues, 266, 267
treatment decisions and, 265
Mondor's disease, 84
Mortality reduction, screening for cancer, 49
Mucinous carcinoma, 209–210
ancillary studies, 210
clinical features, 209
differential diagnosis, 210
glandular (acinar)/tubule formation, 227f
pathologic features, 209
radiologic features, 209
treatment/prognosis, 210
ultrasound, 42–43

Mucinous cystadenocarcinoma, 223
Mucosa-associated lymphoid tissue (MALT), primary breast lymphoma, 284
c-myc gene/protein, DCIS pathology, 186
Myoepithelial cells
lobular carcinoma in situ/atypical lobular hyperplasia in situ, 176
markers See Myoepithelial markers
Myoepithelial markers, 276–279, 277f, 278f, 279f See also specific markers
indications, 276
male breast cancer, 311
Myofibroblastic tumors, primary breast sarcoma vs., 297
Myofibroblastoma, 131–133, 132f
ancillary studies, 132
clinical features, 131
differential diagnosis, 132–133
fibromatosis vs., 129
gynecomastia vs., 306
male breast cancer vs., 310
pathologic features, 131
radiologic features, 131
treatment/prognosis, 132
Myofibroblasts, smooth muscle actin (SMA), 277
Myosin, male breast cancer, 311

N

N-acetyl transferases, familial breast cancer, 247
National Cancer Institute (NCI), FNA diagnosis, 9
National Surgical Adjuvant Breast and Bowel Project (NSABP)
B-32 sentinel node trial, 252–253
micrometastases, clinical significance, 258
Necrosis, 173
angiosarcomas, 292
comedo See Comedo necrosis
fat See Fat necrosis
male breast cancer, 310
medullary carcinoma, 211
nipple adenoma, 145f
primary sarcoma, 294, 295f
as prognostic factor, 238
Needle passes, aspirate maximization in FNA, 5
Needle positioning, breast nodules, deeply placed, 6
Needle-stick injury, 6
Neoplastic cells
lobular carcinoma in situ, 187
syringomatous adenoma, 146
Neoplastic lesions See also specific lesions
benign stromal, 125, 128–133
fibromatosis See Fibromatosis
myofibroblastoma See Myofibroblastoma
lobular See Lobular neoplasia
phyllodes tumor See Phyllodes tumor
Neovascularization, 271
Neuroendocrine differentiation (NED)
breast metastases, 298, 299f
ductal carcinoma in situ (DCIS), 196
immunohistochemistry, 276
male breast cancer, 310
Neuroendocrine tumors
carcinoid, metastatic breast tumors, 299f
carcinoma, 218–219
invasive, 209
Neuron-specific enolase (NSE), neuroendocrine differentiation marker, 276
Nipple(s), 55
discharge, 30
disease See Nipple disease
ducts, 55, 57f
Nipple adenoma, 100, 104f, 142–146, 143f, 144f
ancillary studies, 145
clinical features, 142
differential diagnosis, 145–146
papilloma vs., 100, 104f, 145–146
syringomatous adenoma vs., 147